PEARSON ALWAYS LEARNING

Leslie C. Hendon • Winston C. Lancaster

Complete Introductory Human Anatomy Lab Guide

Custom Eleventh Edition

Cover Art: Front: Courtesy of World History Archive/Alamy Stock Photo. Back: School of Medicine: Students, 1890s, in the University of North Carolina at Chapel Hill Image Collection Collection #P0004, North Carolina Collection Photographic Archives, The Wilson Library, University of North Carolina at Chapel Hill.

Copyright © 2017, 2014, 2013, 2011, 2009, 2007, 2005, 2004, 2003, 2001 by Leslie Hendon and Winston C. Lancaster.
All rights reserved.
Pearson Custom Edition.

This copyright covers material written expressly for this volume by the editor/s as well as the compilation itself. It does not cover the individual selections herein that first appeared elsewhere. Permission to reprint these has been obtained by Pearson Learning Solutions for this edition only. Further reproduction by any means, electronic or mechanical, including photocopying and recording, or by any information storage or retrieval system, must be arranged with the individual copyright holders noted.

All trademarks, service marks, registered trademarks, and registered service marks are the property of their respective owners and are used herein for identification purposes only.

Pearson Learning Solutions, 330 Hudson Street, New York, New York 10013
A Pearson Education Company
www.pearsoned.com

Printed in the United States of America

12 2020

000200010272154619

NH/CM

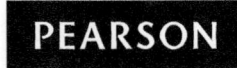

ISBN 10: 1-323-91317-3
ISBN 13: 978-1-323-91317-8

Dedication

This laboratory guide is dedicated to my most excellent husband,
Burt Hendon and to my wonderful Dad, Ted Haddin.

Leslie Hendon

I dedicate this work to my three teachers of anatomy:
O.W. Henson, Jr., Ph.D.
James L. Dobie, Ph.D.
Dorothy H. Lancaster, R.N.

Winston Lancaster

Human Anatomy Laboratory Health Risk Guidelines

HUMAN ANATOMY LABORATORY

STUDENT HEALTH RISK GUIDELINES FOR HUMAN ANATOMY LABORATORY
WITH DONOR BODIES

You have been provided with a unique opportunity to study the human body with the inclusion of human donor bodies as an integral and important instructional tool for the laboratory portion of this course. Few institutions in the country now offer this unique privilege to undergraduate students, therefore to ensure that this opportunity can be continued we want you to be aware of the responsibilities associated with access to donor bodies.

Donor bodies are preserved in a mild solution of **formalin** (which is **formaldehyde** gas dissolved in water) and **phenol**, intended to inhibit the growth of microorganisms. Both of these are toxic and extended exposure should be avoided. Formaldehyde is a colorless, flammable gas at room temperature with a characteristic pungent odor. It has been used by both clinical diagnostic and research laboratories as a preservative or fixative for over a century. It's mechanism of action for fixing lies in its ability to form cross-links between soluble and structural proteins. The resulting structure retains its cellular constituents in their in-vivo relationships to each other, giving it a degree of mechanical strength which enables it to withstand subsequent processing (e.g., immunohisto-staining, micrological sectioning).

Formaldehyde is typically found dissolved in a water and methanol solution called formalin, or in a powder form called paraformaldehyde. Both are capable of releasing formaldehyde gas. The terms formaldehyde and formalin are often used interchangeably, but there are important differences in their concentrations. A fixative labeled **10% buffered formalin** is actually a 4% solution of formaldehyde (i.e., a 10% solution made from a 37–40% solution of formaldehyde). Formaldehyde is typically used as a fixative in 10% formalin or 4% paraformaldehyde solutions. The Alabama Human Donor Program uses formalin to fix gross tissue specimens. The morgues use approximately 20cc of 37% formaldehyde to fix the brains of human donors. Because formaldehyde is water soluble it may irritate the mucous membranes. The effects of formaldehyde exposure can vary from person to person. Typical exposure symptoms are listed below:

CONCENTRATION IN AIR SYMPTOMS

0.1–5 parts per million (ppm): Eye irritation, tears, skin irritation, respiratory tract irritation
5–20 ppm: Burning of eyes and respiratory tract, tears, difficulty in breathing/coughing,
20–100 ppm: Chest tightening, pain, irregular heartbeat, severe lung irritation, pulmonary edema, death in severe cases

In 1992, OSHA established a Federal standard that set the amount of formaldehyde to which workers can be exposed over an 8-hour workday 0.75 ppm. The UAB Office of Occupational Health and Safety annually performs air quality monitoring in Human Anatomy Laboratories A, B, and C (CH 160–164). These laboratories have an externally-directed ventilation system that maintains ambient room exposure levels at well-below the required safe standards. Copies of the annual air quality reports are available on request at (205) 934-2487.

HEALTH EFFECTS OF EXPOSURE TO FORMALDEHYDE

Skin:

Formaldehyde is a severe skin irritant and sensitizer. Contact with formaldehyde solutions, vapor or resins can cause eczema (dry, flaking and itching skin) and in extreme cases can lead to allergic dermatitis or hives. This is a skin disease that can appear as a simple rash to severe skin cracking and blistering, white discoloration, numbness and a drying or hardening of the skin. These symptoms can also be caused by contact with clothing contaminated with formaldehyde.

Eyes:

Exposure to formaldehyde vapor can cause reddening and burning sensations in the eyes, accompanied by tear production. Formaldehyde solutions coming into direct contact with the eye can cause serious damage to the cornea, possibly leading to blindness.

Nose, Throat and Lungs:

Low ambient concentrations of formaldehyde can cause irritation of the upper respiratory tract. At higher concentrations, the effects become more severe, with levels above 10 ppm causing coughing, chest tightness and difficulty breathing, and levels of 25 to 30 ppm causing severe respiratory tract injury. Exposure to 100 ppm is immediately dangerous to life and health leading to death from throat swelling and chemical burns to the lungs.

Respiratory Sensitization:

Repeated exposure to formaldehyde can cause allergic asthma. Symptoms of asthma include chest tightness, shortness of breath, wheezing, and coughing. Formaldehyde's long-term effects on the lungs are not fully understood.

Cancer:

In 2011, the National Toxicology Program, an interagency program of the Department of Health and Human Services, named formaldehyde as a known human carcinogen in its 12th Report on Carcinogens. Exposure has been associated with cancers of the lung, nasopharynx and oropharynx, and nasal passages, and it has been shown to cause cancer in animals.

Mutagenicity:

Formaldehyde is genotoxic in several in vitro test systems, showing properties of both an initiator and a promoter.

Reproductive System:

Scientists have made many attempts to study whether formaldehyde might harm pregnancy or the reproductive system. The results have been mixed and complicated. Studies clearly show that formaldehyde does not cause birth defects. There is some uncertainty whether formaldehyde might cause spontaneous abortions and sperm damage. However, it is believed that exposures in most workplaces probably do not pose any significant risk to pregnancy or the reproductive system.

References

National Toxicology Program (June 2011). Report on Carcinogens, Twelfth Edition. Department of Health and Human Services, Public Health Service, National Toxicology Program. Retrieved June 10, 2011, from: http://ntp.niehs.nih.gov/go/roc12.
https://www.cancer.gov/about-cancer/causes-prevention/risk/substances/formaldehyde/formaldehyde-fact-sheet.

Human Anatomy Laboratory Participation Form for Instruction with Donor Bodies

FORMALIN AND PHENOL

The effect of *formalin* is mostly as an irritant in the respiratory system and mucous membranes. *Phenol* is a caustic substance that also can burn the skin and mucous membranes. The wetting solution used in our donor body lab does not contain these substances. Instead it contains **phenoxyethanol** and **glycerin** in water. These substances retard growth of microorganisms while helping to reduce the desiccation of tissues. Phenoxyethanol is toxic when ingested.

Exposure to all of these substances should be limited in the following ways:

1. Gloves and protective clothing: gloves should be worn at all times when using the donor bodies to avoid skin exposure. **Students must provide their own non-latex gloves (nitrile or poly-vinyl)**. Students should change gloves frequently. It is strongly recommended that students wear **protective clothing** (lab coat OR over-sized long-sleeve shirt) AND protective eyewear when working with the donor bodies or cadaveric specimens to protect skin, eyes, and clothing from contamination and stains.

2. Students wearing contact lenses may find it necessary to remove them when working in the donor body lab. Permeable contact lenses may absorb formalin and cause irritation to the eyes.

If you have *any condition* that might be affected by exposure to any of the above agents, or which may affect your lab participation in any way, do the following:

1. Notify your lab instructor: your instructor can advise you of ways to minimize the impact on lab work. Also, your lab instructor can be prepared for any situation that might arise.

2. If you currently use an inhaler for environment-induced asthma, please bring your inhaler with you to each laboratory session. Inform your lab group members and your Laboratory Instructor of the whereabouts of your inhaler, so that in an emergency, they can provide assistance in locating your inhaler for you.

3. Consult your physician: your physician can give you the best information on what effects the preservatives, etc., may have on your current health status and can help you to make an informed choice regarding continued participation in the lab. If you believe that you have a health condition that would limit or prevent your participation in the laboratory, please contact the office of Disability Support Services located in phone number (934-4205), www.uab.edu/dss for further assistance. Your physician will need to provide documentation of your health condition to DSS personnel.

___

I_____(Name), have read and have been informed of the potential health risks associated with exposure to the vaporized gasses and preservative fluids used in the preparation of human donor bodies on_____(Date).

Contents

Dedication iii
Human Anatomy Laboratory Health Risk Guidelines v
Health Effects of Exposure to Formaldehyde vii
Human Anatomy Laboratory Participation Form for Instruction with Donor Bodies ix
Acknowledgments xix
Preface xxi

ONE

ORIENTATION TO HUMAN ANATOMY AND
GENERAL OVERVIEW OF THE SKELETAL SYSTEM   1

    I.   Anatomical Terms..1
    II. Anatomy of Long Bones 3
    III. Body Language 3
         Study and Review Questions – Orientation to Human Anatomy 5

TWO

THE SKELETAL SYSTEM: AXIAL & APPENDICULAR DIVISIONS   7

    I.   The Axial Skeleton 7
        A. Bones of the Skull 7
        B. The Vertebral Column 18
    II. The Appendicular Skeleton 26
    III. Joints 40
         Study and Review Questions – The Skeletal System 43

THREE

HISTOLOGY   45

    I.   Body Language 45
    II.   Overview of Basic Tissue Types 45
    III. Epithelial Tissue 46
    IV. Connective Tissue 51
    V.   Muscle Tissue 59
    VI. Nervous Tissue 62
    VII. The Integument 62
    VIII. Membranes 66

FOUR

SELECTED MUSCLES OF THE APPENDICULAR & AXIAL SKELETON — 67

- I. Body Language 67
- II. Muscles of the Upper Limb 68
- III. Muscles of the Spine & Neck 77
- IV. Blood Supply to the Upper Limb & Torso 78
- V. Innervation of the Pectoral Region & Upper Limb 80
- VI. Muscles of the Lower Limb 83
- VII. Blood Supply of the Lower Extremities 94
- VIII. Innervation of Muscles of the Lower Extremity 97
- IX. Methods of Naming Muscles 98
- X. Compartments of Skeletal Muscles 99
- Study and Review Questions – Skeletal Muscles 101

FIVE

THE CENTRAL NERVOUS SYSTEM: THE BRAIN & SPINAL CORD — 103

- I. Histology of Neural Tissue 103
- II. Histological Components of the Central Nervous System 105
- III. The Central Nervous System & Related Structures...106
- IV. Spinal Cord & Related Structures..107
- V. Brain...109
- VI. Cranial Nerves 115
- VII. Blood Supply of the Brain 117
- VIII. Autonomic Nervous System 119
- IX. Nervous System Pathways 122
- Study and Review Questions – The Nervous System..125

SIX

ORGANS & MUSCLES OF THE HEAD — 127

- I. Muscles of the Head Region...127
- II. Organs of the Head 129
- III. Selected Special Sense Organs of the Head...132
- IV. Teeth 137
- Study and Review Questions – Organs of the Head 139

SEVEN

THE THORACIC CAVITY & STRUCTURES IN THE NECK — 141

- I. Histology of the Thoracic Cavity..141
- II. Organs and Tissues in the Neck 144
- III. The Thoracic Cavity 146
- IV. Gross Anatomy of the Lungs 148
- V. Gross Anatomy of the Heart 150
- Study and Review Questions – The Thoracic Cavity 159

EIGHT

THE ABDOMINOPELVIC CAVITY: THE DIGESTIVE & URINARY SYSTEMS   163

    I. Histology of Abdominopelvic Organs 163
    II. Boundaries of the Abdominopelvic Cavity 164
    III. Muscles of the Abdominopelvic Cavity 164
    IV. Blood Vessels Inferior to the Diaphragm 168
    V. Nervous Innervation of Abdominal and Pelvic Organs 169
    VI. Organs of the Digestive Tract & Accessory Organs of Digestion 170
    VII. Urinary Organs 173
        Study and Review Questions – The Abdominal Cavity 177

NINE

MALE & FEMALE REPRODUCTIVE SYSTEMS   179

    I. Histology of Reproductive Structures...179
    II. Female Reproductive System 181
    III. Male Reproductive System..184
        Study and Review Questions – The Reproductive System...187

List of Figures

TWO

THE SKELETAL SYSTEM: AXIAL & APPENDICULAR DIVISIONS

Figure 2.1	Human Skull—Anterior and Posterior Views	9
Figure 2.2	Lateral View and Sagittal Section of the Skull	10
Figure 2.3	Inferior View of the Skull	11
Figure 2.4	Cranial Fossae and Foramina	11
Figure 2.5	The Sphenoid Bone	12
Figure 2.6	The Nasal Complex and Paranasal Sinuses	13
Figure 2.7	The Temporal Bone	14
Figure 2.8	The Orbital Complex	15
Figure 2.9	The Mandible	16
Figure 2.10	The Skull of an Infant	19
Figure 2.11a	Atlas and Axis	21
Figure 2.11b	Cervical Vertebrae	22
Figure 2.11c	Thoracic Vertebrae	24
Figure 2.11d	Lumbar Vertebrae	25
Figure 2.11e	The Sacrum and Coccyx	25
Figure 2.12	The Scapula	27
Figure 2.13	The Humerus	28
Figure 2.14	The Radius and Ulna	30
Figure 2.15	Bones of the Wrist and Hand	31
Figure 2.16a	Pelvis, Anterior View	33
Figure 2.16b	Right Coxal Bone, Lateral View	33
Figure 2.16c	Right Coxal Bone, Medial View	34
Figure 2.17	Right Femur	35
Figure 2.18	Right Femur	36
Figure 2.19	Anterior view of the right Tibia and Fibula	37
Figure 2.20	Posterior view of the Right Tibia and Fibula	38
Figure 2.21a	Superior and Inferior views of Right Foot	39
Figure 2.21b	Lateral and medial Views of the Right Foot	39

THREE

HISTOLOGY

Figure 3.1	Simple Squamous Epithelial Tissue	46
Figure 3.2	Simple Cuboidal Epithelial Tissue	46
Figure 3.3	Simple Columnar Epithelial Tissue	47
Figure 3.4	Pseudostratified Ciliated Columnar Epithelial Tissue	47
Figure 3.5	The structure and layers of the epidermis.	48
Figure 3.6	Transitional epithelium	48
Figure 3.7	Glandular Epithelium (Pancreatic Tissue)	49
Figure 3.8	Areolar Connective Tissue	51
Figure 3.9	Adipose Connective Tissue	52
Figure 3.10	Deep Dermis	53

Figure 3.11 Elastic Ligament 54
Figure 3.12 Diagrammatic view of the Histological Organization of
Compact and Spongy Bone. 54
Figure 3.13 The Internal Organization in Representative Bones 55
Figure 3.14 Histology of the Three Types of Cartilage 56
Figure 3.15 White blood cells 58
Figure 3.16 Skeletal Muscle Fibers 60
Figure 3.17 Cardiac Muscle Cells 60
Figure 3.18 Smooth Muscle Cells 60
Figure 3.19 Multipolar Neuron. 61
Figure 3.20a Section of thick skin. 63
Figure 3.20b Meissner Corpuscles in Thick Skin 63
Figure 3.20c Pacinian Corpuscles 64
Figure 3.20d Hair Follicle, Sebaceous Gland & Arrector Pili Muscle 64

FOUR

SELECTED MUSCLES OF THE APPENDICULAR & AXIAL SKELETON

Figure 4.1a, b Muscles That Move the Arm 69
Figure 4.1c Muscles That Move the Arm 70
Figure 4.2 Muscles of the Back & Shoulder 71
Figure 4.3 Muscles That Move the Forearm and Hand, Part I 75
Figure 4.4 Muscles That Move the Forearm and Hand, Part II 76
Figure 4.5 Arteries of the Right Upper Limb and Thorax 79
Figure 4.6 Veins of the Right Upper Limb and Shoulder 80
Figure 4.7a, b The Brachial Plexus 81
Figure 4.7c Schematic of Brachial Plexus 82
Figure 4.8 Muscles That Move the Thigh, Part I 83
Figure 4.9a The Relationships between the Action Lines and the
Axis of the Hip Joint... 85
Figure 4.9b Muscles That Move the Leg, Part I 87
Figure 4.9c Muscles That Move the Leg, Part III 89
Figure 4.9c Muscles That Move the Leg, Part III 90
Figure 4.10a Extrinsic Muscles That Move the Foot and Toes, Part III 92
Figure 4.10b Extrinsic Muscles That Move the Foot and Toes, Part I 93
Figure 4.11 Major Arteries of the Lower Limb, Part I 95
Figure 4.12 Anterior view Showing the Veins of the Right Lower Limb 96

FIVE

THE CENTRAL NERVOUS SYSTEM: THE BRAIN & SPINAL CORD

Figure 5.1 A corresponding view of the cranial cavity with the brain
removed showing the orientation and extent of the falx
cerebri and tentorium cerebelli 107
Figure 5.2 Anatomy of the Spinal Cord 108
Figure 5.3 Sectional Views of the Brain 110

Figure 5.4 The Diencephalon and Brain Stem 112
Figure 5.5 Ventral view of the human brain, showing the cranial nerves 115
Figure 5.6 Major arteries serving the brain (ventral view) 118
Figure 5.7 Parasympathetic (Craniosacral) Division of the Autonomic
Nervous System 120
Figure 5.8 Sympathetic (Thoracolumbar) Division of the Autonomic
Nervous System 121

SIX

ORGANS & MUSCLES OF THE HEAD

Figure 6.1 Muscles of the Head and Neck 127
Figure 6.2 Muscles of Mastication 128
Figure 6.3 The Anatomy of the Upper Respiratory Tract 130
Figure 6.4 The Salivary Glands 131
Figure 6.5 Anatomy of the Ear 133
Figure 6.6 Internal Structure of the Eye 134
Figure 6.7 Extra-ocular Muscles 136

SEVEN

THE THORACIC CAVITY & STRUCTURES IN THE NECK

Figure 7.1 Schematic of lining of pleural and pericardial cavities in a coronal section 147
Figure 7.2 Bronchi and Bronchioles 149
Figure 7.3 Relationships between the heart and the pericardial cavity 150
Figure 7.4a Anterior view of the heart and great vessels 152
Figure 7.4b Posterior view of the heart and great vessels 152
Figure 7.5a Gross Anatomy of the Heart. Anterior view emphasizing the right atrium,
which has been opened; the anterior wall of the atrium has been reflected
to the side..153
Figure 7.5b Gross Anatomy of the Heart. Frontal section of the relaxed heart
showing the major landmarks and the path of blood flow (arrows) through
the atria and ventricles..153
Figure 7.6 Coronary Circulation 156
Figure 7.7 Components of the Conducting System...158

EIGHT

THE ABDOMINOPELVIC CAVITY: THE DIGESTIVE & URINARY SYSTEMS

Figure 8.1 The Oblique and Rectus Muscles 165
Figure 8.2 Muscles of the Pelvic Floor and Perineum 166
Figure 8.3 Major Branches of the Abdominal Aorta 167
Figure 8.4 The Veins of the Hepatic Portal System 169
Figure 8.5 The Duodenum and Related Organs 172
Figure 8.6 The glomerular capsule of the kidney...175

NINE
MALE & FEMALE REPRODUCTIVE SYSTEMS
Figure 9.1　Histological Summary of the Ovarian Cycle 181
Figure 9.2　Female Internal Reproductive Organs 182
Figure 9.3　The Female Reproductive System Sagittal section of female pelvis 183
Figure 9.4　The Male Reproductive System 185

Acknowledgments

The authors thank Dennis Kearns and Frank Hamby for their contributions, and Kris Brostrom, Chris O'Brien, Jill Haber Atkins, Shreiya Madhusoodanan, Jacquita Davis and Christophe Jackson for their support. Leslie Hendon also thanks Burt Hendon for his technical assistance, patience, and understanding. Winston Lancaster thanks Ginger Wyatt for her patience and advice throughout the process.

Preface

USE OF THIS HUMAN ANATOMY LABORATORY GUIDE:

This *Human Anatomy Laboratory Guide* is written and designed for undergraduate anatomy students. Students in an introductory anatomy class will benefit from the depth, detail and clarity of the material presented in this text.

Students using this book will be exposed to all major systems of the body and have hands-on experience with human donor bodies and organs. All laboratory material is presented in manageable sections, with all unfamiliar terms highlighted and defined.

This guide is for students using human donor bodies, anatomical models or virtual dissections. All material is presented in such a way that, whichever method is used in the laboratory, students will be able to analyze and discuss each organ system.

This laboratory guide includes the following helpful features:

- This guide is user-friendly. Instructors will describe the anatomical structures in each section while students follow along examining the appropriate body structure.
- The text is concise and highly descriptive without being wordy or overwhelming.
- Descriptive, easy-to-follow illustrations accompany every major system of the body.
- This guide adapts well for students using prosected donor bodies, virtual "donor bodies" or anatomical models.
- It includes vivid descriptions of every anatomical region, to describe the more difficult concepts.
- A clear format allows students and lab instructors alike to follow through every system or region of the body.
- Tables of each muscle group include origin, insertion, and action, as well as *nerve supply*.
- All content is relevant and presented efficiently; students will use this guide in its entirety.
- Prosected human bodies are used throughout the course.
- Dissections are presented in such a way that groups of students can work independently, but under the close supervision of the laboratory instructor.
- Descriptions of tissues at the microscopic level are included for all major tissue types within the appropriate chapters of this guide.

COURSE GOALS & OBJECTIVES

The objectives of this course are:

- To provide students with knowledge of the normal structure of the human body at both the gross and microscopic levels.
- To meet the needs for pre-professional training in health science programs.
- To prepare students for advanced study in human anatomy.
- Developing practical skills to *analyze* and *synthesize* information concerning one system and apply that knowledge to another organ system.
- Developing skills in studying and critical thinking that will apply to this course and future advanced courses.

- The ability to discuss pertinent topics in clinical anatomy and sports medicine using the appropriate anatomical terms.
- Focusing on learning and understanding relationships between anatomical structures and organ systems from the cellular to the gross level.

SUGGESTIONS FOR STUDENTS

Lecture and lab together form a single course and are designed to complement each other. Any material from lab may be tested on lecture exams.

Always read the lab guide prior to each week's laboratory. Your understanding and your grade will improve by being prepared for each class. New material is clearer if you have read the text first.

Begin studying material during the week in which it is introduced in the laboratory. Knowledge gained from earlier units is frequently called upon, so it is to your advantage to keep up with all material presented in laboratory. In order to clarify and gain depth of understanding, we encourage students to return to the Extended Study lab for independent study.

Material in this course is not conceptually difficult, but the volume of material is great. In order to gain the most from the laboratory, it is best studied over time. Waiting to study until the last minute can make the material feel overwhelming. Keeping your specific goals in mind for taking this course will help you stay focused and motivated.

SUPPLIES FOR EFFECTIVE PARTICIPATION IN LABORATORY

1. *Complete Introductory Human Anatomy Lab Guide*, 10th edition, 2016. Bring this guide with you to every lab and write notes in it.
2. Bring latex or nitrile gloves to lab.
3. Wear a lab coat or old clothes. All students must wear closed-toed shoes to lab.
4. Bring colored pencils for drawing diagrams.

ONE

Orientation to Human Anatomy and General Overview of the Skeletal System

I. ANATOMICAL TERMS

The Language of Anatomy

One of the main goals in studying anatomy is to learn to communicate about the human body on a professional level. This isn't just the names of structures, but also the terminology used to describe how structures relate to each other. These are terms of direction or orientation and are a fundamental part of the language of anatomy. Find the definitions of these terms in your textbook or in a good medical dictionary.

Several chapters of this laboratory guide contain a **Body Language** section, which will assist the student in understanding some of the unfamiliar terms for that particular section.

Each of these terms below will be used exhaustively throughout the laboratory guide. Refer to this introductory list at any time you have a question pertaining to directional terms.

TERMS

1. **Anatomical position**: In anatomical position, the body is standing with lower extremities together; hands are at the sides with palms forward, with head facing forward and eyes straight ahead. Anatomical position is the position of the body from which all other terms of reference are determined.
2. **Dorsal/Posterior**: Toward the back of the organism.
3. **Ventral/Anterior**: Toward the front of the organism.
4. **Medial**: toward the middle, closer to the midline of the body.
5. **Lateral**: Away from the middle, farther from the midline of the body.
6. **Superficial**: Closer to the surface of the body.
7. **Deep**: Farther from the surface of the body, toward the interior of the body.
8. **Superior**: Towards the head, a point of reference higher than the comparison point.
9. **Inferior**: Farther from the head, toward the feet.
10. **Proximal**: Referring to a point on a limb that is closer to the trunk than another point.
11. **Distal**: Referring to a point on a limb that is farther from the trunk than another point.
12. **Cranial**: Toward the head.
13. **Caudal**: Toward the tail.

PLANES IN WHICH A SPECIMEN MAY BE CUT

1. **Sagittal (median):** The plane through the long axis of the body at the midline that divides the body into equal right and left halves.
2. **Parasagittal**: Any plane parallel to the sagittal plane that divides the body into unequal right and left parts.
3. **Frontal/Coronal**: A plane perpendicular to the sagittal plane that bisects the body into anterior and posterior portions.
4. **Transverse/horizontal**: A plane that separates the body into superior and inferior parts, also called a cross-section.

BODY GEOGRAPHY

The following words are **adjectives** that refer to regions of the body. These terms will be used in lecture and lab and will appear on tests throughout the course. Refer to Figure 1.8 of *Human Anatomy* textbook.

1. **Abdominal**—of the abdomen
2. **Antebrachial**—of the forearm (upper extremity distal to the elbow)
3. **Axillary**—of the axilla or armpit
4. **Brachial**— of the upper extremity proximal to the elbow
5. **Capitis (cephalic)**—of the head
6. **Carpal**—of the wrist
7. **Cervical**—of the neck
8. **Clavicular**—of the clavicle
9. **Crural**—of the leg (distal to the knee)
10. **Cutaneous**—of the skin or near the skin
11. **Dorsal**—of or towards the posterior surface of the body
12. **Femoral**—of the thigh
13. **Gluteal**—of the buttocks
14. **Iliac**—of the upper pelvic region relative to the ilium
15. **Inguinal**—of the groin
16. **Lumbar**—of the lower back region
17. **Pectoral**—of the anterior surface of the thorax
18. **Pelvic**—of the pelvis
19. **Popliteal**—of the back of the knee
20. **Tarsal**—of the ankle
21. **Thoracic**—of the chest
22. **Ventral**—of or towards the anterior surface of the body

II. ANATOMY OF LONG BONES

STRUCTURES OF LONG BONES

Define these terms.

(margin note next to 1–2: forms after growth of epiphysis has ended)

1. **Epiphysis** — *above growth* — rounded end part of bone
2. **Epiphyseal line** — marks where the epiphysis meets the metaphysis *(circled)*
3. **Metaphysis** — connects diaphysis to epiphysis
4. **Diaphysis** — long tube part of bone
5. **Compact bone** — solid bone that surrounds tube of spongy bone
6. **Medullary cavity** — cavity inside bones that contains bone marrow
7. **Cancellous bone** (spongy bone) — forms open network of struts & plates w/in compact bone
8. **Yellow bone marrow** — mixture of mature & immature red and white blood cells
9. **Red bone marrow** — stem cells that produce RBCs & WBCs
10. **Periosteum** — connective tissue wrapping that's connected to the deep fascia
11. **Nutrient foramen** — opening in bone for nutrients to enter through diaphysis

III. BODY LANGUAGE

Terms Referring to Openings Through Bones or Depressions on Bones

1. **Alveolus**—a cavity or pit in a bone such as the sockets for teeth of the maxilla and mandible.
2. **Canal**—a long tube-like passage through a bone that is an opening for veins, arteries or nerves.
3. **Fissure**—a slit-shaped opening or separation between two bones for the passage of veins, arteries or nerves.
4. **Foramen**—a hole passing through a bone for the passage of veins, arteries or nerves.
5. **Fossa**—a shallow depression or cavity. The glenoid fossa is a shallow depression in the scapula.
6. **Lamina**—a flattened area of bone, such as the lamina of a vertebra.
7. **Meatus**–a pipe-shaped or tube-like opening, such as the external auditory meatus.
8. **Sinus**—a cavity within a bone.
9. **Sulcus**—a groove or deep depression in a bone.

Bony Structures that Form Articulations or points of muscle attachments

An articulation is a joint; a location where two or more bones make physical contact.

1. **Capitulum**—a small head or eminence on a bone. "Capit" refers to head.
2. **Condyle**—a rounded prominence at the end of a bone, from the Greek for knuckle.
3. **Epicondyle**—a bony prominence usually found proximal to a condyle.

CHAPTER ONE   *Orientation to Human Anatomy*

4. **Head**—a round projection beyond the neck of a bone.
5. **Malleolus**—a process shaped like a small hammerhead, such as the medial malleolus of the tibia.
6. **Olecranon**—the prominent structure on the proximal end of the ulna. From the Greek for elbow.
7. **Process**—a projection from, or a bump on a bone.
8. **Trochlea**—an articular surface shaped like a pulley, from the Latin for pulley.

Bony Structures that Are Sites for Muscle Attachment

1. **Crest**—a rough, bony ridge, such as the iliac crest.
2. **Line**—a prominent ridge along the diaphysis of a bone, such as the linea aspera.
3. **Spine**—a sharp projection or prominent ridge on a bone, such as the spine of the scapula.
4. **Trochanter**—one of two large processes on the femur.
5. **Tubercle**—a rounded enlargement, but smaller and smoother than a trochanter, such as the lesser tubercle of the humerus.
6. **Tuberosity**—a rough, enlarged area, such as the ischial tuberosity.

Study and Review Questions – Orientation to Human Anatomy

CHAPTER ONE

Answers are found in Chapter One of this guide.

1. Define:

    a. Anatomical position: *position of the body from which all other terms of reference are determined*

    b. Inferior: *farther from head, toward feet*

    c. Distal: *point on limb further from trunk than another point*

    d. Cranial: *toward the head*

2. Match the term in **column A** with its definition in **column B**. Write the letter of your answer in the blank by the appropriate term in column A.

    Column A   **Column B**

    _D_ Axillary   A. of the neck

    _C_ Gluteal   B. of the ankle

    _E_ Pectoral   C. of the buttocks area

    _B_ Tarsal   D. of the "armpit" region

    _A_ Cervical   E. of the front of the chest

3. Where in/on the body are the following located:

    a. **Yellow bone marrow** is located *in medullary cavity*

    b. **Cancellous bone** is located *beneath compact bone, surrounding medullary cavity*

    c. A **lamina** is located *on vertabrae*

4. Define the following terms:

    a. Foramen: *hole passing through bone for veins, arteries, or nerves*

    b. Sulcus: *groove or deep depression in bone*

    c. Tuberosity: *rough, enlarged area*

    d. Condyle: *rounded prominence at end of bone*

    e. Fissure: *slit-shaped opening b/t two bones for veins, arteries, or nerves*

    f. Canal: *long, tube-like passage through bone that's an opening for veins, arteries, or nerves*

EXERCISES IN HUMAN ANATOMY   5

5. Describe the relationships of the following structures in correct anatomical position.
    a. The knee is __proximal__ to the ankle.
    b. The elbow is __distal__ to the shoulder.
    c. The knee is __inferior__ to the hip.
    d. The head is __superior__ to the naval.

6. Define the following anatomical terms.
    a. Brachial __of the upper extremity proximal to the elbow__
    b. Inguinal __of the groin__
    c. Iliac __of the upper pelvic region, relative to the ilium__
    d. Pelvic __of the pelvis__
    e. Popliteal __of the back of the knee__

TWO

The Skeletal System: Axial & Appendicular Divisions

In the laboratory on the skeletal system, you will learn all 206 bones of the human body. Additionally, you will learn definitions of terms critical to your complete understanding of the human skeletal system. Study the names of bones as well as their landmarks. You are learning these bony landmarks in preparation for learning origins and insertions for skeletal muscles in Chapter Four of this Lab Guide.

The skeletal system is comprised of the **axial skeleton** and the **appendicular skeleton**. The axial skeleton includes the skull, vertebrae, and the thoracic cage. The appendicular skeleton consists of the bones of the upper and lower limbs, including the pectoral and pelvic girdles. The pectoral girdle is the framework to which the upper limbs attach and it is made up of the scapulae and clavicles. The pelvic girdle provides the framework by which the lower limbs are attached to the axial skeleton and is made up of the two coxal bones.

I. THE AXIAL SKELETON

A. BONES OF THE SKULL

The skull is formed from both cranial and facial bones. The cranium forms the "brain case" surrounding the delicate brain. Bones of the face form facial structures such as the cheeks, portions of the orbit (eyes sockets), the chin and bridge of the nose.

In addition to the cranium's protective role and the facial bones' structural roles, the skull has several other important functions. As you study each bone of the skull, look for the features that distinguish each bone.

1. Openings within individual skull bones allow passage of nerves and blood vessels. You will identify many of these foramina during your study of the skull.

2. Internally the cranial cavity is divided into three shelf-like sections:

    a. The **anterior cranial fossa** – formed by the frontal bone and part of the sphenoid bone

    b. The **middle cranial fossa** – formed by part of the sphenoid bone and the temporal bone

    c. The **posterior cranial fossa** – formed by the occipital bone and part of the temporal bone.

SELECTED SUTURES OF THE HUMAN SKULL

Skull bones come together at immovable joints called sutures. Four of the most prominent sutures are described here (Figs. 2.1 & 2.2).

1. The **coronal suture** separates the frontal bone from the two parietal bones.

2. The **sagittal suture** separates the two parietal bones from each other.

3. The **lambdoidal suture** separates the occipital bone from the two parietal bones.

4. The **squamosal suture** separates each temporal bone from the adjacent parietal bone.

STRUCTURES OF CRANIAL BONES

Frontal Bone

Externally, the frontal bone forms the forehead and the superior surface of the **orbit**. Internally, the frontal bone forms the anterior part of the **anterior cranial fossa**. The frontal bone has articulations (joints) with the **ethmoid bone** and the **sphenoid bone**, as well as the **zygomatic, nasal and parietal bones** (Figures 2.1, 2.2, and 2.4). Some of the important structures of the frontal bone are described below.

1. The **supraorbital margins** are the ridges at the superior border of the orbits.

2. The **frontal sinuses** are air-filled cavities within the frontal bone superior to the orbit.

3. The **supraorbital foramen** is a tiny opening within each supraorbital region for the passage of nerves and blood vessels. It is a variable structure and may be a small notch.

Sphenoid Bone

The **sphenoid bone** forms part of the floor of the middle cranial fossa and lateral walls of the cranium. The sphenoid bone has been described as looking like a bat or butterfly. Some prominent structures of the sphenoid bone are discussed below (Figs. 2.1 & 2.2; 2.4 & 2.5).

The sphenoid bone is considered the "keystone" (foundation) bone of the skull. As such, it has articulations with *nearly every skull bone*, including the frontal bone, ethmoid bone, occipital bone and parietal bones of the cranium and the maxillae, vomer, palatine bones, and zygomatic bones of the face.

1. **Greater wings of the sphenoid bone** help give the sphenoid bone its characteristic "bat" shape. The **greater wings** of the sphenoid bone extend laterally and can be seen in the lateral view of an articulated skull. The greater wings articulate with the frontal bone and the parietal bone on each side of the skull. A portion of the greater wings of the sphenoid bone also forms the posterior wall of the orbits.

2. **Lesser wings of the sphenoid bone** are small, wing-shaped structures located superior and medial to the greater wings. The lesser wings also form the superior border of the superior orbital fissures.

3. **Optic canals** pass through the **lesser wings of the sphenoid bones.** The **optic canals** are the openings through which the optic nerves pass.

4. **Superior orbital fissures** are diagonal slits located lateral to the optic canals. The lesser and greater wings of the sphenoid bone form the borders of the superior orbital fissure. The superior orbital fissures are passageways for blood vessels and cranial nerves III, IV, V_1 and VI.

5. The **body of the sphenoid bone** is the central portion of the sphenoid located medial to the greater wings. The body of the sphenoid contains the **sphenoid sinuses**.

6. The **sella turcica** is a deep depression in the superior portion of the body of the sphenoid. The sella turcica houses the pituitary gland.

7. The **foramen rotundum** is a small opening located within the medial region of the greater wing. It serves as an opening for the passage of the maxillary division of cranial nerve V.

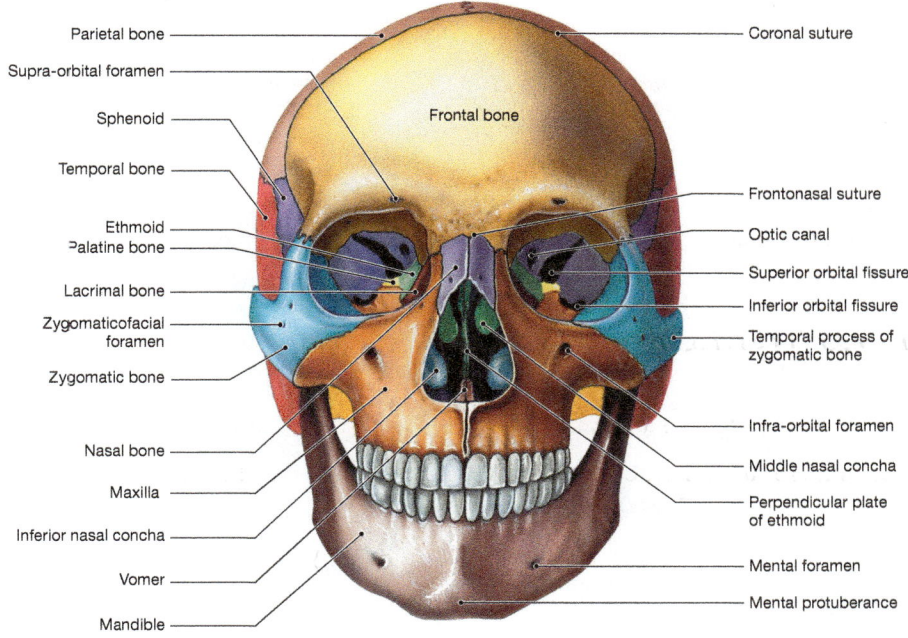

(a) Anterior view of the bones of the adult skull

From *Human Anatomy*, Ninth Edition, by Frederic H. Martini, Robert B. Tallitsch, and Judi L. Nath (2018), reproduced by permission of Pearson Education.

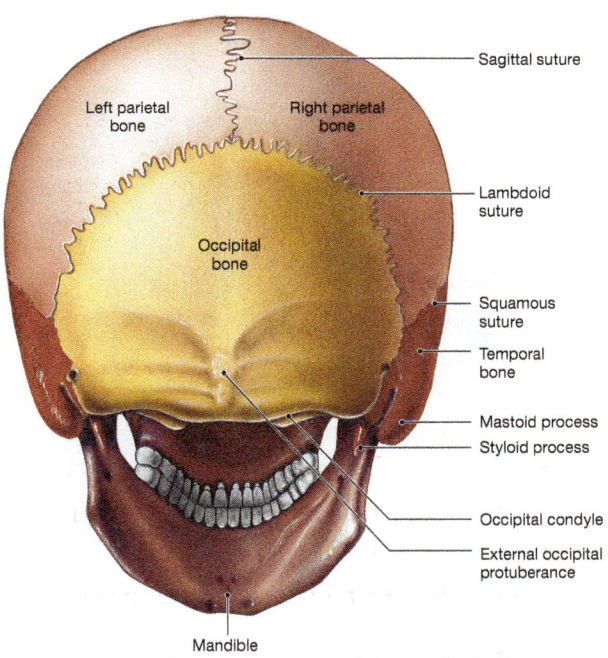

(b) Posterior view of the bones of the adult skull

From *Human Anatomy*, Ninth Edition, by Frederic H. Martini, Robert B. Tallitsch, and Judi L. Nath (2018), reproduced by permission of Pearson Education.

Figure 2.1 **Human Skull**—Anterior and Posterior Views.

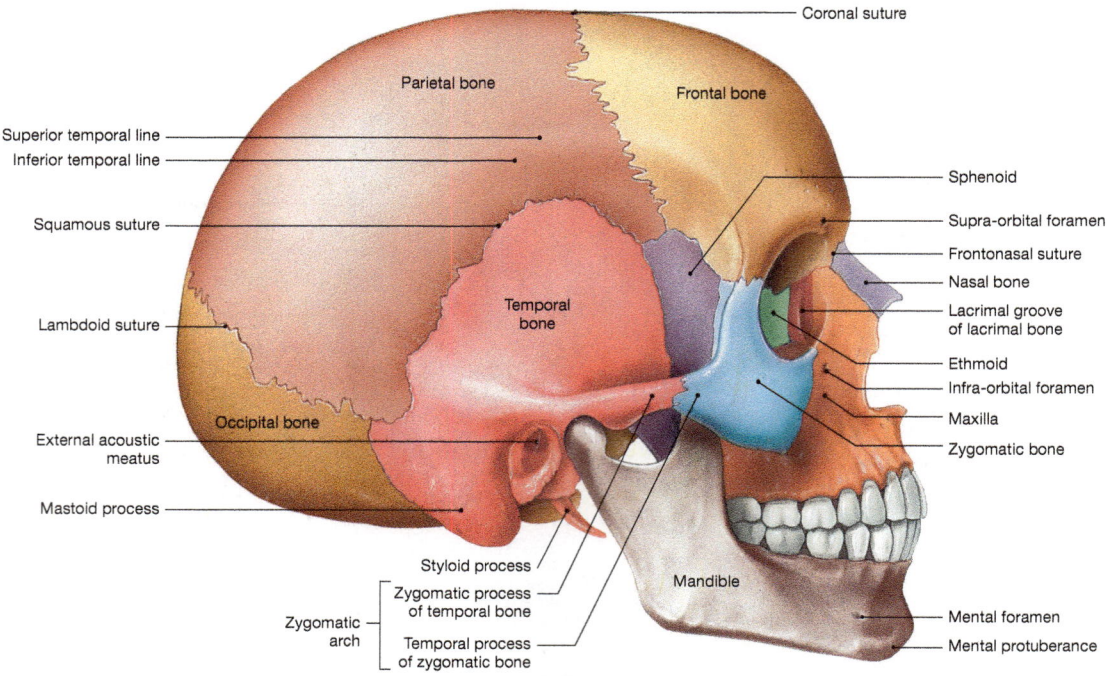

(a) Lateral view of the bones of the adult skull

From *Human Anatomy*, Ninth Edition, by Frederic H. Martini, Robert B. Tallitsch, and Judi L. Nath (2018), reproduced by permission of Pearson Education.

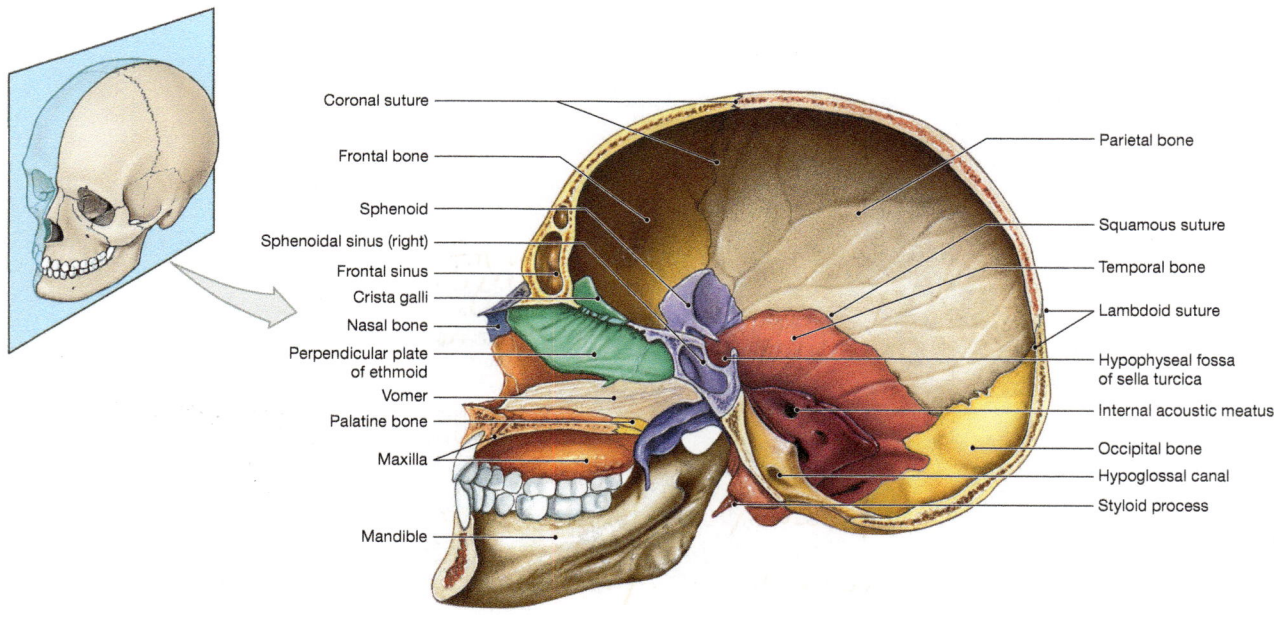

(b) Sagittal Section of the Adult Skull

From *Human Anatomy*, Ninth Edition, by Frederic H. Martini, Robert B. Tallitsch, and Judi L. Nath (2018), reproduced by permission of Pearson Education.

Figure 2.2 **Lateral View and Sagittal Section of the Skull.**

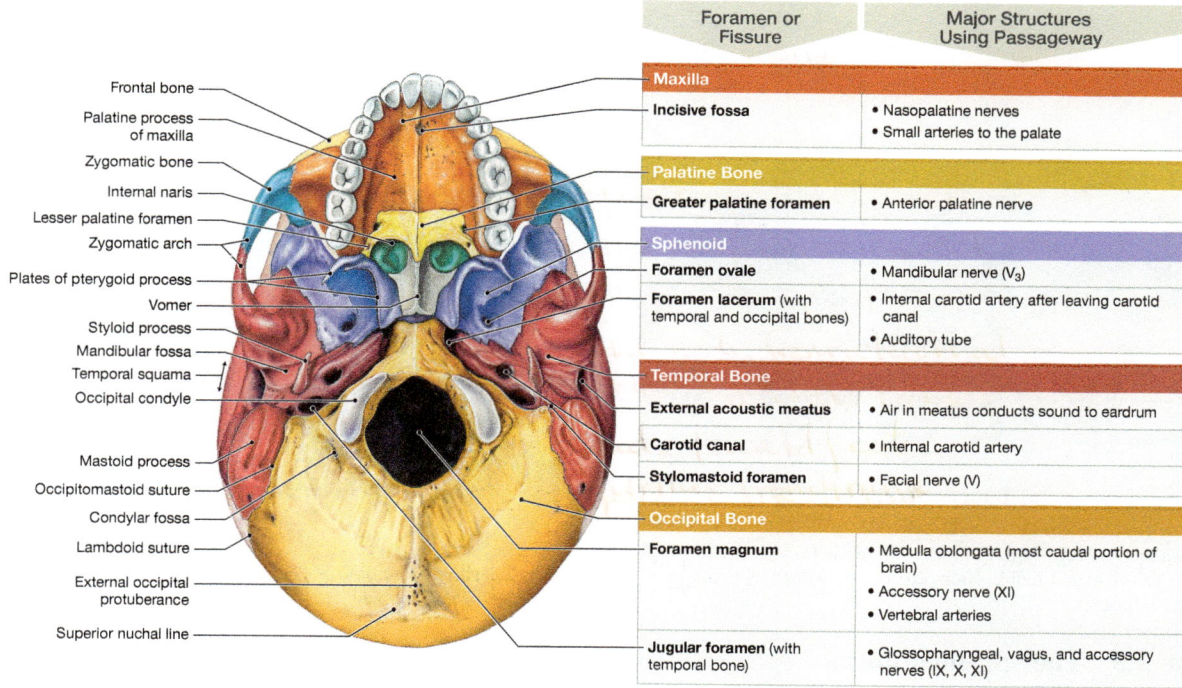

From *Human Anatomy*, Ninth Edition, by Frederic H. Martini, Robert B. Tallitsch, and Judi L. Nath (2018), reproduced by permission of Pearson Education.

Figure 2.3 Inferior View of the Skull.

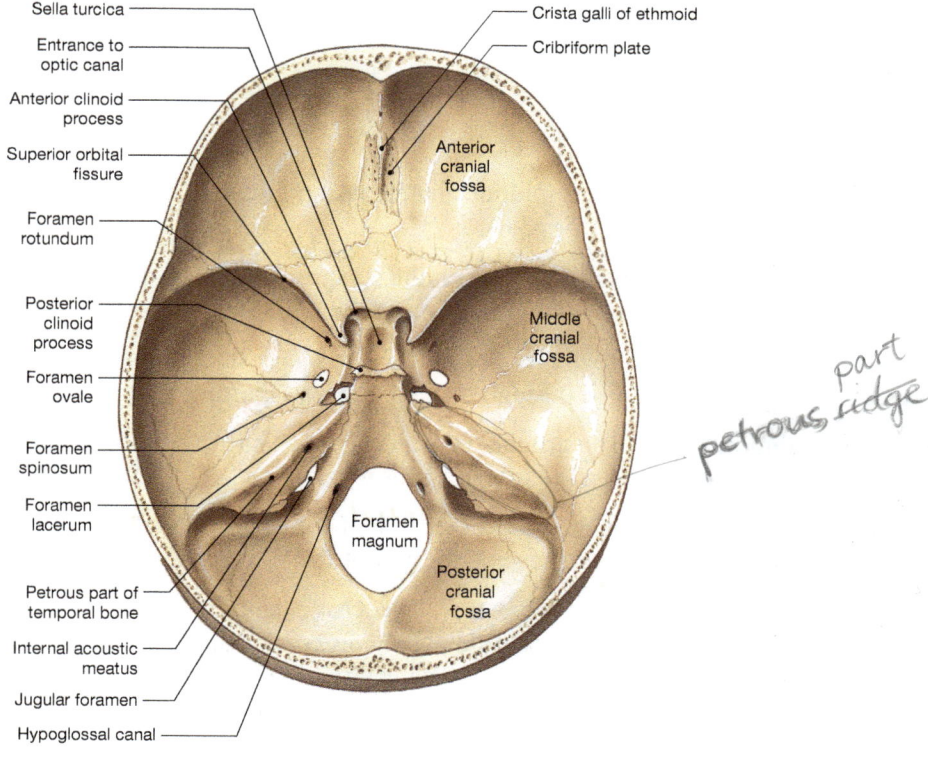

From *Human Anatomy*, Ninth Edition, by Frederic H. Martini, Robert B. Tallitsch, and Judi L. Nath (2018), reproduced by permission of Pearson Education.

Figure 2.4 Cranial Fossae and Foramina.

CHAPTER TWO   *The Skeletal System: Axial & Appendicular Divisions*   11

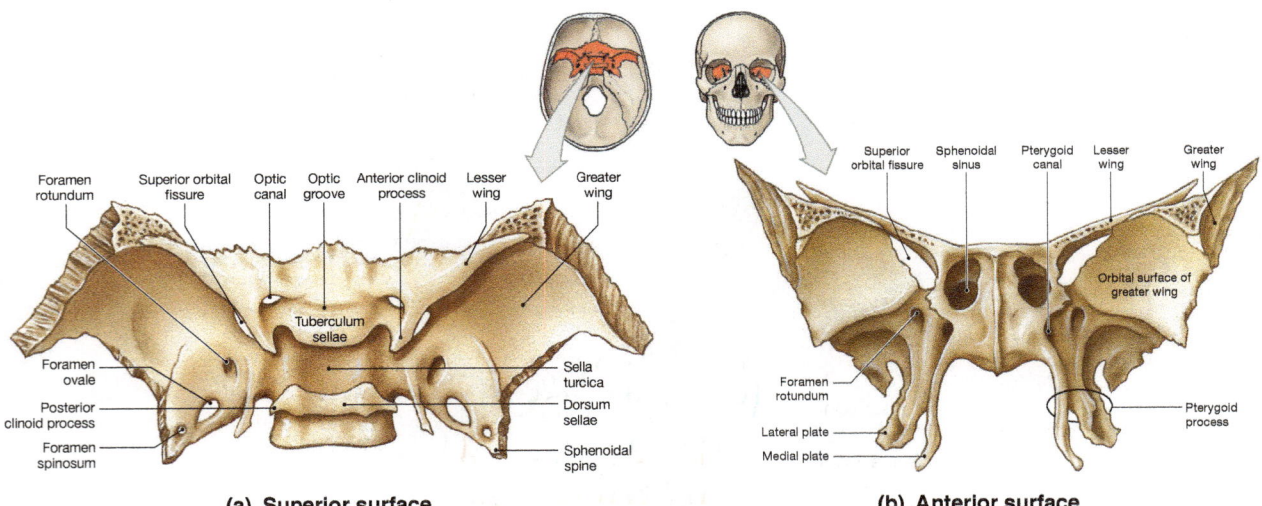

(a) Superior surface

From *Human Anatomy*, Ninth Edition, by Frederic H. Martini, Robert B. Tallitsch, and Judi L. Nath (2018), reproduced by permission of Pearson Education.

(b) Anterior surface

From *Human Anatomy*, Ninth Edition, by Frederic H. Martini, Robert B. Tallitsch, and Judi L. Nath (2018), reproduced by permission of Pearson Education.

Figure 2.5 The Sphenoid Bone.

8. The **foramen ovale** is slightly larger than and more laterally and posteriorly located than the foramen rotundum. The foramen ovale is the passageway for the mandibular division of cranial nerve V.

9. **Pterygoid plates** (pterygoid processes) project from the inferior surface of the sphenoid bone. The pterygoid plates (pterygoid processes) are located behind the upper 3rd molar in an articulated skull.

Ethmoid Bone

The **ethmoid bone** is located at the midline and forms a portion of the anterior floor of the cranium and the roof of the nasal cavity. (Fig. 2.6).

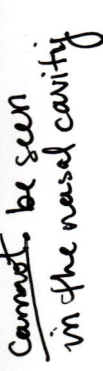
cannot be seen in the nasal cavity

1. The **crista galli** is the pointed structure on the superior surface of the ethmoid bone. A portion of the dura mater (one of the membranes covering the brain) attaches to the crista galli. → *shark fin where dura mater attaches*

2. The **cribriform plate** is a region of porous bone to either side of the crista galli. **Olfactory nerves** (cranial nerves I) pass through the **cribriform foramina** of the ethmoid bone. → *only part of brain that's outside skull*

3. Study the ethmoid bone on an articulated skull. Find its surfaces in the intracranial cavity (anterior cranial fossa) and in the orbit and nasal cavity.

4. The **perpendicular plate** is the vertical portion of the ethmoid located at the midline of the bone. The perpendicular plate forms the superior part of the bony nasal septum (Fig. 2.2b and 2.6a).

5. **Superior** and **middle nasal conchae** are bony scroll-shaped structures extending into the nasal cavity. Locate the **superior and middle nasal conchae** on a disarticulated ethmoid. Also locate the **middle nasal conchae** through the nasal cavity of an articulated skull; the superior nasal conchae cannot be seen in this view (Fig. 2.6b).

6. **Ethmoid sinuses** (ethmoid cells) are small cavities within the ethmoid bone.

7. **Lateral masses** (ethmoidal labyrinth) are located lateral to the nasal conchae. The lateral masses form the medial wall of the orbit (Fig. 2.7).

Complete Introductory Human Anatomy Lab Guide

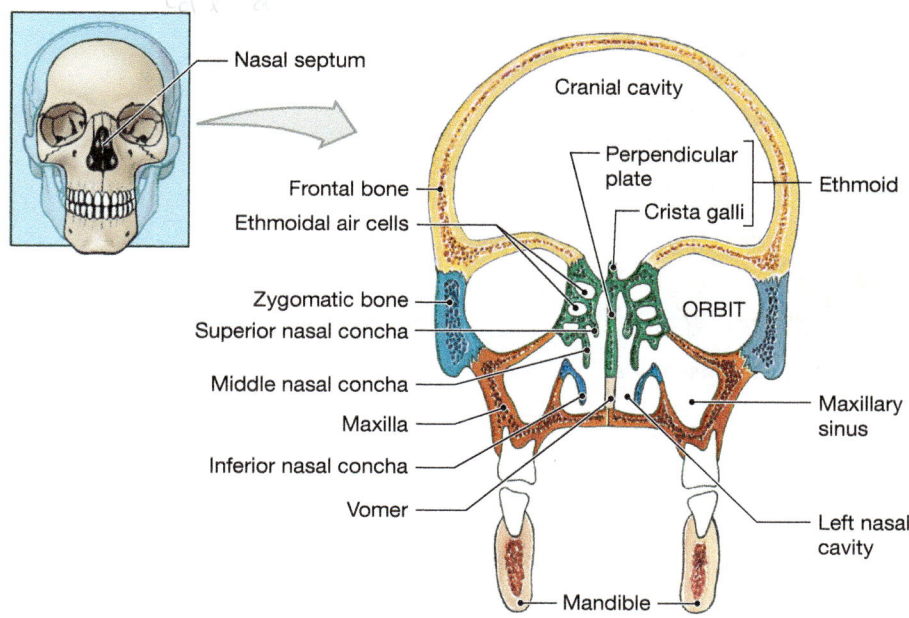

(a) A diagrammatic frontal section showing the positions of the paranasal sinuses

From *Human Anatomy*, Eighth Edition, by Frederic H. Martini and Robert B. Tallitsch (2015), reproduced by permission of Pearson Education.

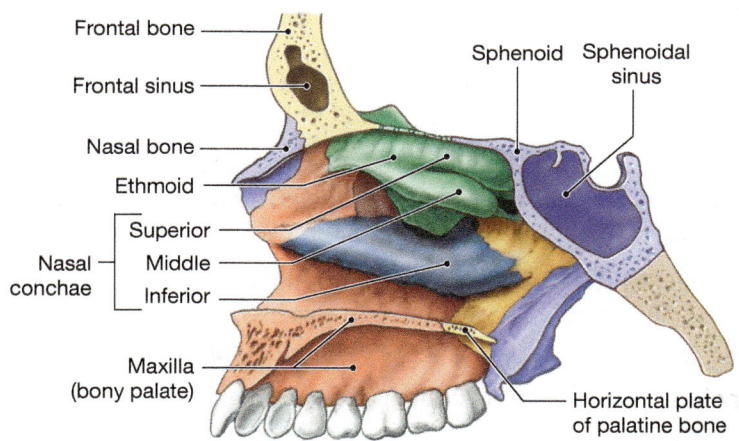

(b) Diagrammatic sagittal section with the nasal septum removed to show major features of the wall of the right nasal cavity

From *Human Anatomy*, Eighth Edition, by Frederic H. Martini and Robert B. Tallitsch (2015), reproduced by permission of Pearson Education.

Figure 2.6 **The Nasal Complex and Paranasal Sinuses.** Sections through the skull and head showing relationships among the bones of the nasal complex and the positions of the paranasal sinuses.

CHAPTER TWO   *The Skeletal System: Axial & Appendicular Divisions*

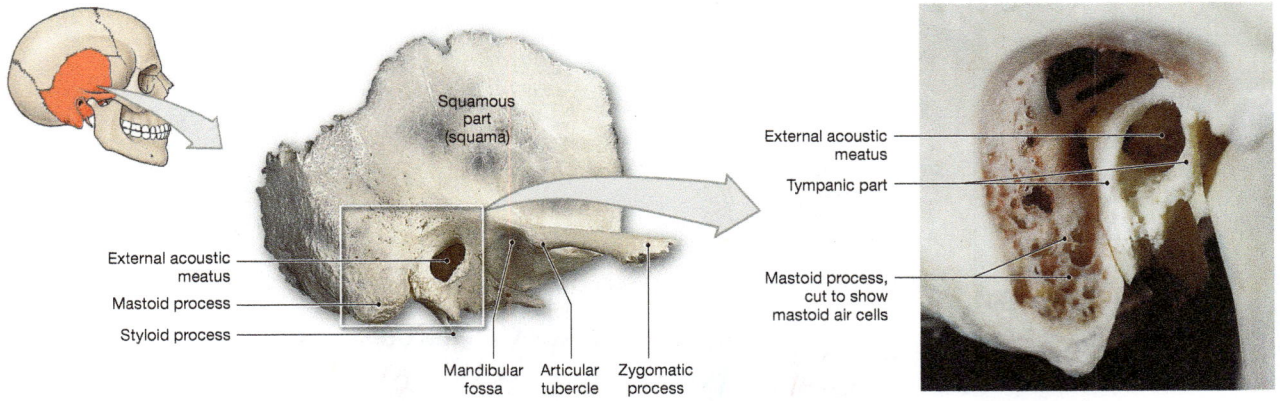

(a) Right temporal bone, lateral view

(b) Cutaway view of the mastoid air cells

From *Human Anatomy*, Ninth Edition, by Frederic H. Martini, Robert B. Tallitsch, and Judi L. Nath (2018), reproduced by permission of Pearson Education.

From *Human Anatomy*, Ninth Edition, by Frederic H. Martini, Robert B. Tallitsch, and Judi L. Nath (2018), reproduced by permission of Pearson Education.

Figure 2.7 The Temporal Bone.

Temporal Bone

The **temporal bone** forms part of the lateral walls and part of the floor of the middle cranial fossa (Figs. 2.2, 2.3 & 2.7).

1. The **mastoid process of the temporal bone** is a large, blunt process located posterior and inferior to the external ear. The mastoid process is an attachment site for the sternocleidomastoid muscle.

2. The **styloid process** is the pointed structure located anterior to the mastoid process. Tendons and ligaments connect this structure with the **hyoid bone**.

3. The **petrous part** of the temporal bone is a bony ridge that forms part of the floor of the cranium. It contains the **auditory ossicles** (**malleus, incus,** and **stapes**) as well as structures of the inner ear. The petrous ridge forms the posterior border of the middle cranial fossa.

4. The **external acoustic meatus** is the opening for the external ear canal. The external acoustic meatus is anterior and superior to the **mastoid process.**

5. The **carotid canal** is the passageway for the **internal carotid artery.** Within the cranial cavity, the carotid canal opens near the sella turcica of the sphenoid bone. On the base of the skull, the carotid canal opens just *anterior* to the jugular foramen.

6. The **zygomatic process of the temporal bone** meets the **temporal process of the zygomatic bone** and it is anterior to the external acoustic meatus.

7. The **mandibular fossa** is a depression on the proximal, inferior surface of the zygomatic process of the temporal bone, just anterior to the external acoustic meatus. The mandibular fossa is the articular site for the mandibular condyle (see mandible).

8. The **internal acoustic meatus** is located on the medial surface of the petrous part of the temporal bone. The internal acoustic meatus is the passageway for cranial nerves VII and VIII.

9. The jugular foramen is inferior to the internal acoustic meatus, along the border with the occipital bone.

Bones of the Orbital

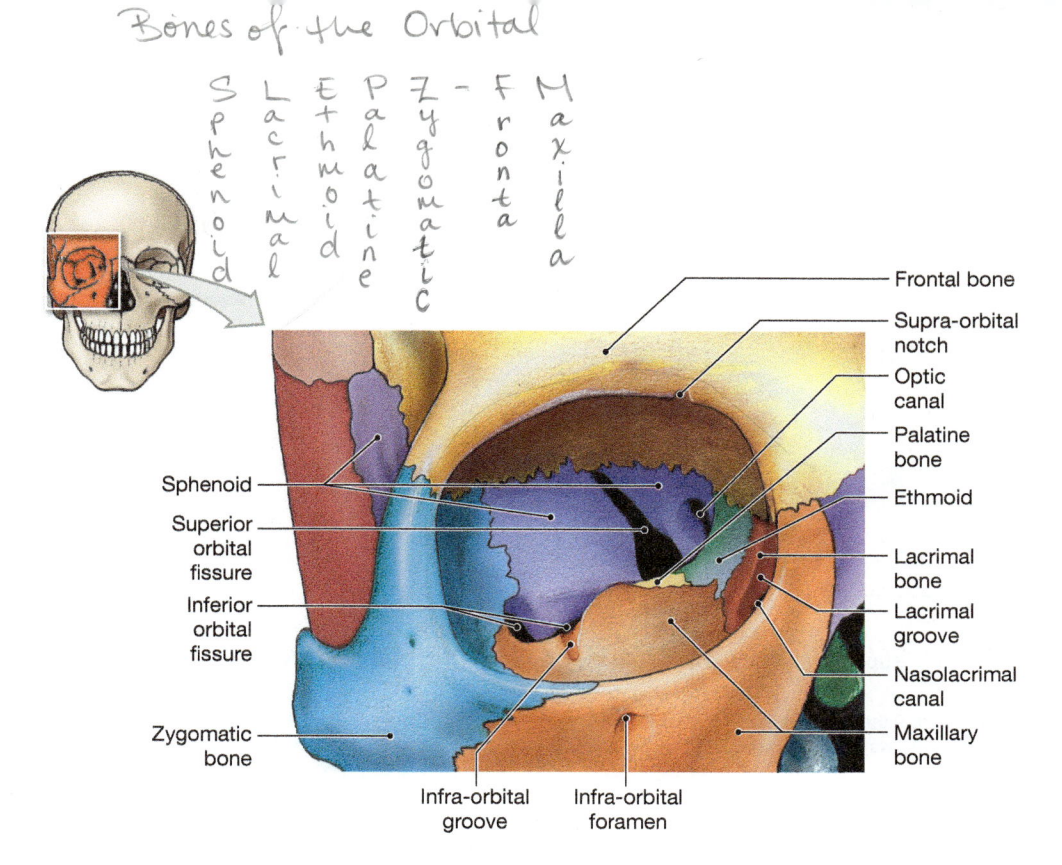

S - Sphenoid
L - Lacrimal
E - Ethmoid
P - Palatine
Z - Zygomatic
F - Frontal
M - Maxilla

Figure 2.8 **The Orbital Complex**. The structure of the orbital complex on the right side. Seven bones form the bony orbit that encloses and protects the right eye.

From *Human Anatomy*, Ninth Edition, by Frederic H. Martini, Robert B. Tallitsch, and Judi L. Nath (2018), reproduced by permission of Pearson Education.

Parietal Bone

The **parietal bone** forms the lateral walls and roof of the cranium. Each parietal bone articulates with the **frontal** and **occipital bone** and also with the **sphenoid** and **temporal bone** on the same side of the skull (Figs. 2.1, 2.2). Note the grooves on the internal surface of the parietal bone for the meningeal arteries.

Occipital Bone

The **occipital bone** forms the posterior and inferior portion of the skull (Figs. 2.1, 2.2 & 2.3). Inside the cranial cavity it forms the floor of the posterior cranial fossa.

1. The **foramen magnum** is the large opening in the inferior portion (base) of the occipital bone through which the brainstem passes.

2. The **occipital condyles** are the smooth bumps located laterally (to either side) of the foramen magnum. The concave facets of the **atlas** (1st cervical vertebra) articulate with the occipital condyles.

3. The **jugular foramina** are small, oval openings formed along the suture between the occipital bone and temporal bone. The jugular foramina are the openings through which blood drains from the intracranial cavity and the beginning of the **internal jugular veins**. Cranial nerves IX, X and XI pass through the jugular foramen.

4. The **hypoglossal canal** is the small opening that passes through the occipital bone just above each occipital condyle. Cranial nerve XII (the hypoglossal nerve) passes through this canal. *(tongue-related)*

5. The **basioccipital** is the thick region of the occipital bone anterior to the foramen magnum where the occipital bone articulates with the sphenoid bone.

CHAPTER TWO   *The Skeletal System: Axial & Appendicular Divisions*   15

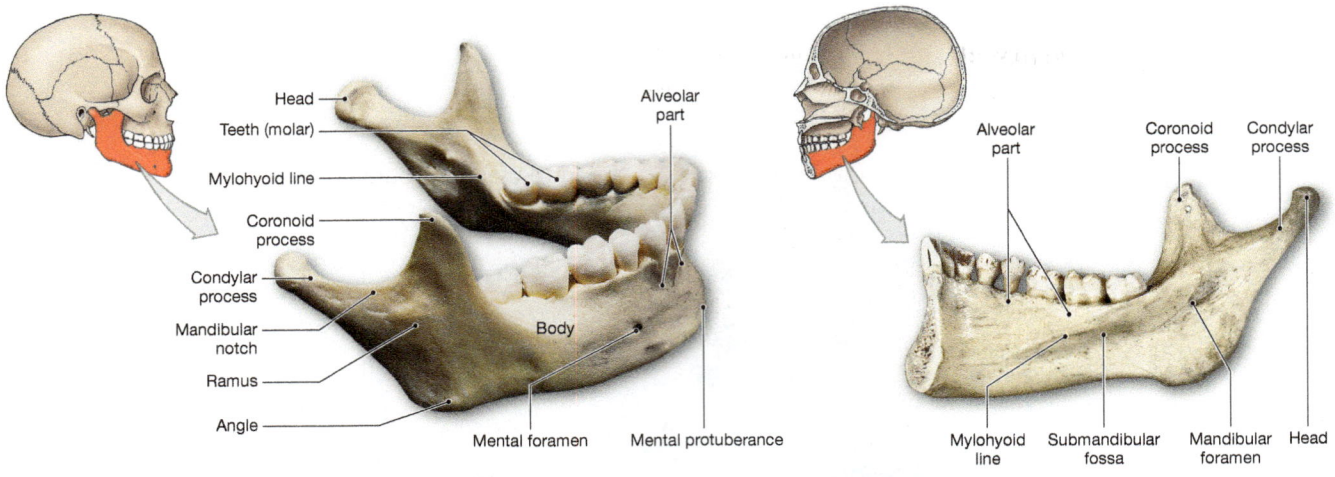

Nasal Septum = perpendicular plate + vomer + septal cartilage

Figure 2.9 **The Mandible.** Views of the mandible showing major anatomical landmarks.

STRUCTURES OF FACIAL BONES

Vomer

The **vomer** articulates with the perpendicular plate of the ethmoid bone to form the posterior, inferior portion of the bony nasal septum (Fig. 2.1, 2.2).

Mandible

The **mandible** is the bone of the jaw and is the only movable bone in the skull (Figs. 2.1, 2.2, 2.9).

1. The **mandibular condyle** is the articular surface on the condylar process that articulates with the **mandibular fossa of the temporal bone** to form the temporomandibular joint.

2. The **coronoid process** is anterior to the condylar process. The coronoid process is the site of attachment for the temporalis muscle.

3. The **alveolar process** is the area of the mandible that houses tooth sockets (alveoli) for the lower dentition.

4. The **angle** of the mandible is the prominent point on the posterior side of the mandible just below the ear.

5. **Mental foramina** are small openings on the anterior surface of the mandible for the passage of blood vessels and nerves.

Hyoid Bone

The **hyoid bone** does not articulate with any bone *directly*, but is still included in the study of the skull. The **hyoid bone** is attached to the **styloid process of the temporal bone,** the **inferior border of the mandible** and to the **manubrium of the sternum** by muscles and ligaments.

Maxilla

Together the two **maxillae** form the "upper jaw." The two maxillae articulate with each other along the midline between the two front incisors and through the hard palate. Each maxilla also forms parts of the orbit and hard palate and nasal cavity (Figs. 2.1 & 2.2).

1. The **frontal process of the maxilla** is a pointed structure that articulates with the frontal bone. The frontal process also forms the medial border and most of the floor of the orbit.

2. The **alveolar process** is the area of the maxilla that houses alveoli for the upper dentition.

3. The **palatine process of the maxilla** is the anterior portion of the hard palate, which articulates with the **horizontal plate of the palatine bone.** The largest part of the hard palate is contributed by the maxilla (Figs. 2.2, 2.3 & 2.6).

4. **Maxillary sinuses** are cavities within the maxilla (Fig. 2.6).

Palatine Bones

The **palatine bones** form the smaller, posterior portion of the hard palate and a small portion of the orbit. Observe the **horizontal plate of the palatine bone,** which is located at the posterior boundary of the **palatine process of the maxilla.**

Zygomatic Bones

The **zygomatic bones** form the lateral wall of the orbit (Figs. 2.1, 2.2 & 2.7).

1. The **temporal process of the zygomatic bone** points posteriorly and articulates with the zygomatic process of the temporal bone.

2. The **zygomatic arch** is a composite structure formed by union of the **zygomatic process of the temporal bone** and the **temporal process of the zygomatic bone.** The zygomatic arch forms the "cheekbone."

3. The **frontal process of the zygomatic bone** forms the lateral wall of the orbit and it articulates with the frontal bone.

Nasal Bones

Nasal bones form part of the bridge of the nose. The nasal bones articulate with both the **frontal bone** and **maxilla.**

Lacrimal Bones

Lacrimal bones form a portion of the orbit and contain the opening for the nasolacrimal duct. The nasolacrimal duct conducts tears from the orbit into the nasal cavity (Fig. 2.7).

Inferior Nasal Conchae

Inferior nasal conchae are connected to the walls of the maxilla and are visible through the nasal cavity. Note: Inferior nasal conchae are separate bones that are **not** part of the ethmoid bone.

Auditory Ossicles

Auditory Ossicles are the smallest bones in the body. The **malleus, incus,** and **stapes** are located within the middle ear cavity in the petrous part of the temporal bone.

Bones and Structures Forming Regions of the Skull

Bones Forming the Orbit of the Eye

Seven bones form each orbital fossa. These bones are the **maxilla**, **palatine**, **zygomatic**, **lacrimal**, **frontal**, **sphenoid** and **ethmoid bones**. The **optic canals**, **superior** and **inferior orbital fissures** are also included as part of the orbital fossae (Fig. 2.1, 2.7). The **inferior orbital fissure** is between the sphenoid and the maxilla.

Framework & Structure of the Nose

1. The lateral walls of the nasal cavity are framed by the three sets of nasal conchae. The middle and superior nasal conchae are part of the ethmoid bone; the inferior nasal concha is an independent bone attached to the wall of the maxilla.

2. The **nasal septum** divides the nose internally into right and left passageways. Structures forming the nasal septum include the **perpendicular plate of the ethmoid bone, vomer** and **septal cartilage.**

3. The superior part of the **palatine process of the maxilla** forms the floor of the nasal cavity.

4. The **cribriform plate of the ethmoid** defines the superior boundary of the nasal cavity.

Sinuses

Sinuses are cavities found within several bones of the skull. We have studied four sinuses: the **frontal, sphenoid, ethmoid** and **maxillary** sinuses. Paranasal sinuses are always named for the skull bone in which they lie.

Fontanels of the Infant Skull

Fontanels ("soft spots") begin as membranous portions of the infant skull at the places where the parietal bones fuse with their adjoining bones. The six fontanels are: the **frontal (or anterior)**, **occipital (or posterior)**, **two sphenoid** and **two mastoid fontanels**. Identify these fontanels on an anatomical model or using virtual images on the computer.

B. THE VERTEBRAL COLUMN

Features Common to Most Vertebrae

1. The **body** is the cylindrical, anterior portion of a vertebra. Vertebral bodies bear the weight of the vertebrae superior to them, and become progressively larger from the second cervical vertebra inferiorly through the lower lumbar vertebrae.

2. The **vertebral arch** protects the spinal cord. It is made up of laminae and pedicles on each vertebra.

    - The **laminae** (singular lamina) form the roof of the vertebral canal. They extend medially from the pedicles to the spinous process at the midline.
    - Right and left **pedicles** form pillars between the body and the laminae.

3. The **vertebral foramen** is the opening encircled by the vertebral arch and body of each vertebra.

4. The **vertebral canal** is formed in the intact vertebral column by joining all of the adjacent vertebral foramina. The spinal cord is protected within the vertebral canal.

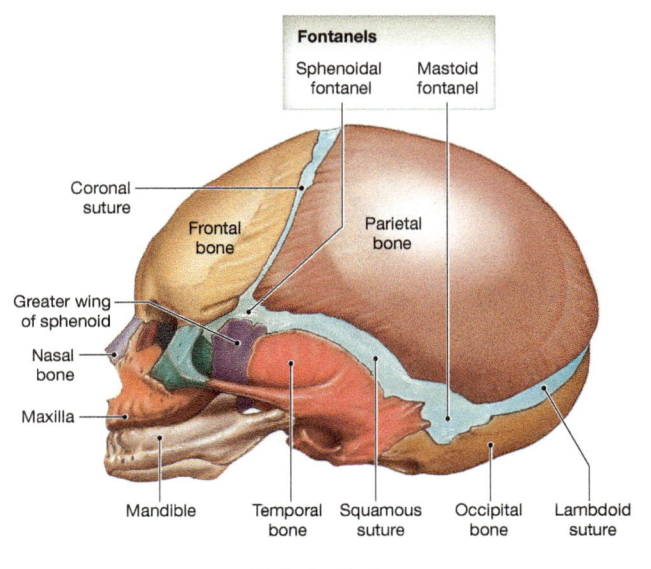

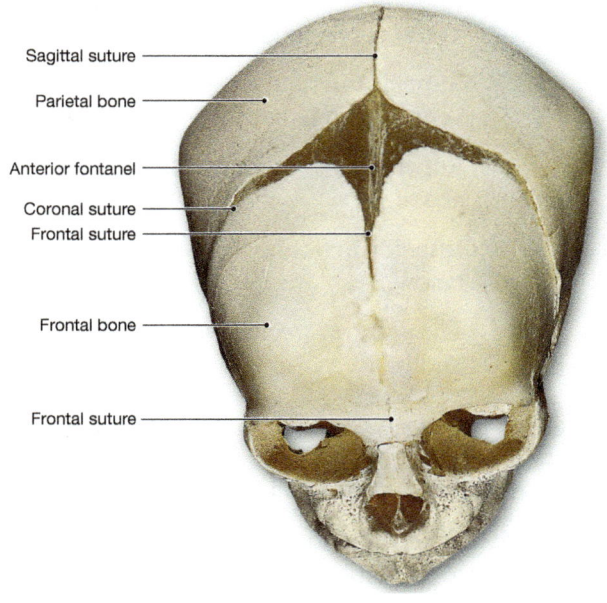

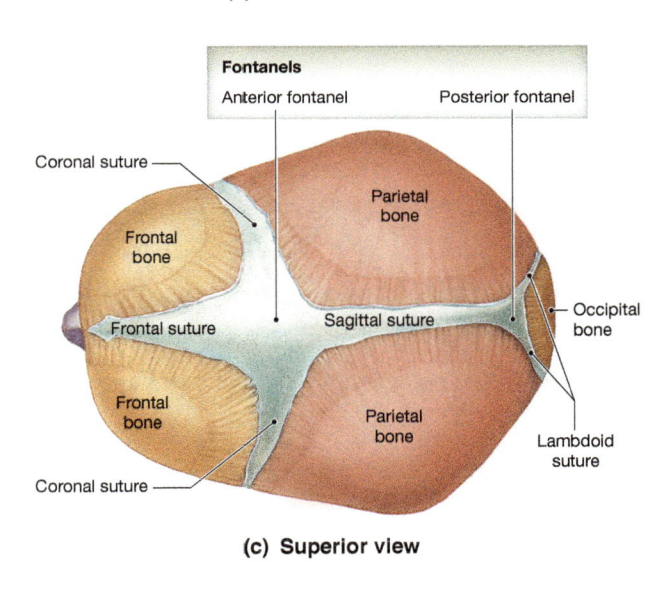

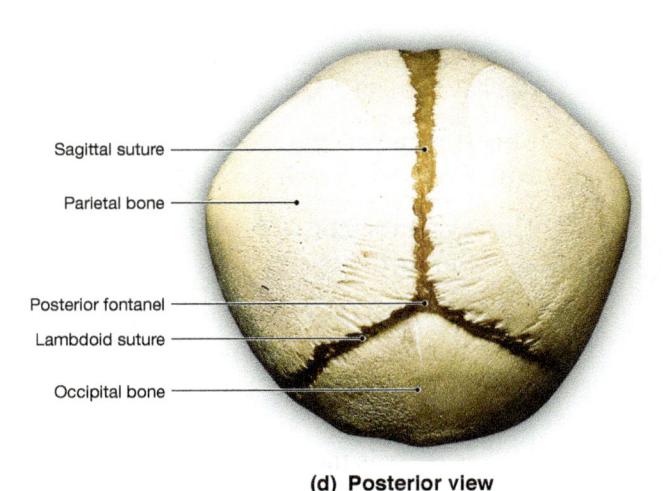

Figure 2.10 **The Skull of an Infant.** The flat bones in the infant skull are separated by fontanels, which allow for cranial expansion and the distortion of the skull during birth. By about age 5 these areas will disappear, and skull growth will be completed.

CHAPTER TWO   *The Skeletal System: Axial & Appendicular Divisions*   19

CHARACTERISTICS OF VERTEBRAE

Processes Found on Vertebrae

1. **Transverse processes** are projections from the sides of cervical, thoracic and lumbar vertebrae.
2. **Superior articular processes** and **inferior articular processes** are the bony projections from the vertebral arch that bear the superior and inferior articular facets.
3. **Superior articular facets** articulate with the inferior articular facets of the adjacent vertebra above.
4. **Inferior articular facets** articulate with the superior articular facets of the adjacent vertebra below.
5. The **spinous process** is the dorsally directed process of bone from the vertebral arch at the midline.

CHARACTERISTICS OF THE VERTEBRAL COLUMN

The human vertebral column is divided into five regions (Fig. 2.11).

Seven **cervical vertebrae** form the neck region. The first two cervical vertebrae are named the **atlas** and **axis**, respectively. The remaining five cervical vertebrae are simply numbered 3–7.

The twelve **thoracic vertebrae** are inferior to the cervical region. Thoracic vertebrae have articular surfaces for the ribs. The head of the rib articulates with the body of the thoracic vertebra and the tubercle of the rib articulates with the transverse process.

The five **lumbar vertebrae** are inferior to the thoracic vertebrae. They have larger bodies and they do not have articular sites for ribs.

Sacral vertebrae fuse to form a single bone called the **sacrum,** in the adult. The sacrum articulates with the ilium of each coxal bone.

Coccygeal vertebrae 3–5 coccygeal vertebrae form the "tail bone." They are usually fused into a single bone, the **coccyx**.

The **intervertebral foramen** is the opening formed between the pedicles of adjacent vertebrae through which the spinal nerves branch off from the spinal cord.

Intervertebral discs are shock-absorbing cushions between each vertebra made mostly of fibrocartilage.

Curvatures of the Vertebral Column

From a lateral view, the adult vertebral column is not straight, but rather has four curvatures. The thoracic and sacral regions are concave anteriorly and the cervical and lumbar curvatures are concave posteriorly. The thoracic and sacral curvatures are **primary curvatures** that form during embryonic development, while the cervical and lumbar curvatures are secondary curvatures. The **secondary curvatures** form several months after birth and help distribute body weight over the feet. These curvatures help distribute the body's weight evenly over the feet, and function to absorb the impact of walking.

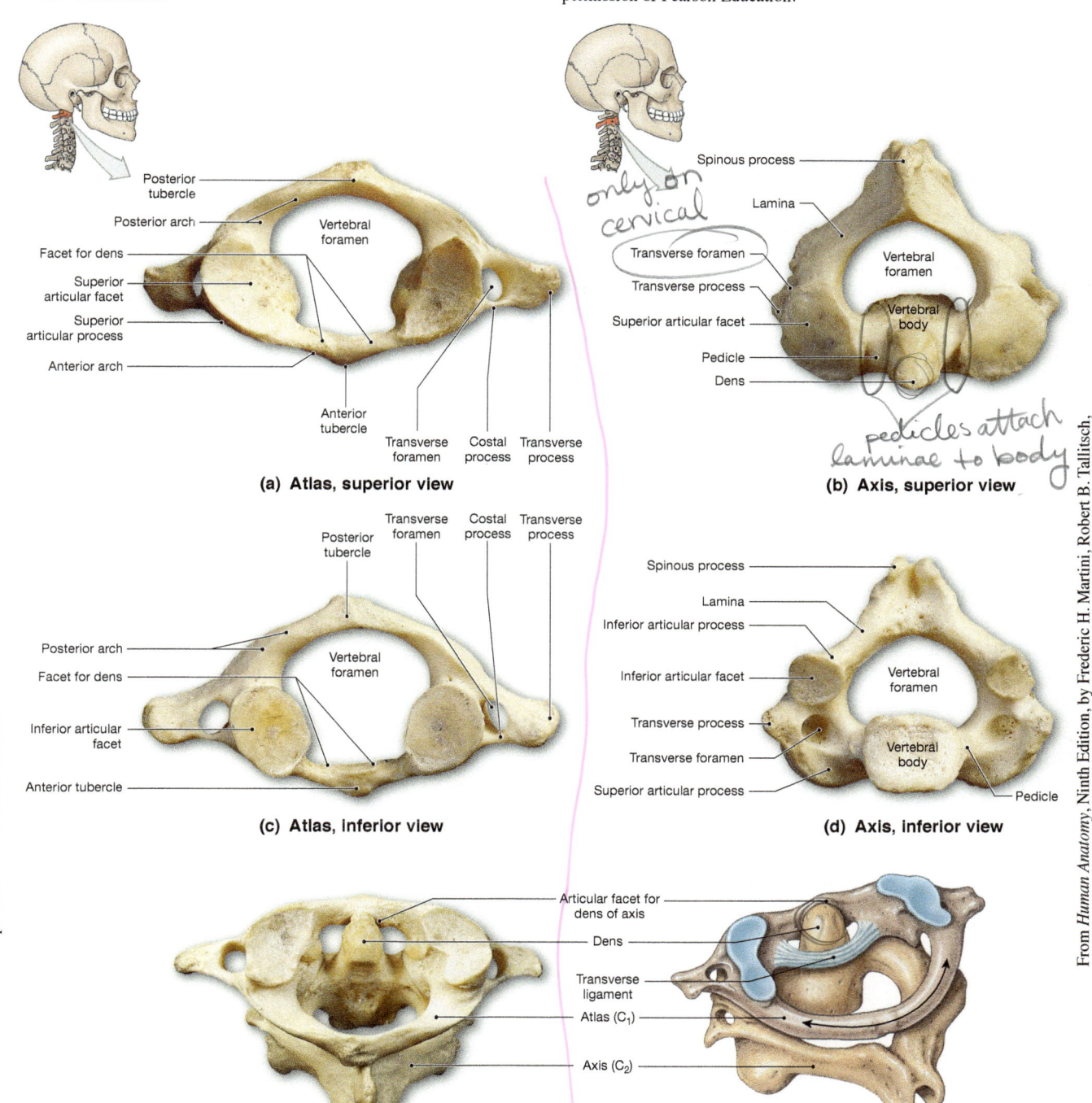

Figure 2.11a Atlas and Axis.

CHAPTER TWO   *The Skeletal System: Axial & Appendicular Divisions*   21

(a) Lateral view of the cervical vertebrae

From *Human Anatomy*, Ninth Edition, by Frederic H. Martini, Robert B. Tallitsch, and Judi L. Nath (2018), reproduced by permission of Pearson Education.

(b) Lateral view of a typical (C_3–C_6) cervical vertebra

(c) Superior view of the same vertebra

From *Human Anatomy*, Ninth Edition, by Frederic H. Martini, Robert B. Tallitsch, and Judi L. Nath (2018), reproduced by permission of Pearson Education.

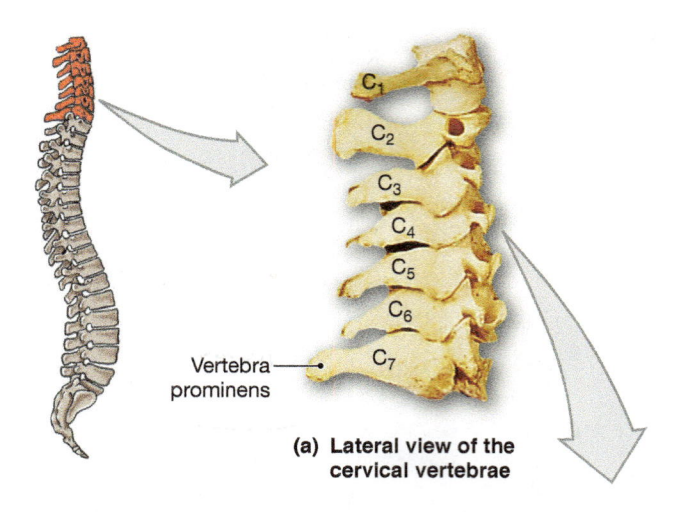

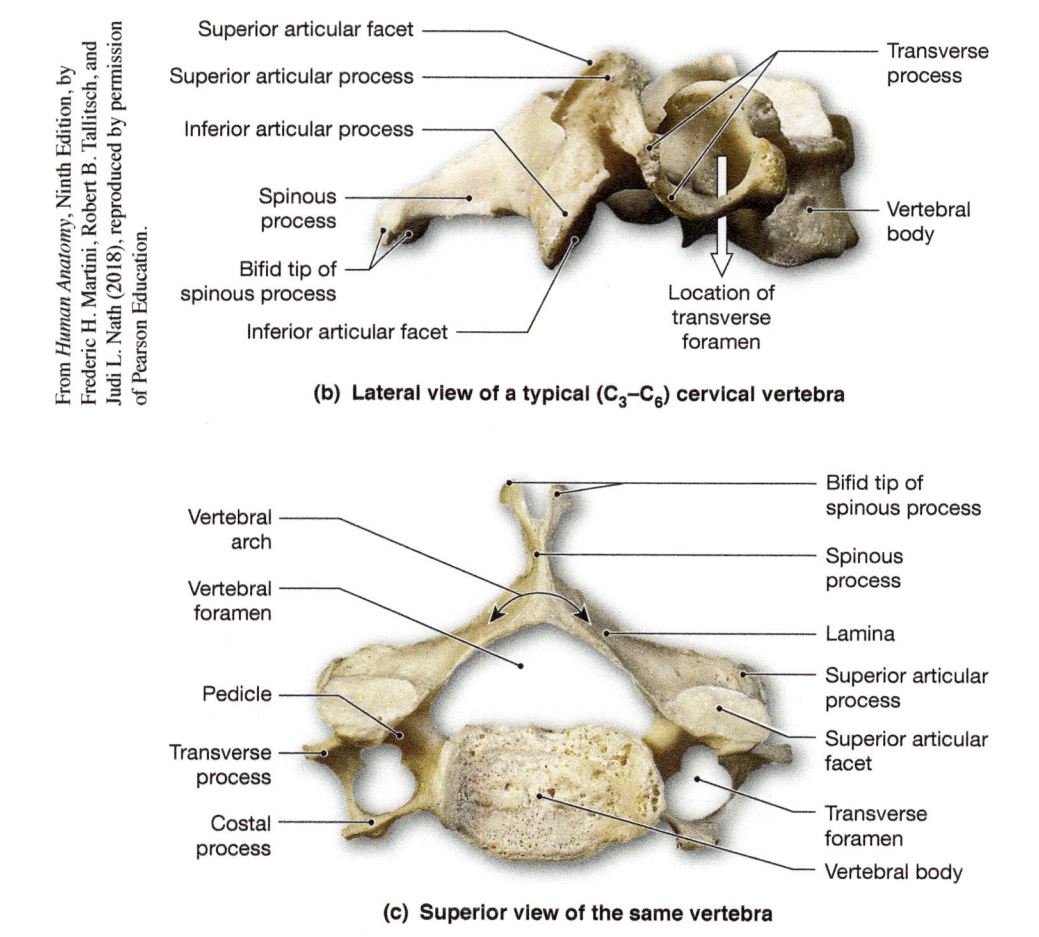

Figure 2.11b **Cervical Vertebrae.**

CHARACTERISTICS OF SPECIFIC TYPES OF VERTEBRAE

Cervical Vertebrae

The first two cervical vertebrae, the **atlas** and the **axis**, have unique characteristics and will be considered separately from the remaining five cervical vertebrae.

1. The **atlas** is the first cervical vertebra and has the following characteristics. (Fig. 2.11a)

    - The atlas has two lateral masses connected by an anterior and posterior arch. The atlas does not have a body.
    - At the midline there are tubercles on the anterior and posterior arches; the atlas does not have a spinous process.
    - The lateral masses of the atlas bear **superior articular facets** (concave facets) on their superior surfaces for articulation with the occipital condyles of the occipital bone.
    - The lateral masses of the atlas bear **inferior articular facets** on their inferior surfaces for articulation with the superior articular facets of cervical vertebra two, the axis.
    - Articulation of the **atlas** with the occipital condyles allows nodding of the head up and down.

2. The **axis** is the second cervical vertebra and has the following characteristics.

    - The **dens** (odontoid process) **of the axis** is a tooth-shaped structure that points superiorly and articulates with the atlas.
    - The dens is formed by the fusion of the **body of the atlas** and the **body of the axis.**
    - Articulation of the **dens** of the axis with the anterior arch of the **atlas** allows the atlas to pivot on the axis and permits rotational movement of the head.

3. Cervical vertebrae, including the atlas and axis, have **transverse foramina** within their transverse processes for the passage of the paired **vertebral arteries** and **veins**.

4. Typically, cervical vertebrae numbers 2–6 have short, bifid spinous processes.

5. Cervical vertebra seven (C7), has a long, prominent spinous process and so is called the vertebra prominens. This process is easily palpated on a living subject.

Thoracic Vertebrae

(Fig. 2.11c)

1. Thoracic vertebrae articulate with ribs. **Bodies** of thoracic vertebrae have **facets** or **demifacets** (half a facet) for articulation with the head (capitulum) of the ribs. Ribs 11 and 12 articulate only with the bodies of the 11th and 12th thoracic vertebrae.

2. **Transverse processes** of T_{1-10} have articular facets for articulation with tubercles of the ribs.

3. **Spinous processes** of thoracic vertebrae are **slender,** point inferiorly, and in some areas overlap the spinous processes of vertebrae inferior to them.

4. **Superior articular facets** face posteriorly on thoracic vertebrae, which helps distinguish thoracic vertebrae from lumbar vertebrae.

Lumbar Vertebrae

(Fig. 2.11d)

1. **Bodies** of lumbar vertebrae are large and sturdy (robust).

2. **Spinous processes** are large, blunt and robust, and point directly posterior.

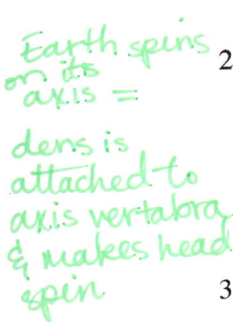

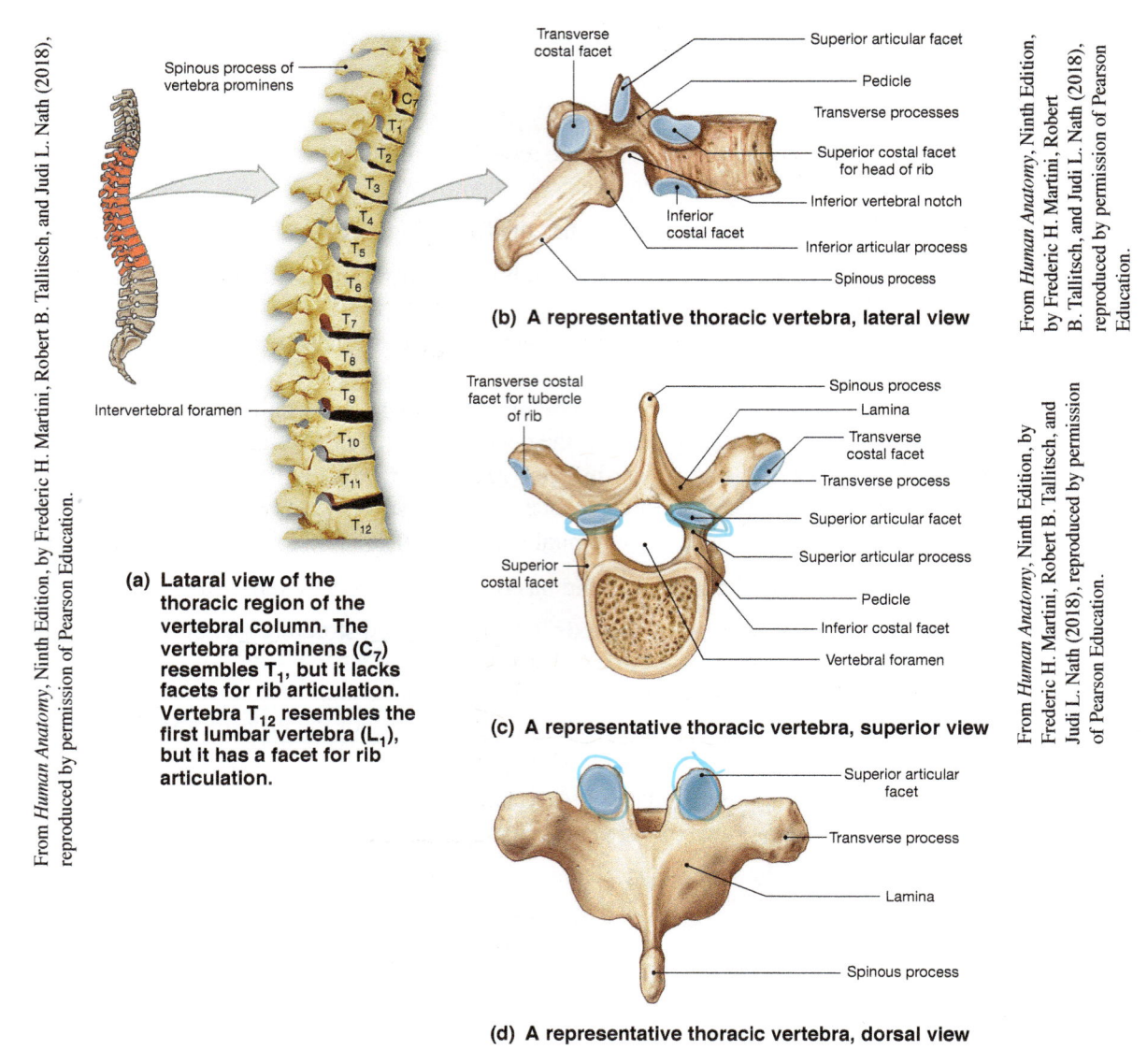

Figure 2.11c Thoracic Vertebrae.

3. **Transverse processes** are thick and heavy.

4. **Superior articular** facets of lumbar vertebrae face medially, which aids in distinguishing lumbar from thoracic vertebrae.

Sacral Vertebrae

(Fig. 2.11e)

1. The five sacral vertebrae are fused into a single unit to form the **sacrum** in the adult skeleton.

2. The **sacral canal** is the continuation of the vertebral canal that passes through the sacrum from superior to inferior. It is through this opening that the spinal nerves pass *before* exiting the sacral foramina.

Complete Introductory Human Anatomy Lab Guide

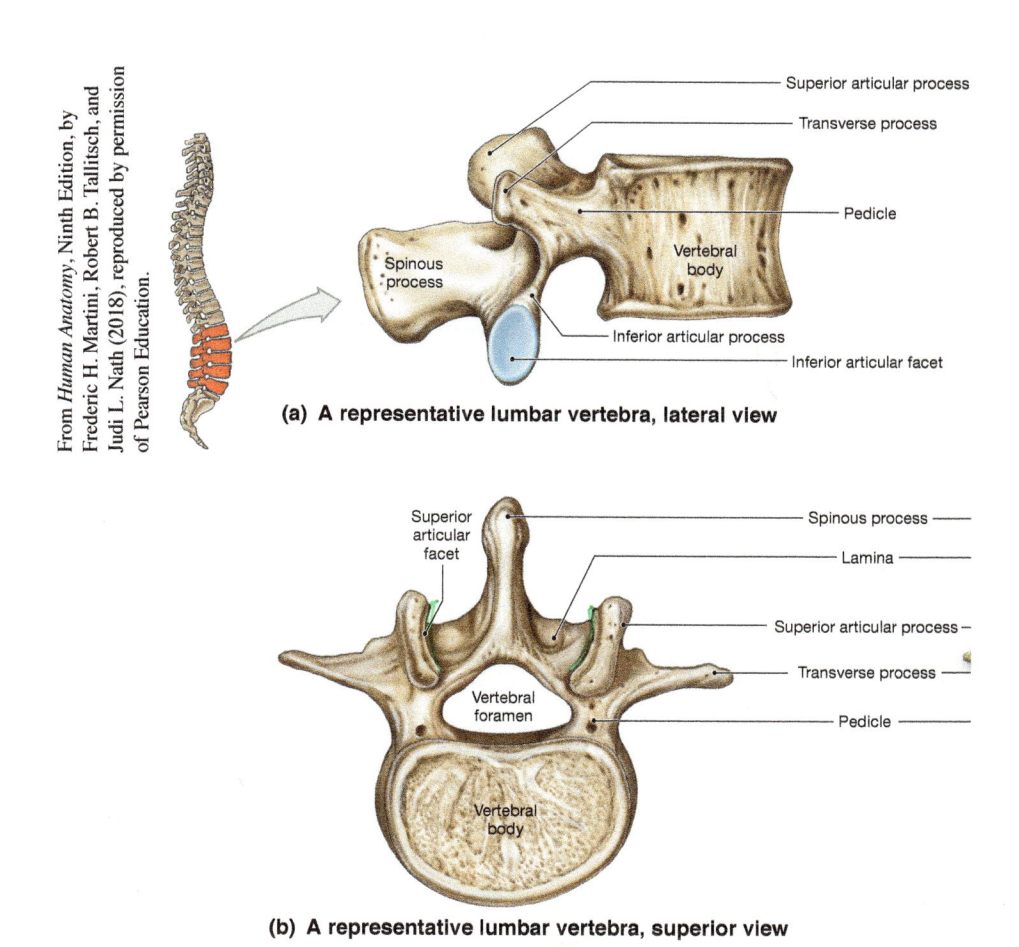

(a) A representative lumbar vertebra, lateral view

(b) A representative lumbar vertebra, superior view

From *Human Anatomy*, Ninth Edition, by Frederic H. Martini, Robert B. Tallitsch, and Judi L. Nath (2018), reproduced by permission of Pearson Education.

Figure 2.11d Lumbar Vertebrae.

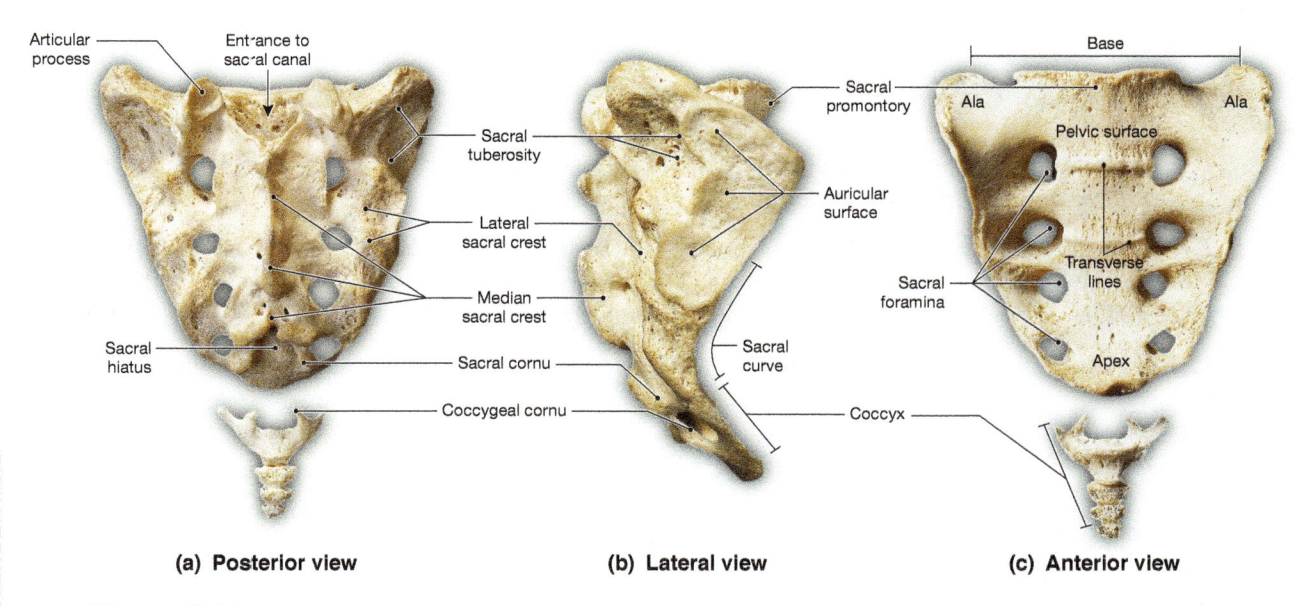

(a) Posterior view (b) Lateral view (c) Anterior view

Figure 2.11e **The Sacrum and Coccyx.** Fused vertebrae form the adult sacrum and coccyx.

CHAPTER TWO   *The Skeletal System: Axial & Appendicular Divisions*

3. **Sacral foramina** are openings that pass through the sacrum anteriorly and posteriorly for the exit of spinal nerves.
4. The **ala** form from the union of transverse processes of the upper sacral vertebrae. The lateral surfaces of the ala form the sacroilial articulation with the ilium of the coxal bone.

Coccygeal Vertebrae

1. The **coccygeal vertebrae** develop as 3–5 separate vertebrae, but fuse into one structure between the ages of twenty and thirty.
2. The coccygeal vertebrae are located inferior to the sacrum.

C. THE THORACIC CAGE

The thoracic cage is made up of the **ribs**, **sternum** and **costal cartilages**. Locate each of the following structures.

The Sternum Has the Following Components

1. The **manubrium** articulates at its superolateral surface with the clavicle. The articulation of the manubrium and clavicle forms the **sternoclavicular joint.**
2. The **body** of the sternum has articulations with costal cartilages of ribs. It also articulates directly with the inferior end of the manubrium and the superior surface of the xiphoid process.
3. The **xiphoid process** is the pointed inferior end of the sternum. It articulates with the inferior end of the body.

Ribs Articulate with Thoracic Vertebrae

1. The **head** of a rib articulates with the demifacets of the **body** of a thoracic vertebra.
2. **Tubercles** of each rib articulate with **transverse processes** of the 10 superior thoracic vertebrae.

Ribs and Costal Cartilages

1. Ribs 1–7 are classified as vertebrosternal ribs (often called "true ribs") because they span between vertebrae and the body of the sternum via costal cartilages.
2. Ribs 8–10 are classified as vertebrochondal ribs (often called "false ribs") because they span between vertebrae and the costal margin. The costal margin is formed by the fusion of the costal cartilages of ribs 8–10 that connects to the costal cartilage of rib 7.
3. Ribs 11–12 are vertebral ribs (often called floating ribs) and do not articulate with the sternum.

II. THE APPENDICULAR SKELETON

The **appendicular skeleton** includes the bones of both upper and lower limbs including the limb girdles. The upper limbs are attached to the axial skeleton by the **pectoral girdle** and the lower limbs are attached by the **pelvic girdle**.

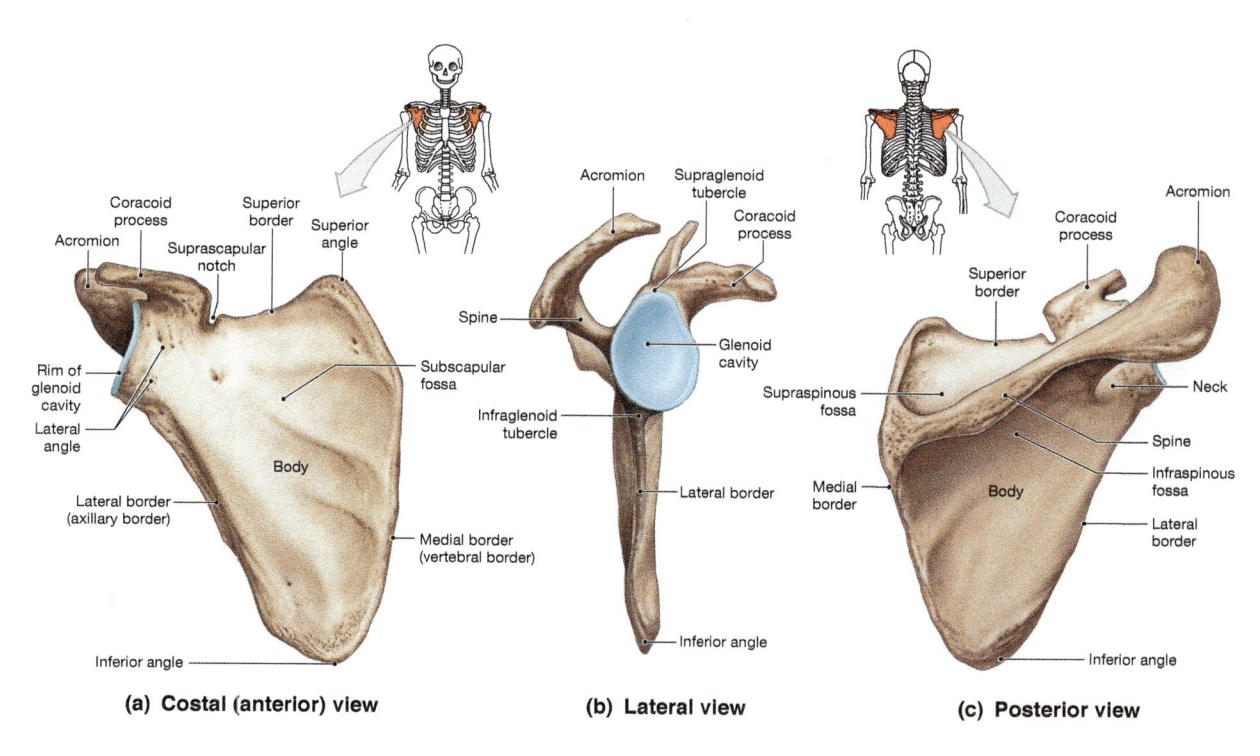

Figure 2.12 The Scapula.

A. COMPONENTS OF THE PECTORAL GIRDLE

Scapula

(Fig. 2.12)

The **scapula** forms part of the pectoral girdle. It is a triangle-shaped bone that serves as a site of attachment for many muscles that move the upper extremity.

1. The **glenoid cavity** (glenoid fossa) is the shallow depression on the superior, lateral side of the scapula. The glenoid cavity is the articular site for the **head of the humerus.** The **glenohumeral joint** is a synovial ball-and-socket joint formed between the head of the humerus and the glenoid cavity of the scapula.

2. The **coracoid process** is a beak-shaped projection on the scapula, located superiorly and anteriorly to the **glenoid cavity.**

3. The **spine of the scapula** is the bony ridge coursing diagonally along the posterior surface of the scapula.

4. The **acromion process of the scapula** is the lateral, expanded end of the spine of the scapula. The acromion process forms the lateral-most extremity of the scapula.

5. The **medial border of the scapula** (vertebral border) faces the vertebral column.

6. The **supraspinous fossa** is a depression located above the spine of the scapula.

7. The **infraspinous fossa** is a depression located below the spine of the scapula.

8. The **subscapular fossa** is on the anterior surface of the scapula.

9. Superior angle and inferior angle.

Clavicle

The **clavicle** articulates at its medial end with the **manubrium of the sternum,** forming the **sternoclavicular joint**. At its lateral end, the clavicle articulates with the acromion process of the scapula, forming the **acromioclavicular joint**.

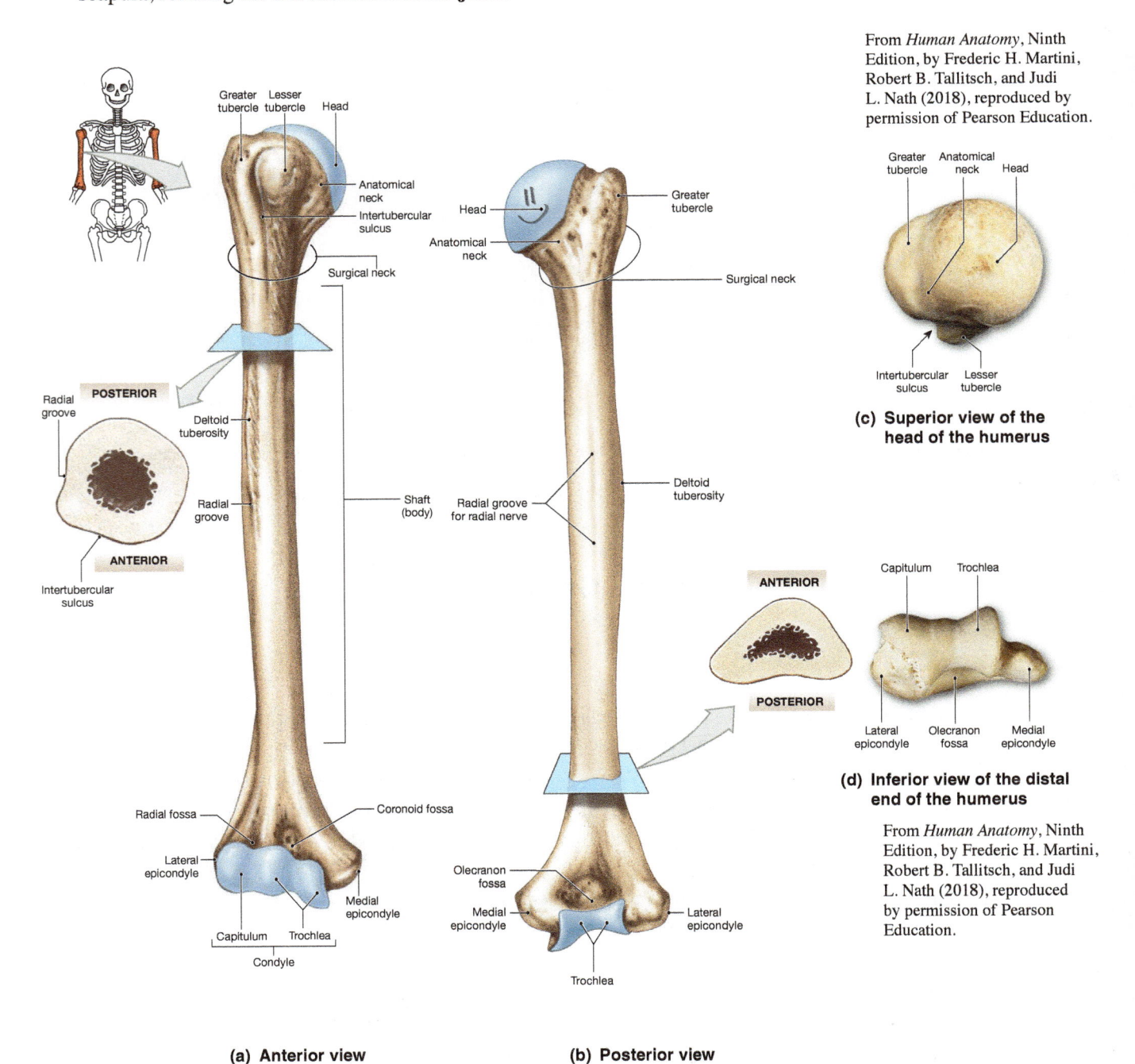

From *Human Anatomy*, Ninth Edition, by Frederic H. Martini, Robert B. Tallitsch, and Judi L. Nath (2018), reproduced by permission of Pearson Education.

(c) **Superior view of the head of the humerus**

(d) **Inferior view of the distal end of the humerus**

From *Human Anatomy*, Ninth Edition, by Frederic H. Martini, Robert B. Tallitsch, and Judi L. Nath (2018), reproduced by permission of Pearson Education.

(a) Anterior view

(b) Posterior view

From *Human Anatomy*, Ninth Edition, by Frederic H. Martini, Robert B. Tallitsch, and Judi L. Nath (2018), reproduced by permission of Pearson Education.

From *Human Anatomy*, Ninth Edition, by Frederic H. Martini, Robert B. Tallitsch, and Judi L. Nath (2018), reproduced by permission of Pearson Education.

Figure 2.13   The Humerus.

B. THE UPPER LIMB

Humerus

The **humerus** is the single bone of the arm (Fig. 2.13). The "arm" is the region located between the shoulder and elbow. Several structures of the humerus listed below are sites of muscle attachment.

1. The **head of the humerus** is the large, rounded structure at the proximal end of the humerus.

2. The **greater tubercle of the humerus** is the raised area at the proximal end of the humerus, laterally.

3. The **lesser tubercle of the humerus** is a small raised area near the greater tubercle at the proximal end of the humerus on the anterior side.

4. The **intertubercular groove of the humerus** (intertubercular sulcus) is located between the greater and lesser tubercles.

5. The **deltoid tuberosity** is a rough, raised area along the middle of the diaphysis of the humerus.

6. The **olecranon fossa** is a depression at the distal end of the **posterior** surface of the humerus.

7. The **coronoid fossa** is a small depression at the distal end of the **anterior** surface of the humerus. The **coronoid process** of the ulna articulates at the coronoid fossa of the humerus when the forearm is flexed.

8. The **trochlea** is a spool-shaped structure located at the distal, posterior humerus that articulates with the **trochlear notch of the ulna.** It forms part of the hinge joint at the elbow. Trochlea is the Latin term for pulley.

9. The **capitulum** is the rounded, hemispherical structure on the lateral side of the distal end of the humerus. The capitulum articulates with the **head of the radius.**

10. **Medial** and **lateral epicondyles** are processes located just proximal to the capitulum and trochlea.

Ulna

The **ulna** is the medial bone of the forearm (Figs. 2.13 & 2.14). The "forearm" is the region between the elbow and the wrist. Several structures on the ulna serve as sites for muscle attachment.

1. **Trochlear notch of the ulna** is a "U"- shaped depression at the proximal end of the ulna. The trochlear notch articulates with the **trochlea of the humerus.** The **humeroulnar** joint is a synovial hinge-type joint located between the trochlea of the humerus and the trochlear notch of the ulna.

2. The **olecranon process of the ulna** is the proximal process of the ulna. The olecranon process articulates with the olecranon fossa of the humerus.

3. The **coronoid process of the ulna** is a small process on the anterior side of the ulna that articulates with the coronoid fossa of the humerus.

4. The **radial notch** is a small articular surface at the proximal end of the ulna. The **head of the radius** articulates with the ulna at this site.

5. The **ulnar styloid process** is the pointed structure at the distal end of the ulna.

6. The **head of ulna** is located at the distal end of the ulna, just proximal to the styloid process.

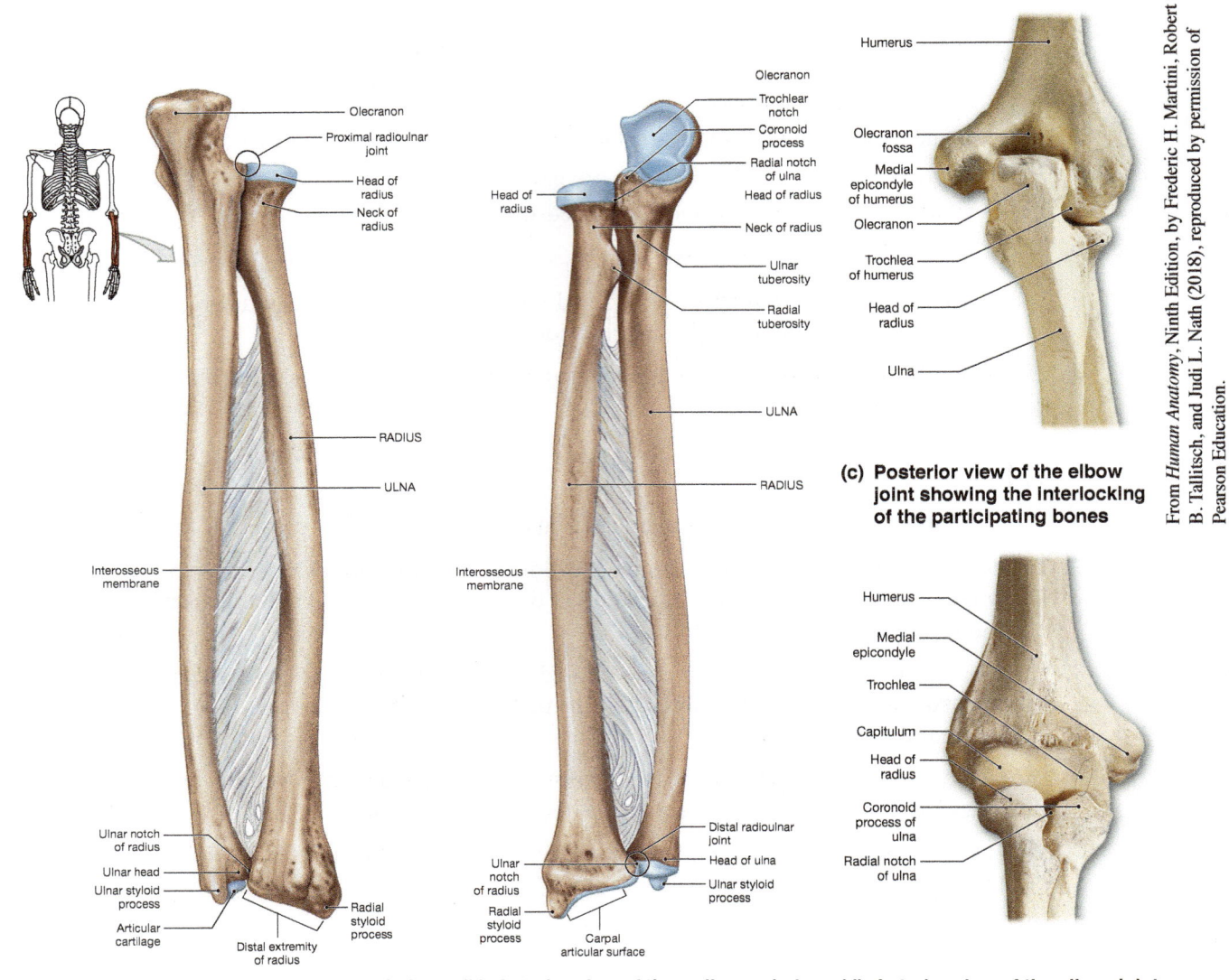

(a) Posterior view of the right radius and ulna

From *Human Anatomy*, Ninth Edition, by Frederic H. Martini, Robert B. Tallitsch, and Judi L. Nath (2018), reproduced by permission of Pearson Education.

(b) Anterior view of the radius and ulna

From *Human Anatomy*, Ninth Edition, by Frederic H. Martini, Robert B. Tallitsch, and Judi L. Nath (2018), reproduced by permission of Pearson Education.

(c) Posterior view of the elbow joint showing the interlocking of the participating bones

From *Human Anatomy*, Ninth Edition, by Frederic H. Martini, Robert B. Tallitsch, and Judi L. Nath (2018), reproduced by permission of Pearson Education.

(d) Anterior view of the elbow joint

From *Human Anatomy*, Ninth Edition, by Frederic H. Martini, Robert B. Tallitsch, and Judi L. Nath (2018), reproduced by permission of Pearson Education.

Figure 2.14   The Radius and Ulna.

Radius

The **radius** is the more lateral of the two bones of the forearm (Fig. 2.14). The radius also serves as a site of attachment for several muscles.

1. The **radial tuberosity** is a roughened, raised area at the proximal end of the radius.

2. The **radial styloid process** is the pointed structure at the distal end of the radius.

3. The **head of radius** is a rounded structure at the proximal end of the radius. It articulates with the **capitulum of the humerus** and the **radial notch of the ulna.** The **radioulnar** joint is a synovial pivot-type joint located between the head of the radius and the radial notch of the ulna.

Bones of the Wrist and Hand

An easy way to remember the carpal bones is either the mnemonic device; "Sam left the party to take Cathy home" or "Students love to party, then tomorrow call home." (Fig. 2.15)

1. **The proximal row of carpals from lateral to medial:**

    - The **scaphoid** is the most lateral of the carpal bones when the hand is in correct anatomical position. It articulates with the distal radius and the lunate.
    - The **lunate** is located medial to scaphoid and articulates with the distal radius. The lunate also articulates with the triquetrum, hamate and capitate.
    - The **triquetrum** is located medial to the lunate. It also has articulations with the pisiform and hamate.
    - The **pisiform** is located at the base of the palm on its medial side. The pisiform is a sesamoid bone, meaning that it is a bone embedded in a tendon; it articulates with the triquetrum and no other bones.

2. **The distal row of carpals from lateral to medial:**

    - The **trapezium** articulates with the scaphoid and trapezoid. The trapezium has distal articulations primarily with metacarpal I, and a small articulation with metacarpal II.
    - The **trapezoid** lies between the trapezium and capitate. The trapezoid has a distal articulation with metacarpal II.
    - The **capitate** is located between the trapezoid and hamate. The capitate has a proximal articulation with the scaphoid and lunate and a distal articulation with metacarpal III.

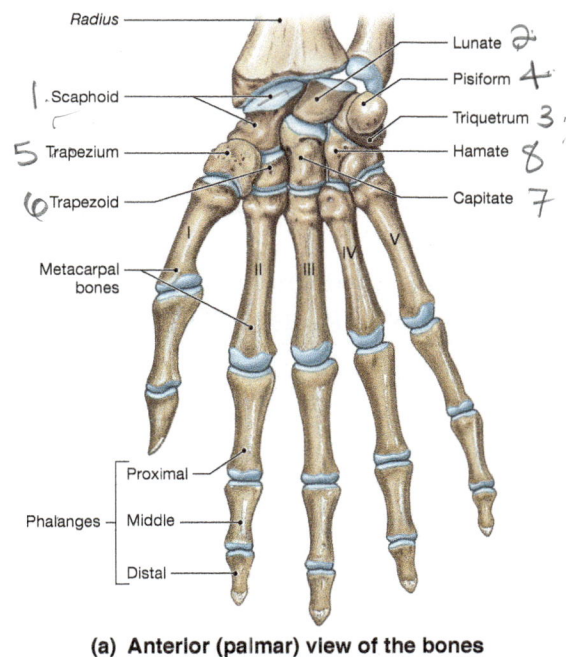

(a) Anterior (palmar) view of the bones of the right wrist and hand

(b) Posterior (dorsal) view of the bones of the right wrist and hand

From *Human Anatomy*, Ninth Edition, by Frederic H. Martini, Robert B. Tallitsch, and Judi L. Nath (2018), reproduced by permission of Pearson Education.

From *Human Anatomy*, Ninth Edition, by Frederic H. Martini, Robert B. Tallitsch, and Judi L. Nath (2018), reproduced by permission of Pearson Education.

Figure 2.15 Bones of the Wrist and Hand.

CHAPTER TWO   *The Skeletal System: Axial & Appendicular Divisions*

- The **hamate** is the most medial carpal of the distal row. The hamate has a hook-shaped structure called the *hamulus of the hamate*. The hamate has a proximal articulation with the triquetral and lunate. The hamate has distal articulations with metacarpals IV and V and a lateral articulation with the capitate.

3. **Metacarpals** are numbered I–V beginning with the thumb (pollex).

4. **Phalanges** (singular: phalanx) The phalanges of each finger are named proximal, middle and distal phalanx. Each finger has three phalanges except the thumb, which has only two: the proximal and distal phalanx.

C. The Pelvic Girdle

The **pelvic girdle** is composed of the two coxal bones. The three regions of the coxal bones are formed by the fusion of the **ilium**, **ischium** and **pubis**. These three bones fuse at the **acetabulum**, which is a cup-like depression on the lateral side of each coxal bone and is the site of articulation for the head of the femur. (Fig. 2.16)

Coxal Bones

Ilium

(Fig. 2.16)

1. The **iliac crest** is the ridge along the superior edge of the ilium.
2. The **anterior superior iliac spine** is a bony prominence that forms the anterior end of the iliac crest.
3. The **anterior inferior iliac spine** is a bony prominence located just inferior to the anterior superior iliac spine.
4. The **posterior superior iliac spine** is a prominent structure that forms the posterior end of the iliac crest.
5. The **posterior inferior iliac spine** is a bony projection located inferior to the posterior superior iliac spine.
6. The **greater sciatic notch** is a conspicuous groove located below the posterior inferior iliac spine. The greater sciatic notch is the groove through which the sciatic nerve passes from the hip into the thigh.

Ischium

(Fig. 2.16)

1. The **ischial tuberosity** is a rough area on the inferior surface of the ischium. The ischial tuberosity is a site of attachment for the "hamstring" muscles.
2. The **obturator foramen** is a large, oval opening in the coxal bone formed from parts of the ischium and pubis. The obturator foramen is covered by the obturator membrane which is the attachment site for muscles. A small gap in the membrane, the obturator canal, allows passage of the obturator nerve, artery and vein.
3. The **ischial spine** is a small process on the posterior surface of the ischium. It separates the greater and lesser sciatic notches.

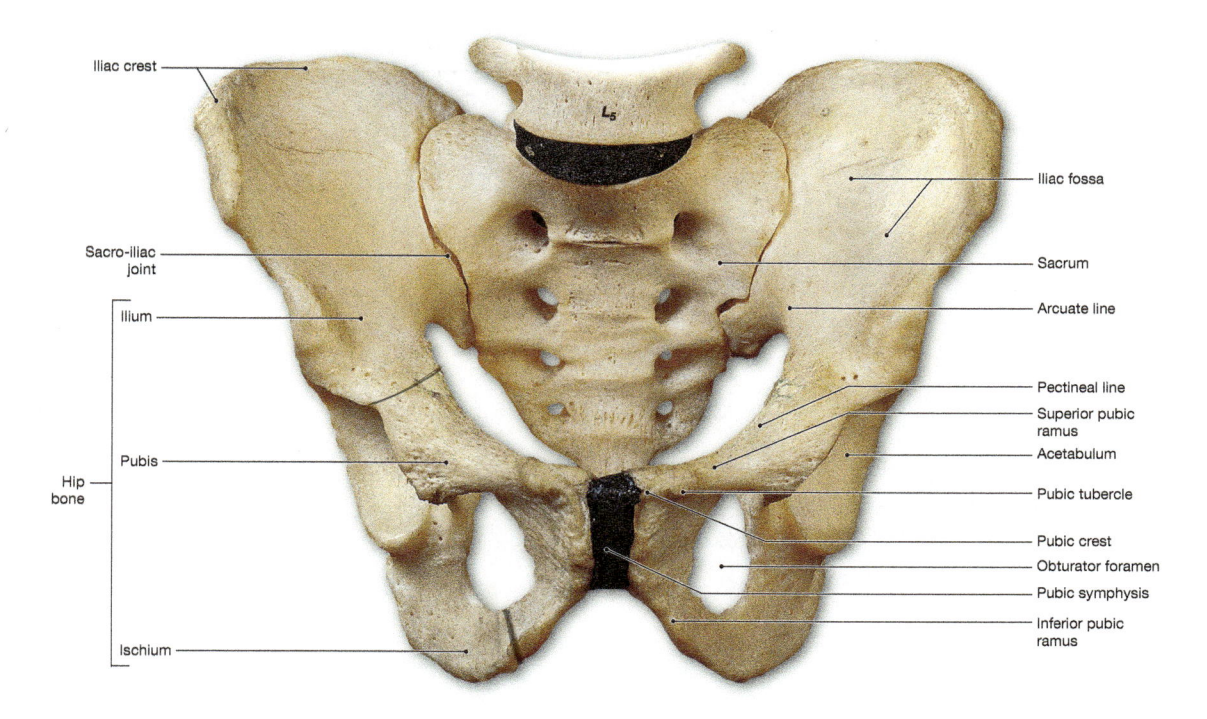

Figure 2.16a   Pelvis, Anterior View.

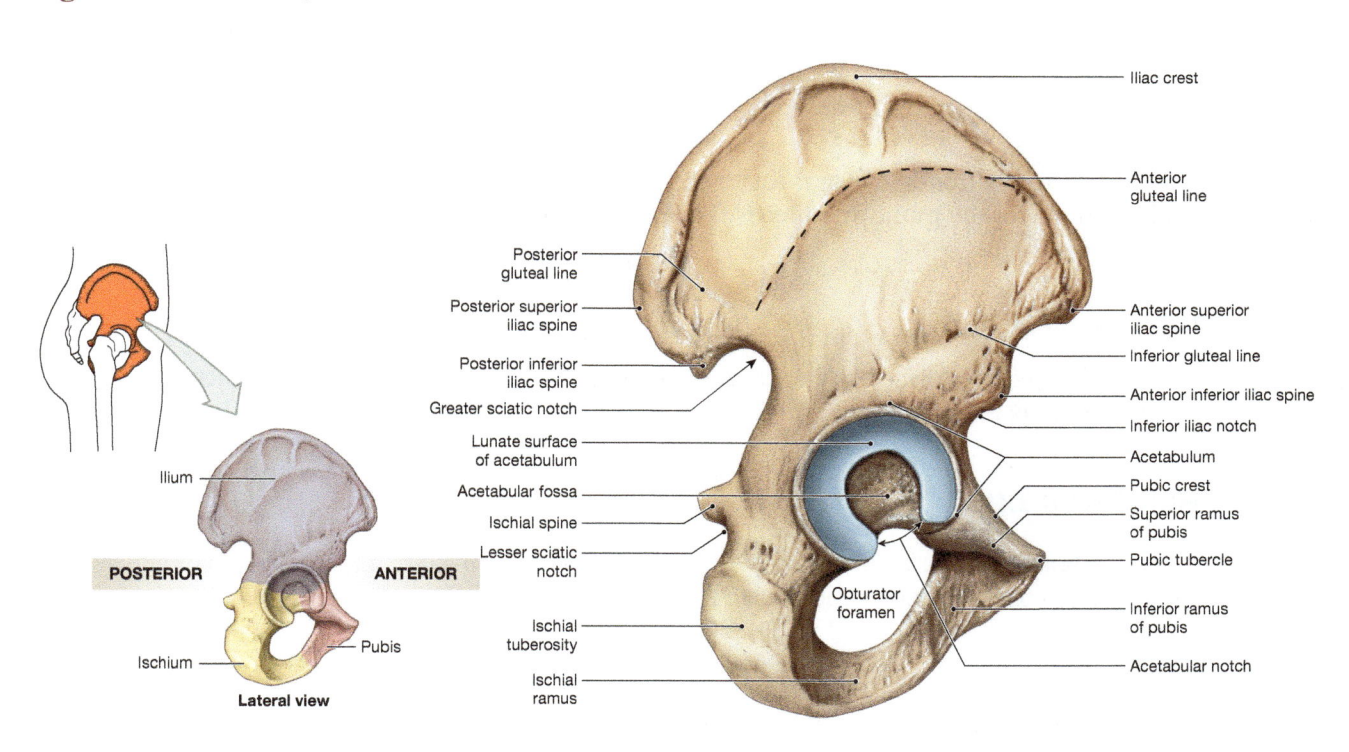

Figure 2.16b   Right Coxal Bone, Lateral View.

CHAPTER TWO   *The Skeletal System: Axial & Appendicular Divisions*   33

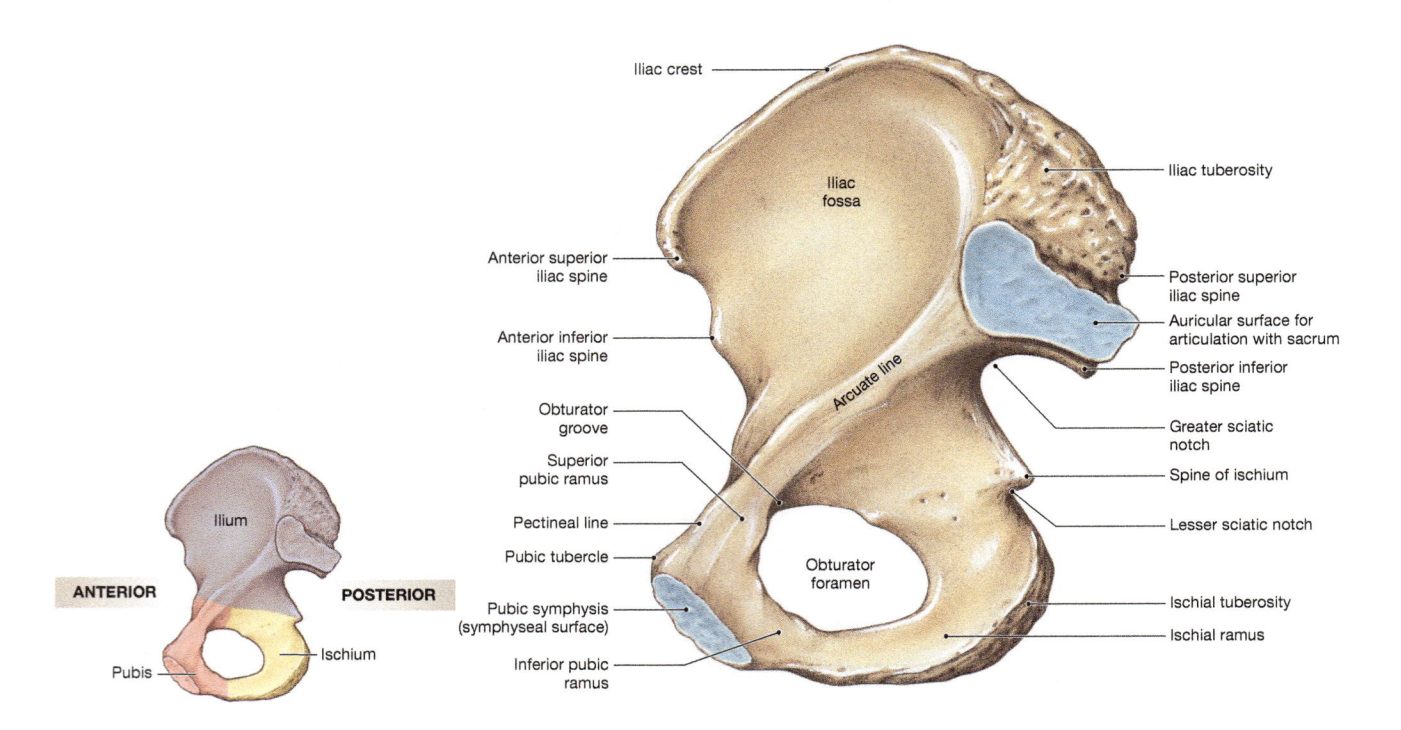

Figure 2.16c Right Coxal Bone, Medial View.

Pubis

(Fig. 2.16)

The **pubis** is the anterior bone that meets with the pubis of the opposite side at the midline. This is the articular surface for the **pubic symphysis**. The pubis also serves as a site of attachment for several muscles of the thigh.

Sacroiliac Joint

The **sacroiliac joint** is formed by the articulation of the sacrum with the ilium on either side of the body. This joint is important in weight bearing and is both cartilaginous and synovial.

D. THE LOWER LIMB

Learn these bony landmarks of the lower limbs so that when you study muscles, you will understand the relationship of these bony structures to the muscles to which they attach.

Femur

The **femur** is the single bone of the thigh (Figs. 2.17 & 2.18). Several muscles that move the thigh have attachments on the femur. The "thigh" is the region located between the hip and the knee.

(a) Landmarks on the anterior surface of the right femur

(b) Landmarks on the posterior surface of the right femur

(c) Medial view of the femoral head

(d) Lateral view of the femoral head

From *Human Anatomy*, Ninth Edition, by Frederic H. Martini, Robert B. Tallitsch, and Judi L. Nath (2018), reproduced by permission of Pearson Education.

From *Human Anatomy*, Ninth Edition, by Frederic H. Martini, Robert B. Tallitsch, and Judi L. Nath (2018), reproduced by permission of Pearson Education.

From *Human Anatomy*, Ninth Edition, by Frederic H. Martini, Robert B. Tallitsch, and Judi L. Nath (2018), reproduced by permission of Pearson Education.

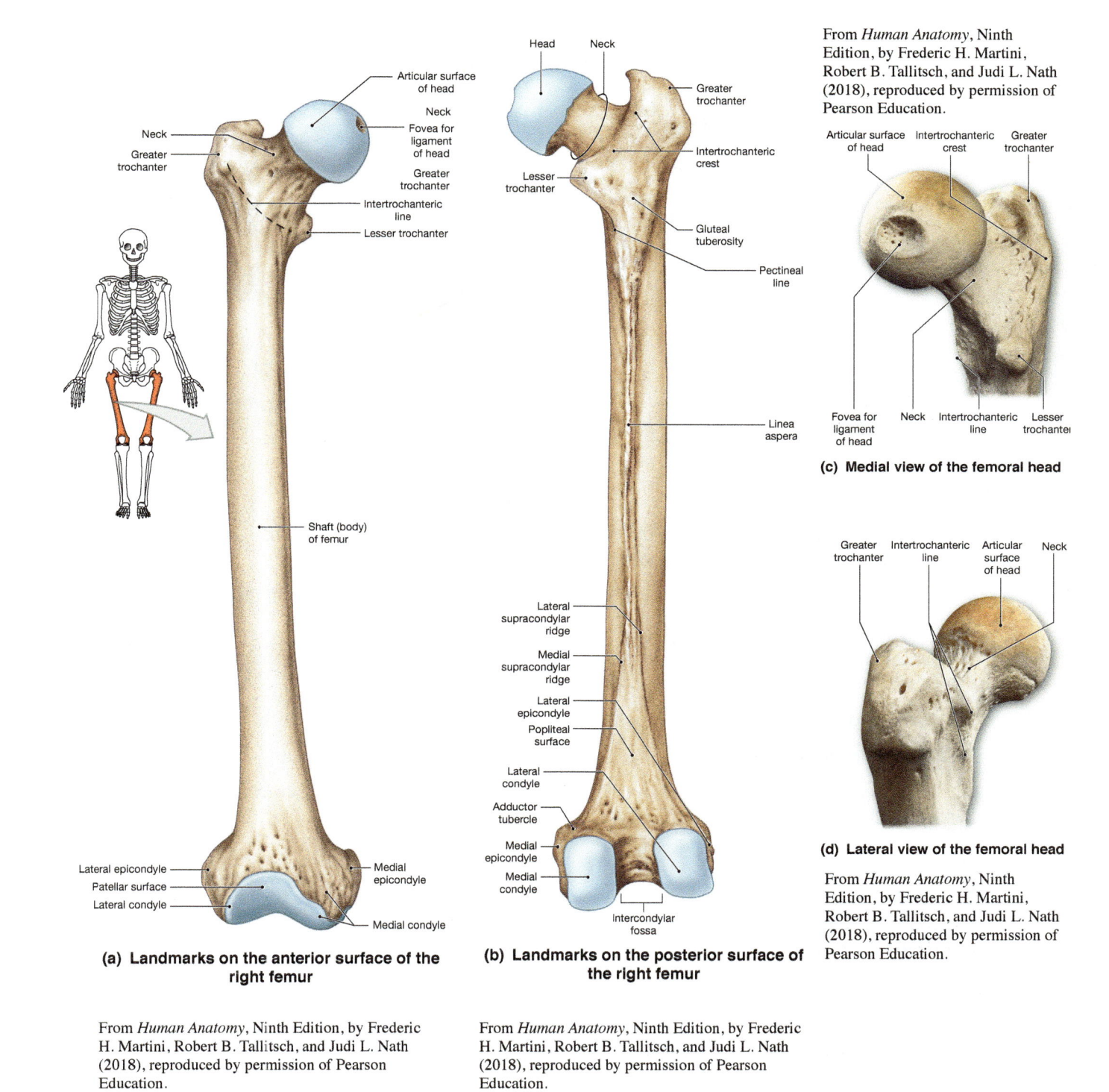

Figure 2.17 Right Femur.

1. The **head of the femur** is the rounded structure at the proximal end of the femur. The head of the femur articulates with the **acetabulum.**

2. The **neck of the femur** is the narrowed portion of the femur that joins the head with the diaphysis (shaft).

CHAPTER TWO   *The Skeletal System: Axial & Appendicular Divisions*

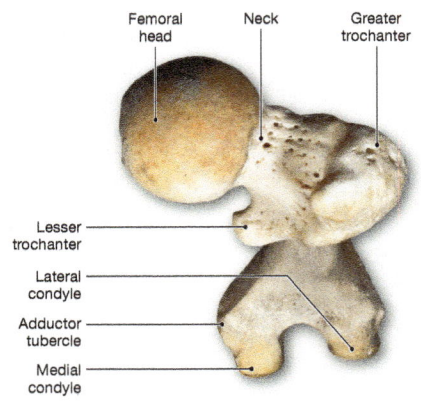

(a) A superior view of the femur

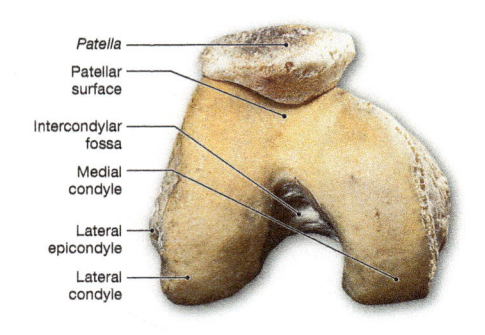

(b) An inferior view of the right femur showing the articular surfaces that participate in the knee joint

From *Human Anatomy*, Ninth Edition, by Frederic H. Martini, Robert B. Tallitsch, and Judi L. Nath (2018), reproduced by permission of Pearson Education.

From *Human Anatomy*, Ninth Edition, by Frederic H. Martini, Robert B. Tallitsch, and Judi L. Nath (2018), reproduced by permission of Pearson Education.

Figure 2.18   Right Femur.

3. The **greater trochanter** of the femur is a large, rough raised area at the proximal end of the femur that forms the most lateral part of the femur.

4. The **lesser trochanter** of the femur is the smaller bony prominence located on the medial side of the proximal femur.

5. **Medial** and **lateral condyles** are located at the distal end of the femur. They are the smooth surfaces that articulate with the condyles of the tibia.

6. **Medial** and **lateral epicondyles** are the rough areas proximal to the condyles of the femur.

7. The **linea aspera** is a prominent ridge along the posterior surface of the femur.

8. The **gluteal tuberosity** is a small, rough structure located lateral to the lesser trochanter and inferior to the greater trochanter.

Patella

The **patella** lends stability to the knee. It slides along the patellar surface of the femur, which is between the condyles of the femur. The patella is a **sesamoid bone**, meaning that it is a bone embedded in a tendon.

Tibia

The **tibia** is the larger of the two bones of the leg and articulates with the distal femur. The tibia is the more medial of the two leg bones (Figs. 2.19 & 2.20). Recall that the "leg" is defined as the region between the knee and ankle.

1. The **tibial tuberosity** is the bony prominence on the anterior surface of the proximal tibia.

2. **Medial** and **lateral condyles** articulate with the condyles of the femur.

3. The **medial malleolus** is a prominent structure of the distal tibia on its medial surface. The **medial malleolus** forms the "inner ankle."

Fibula

The **fibula** is the smaller of the two bones of the leg and is located lateral to the tibia (Figs. 2.19 & 2.20)

1. The **head** of the fibula articulates with the proximal end of the tibia.
2. The **lateral malleolus** is a prominent structure of the distal fibula on its lateral surface. The lateral malleolus forms the "outer ankle."

Bones of the Ankle and Foot

1. Seven **tarsal** bones make up the ankle (Fig. 2.21).
   - The **talus** articulates with distal tibia and fibula.
   - The **calcaneus** articulates inferior to talus. The calcaneal tendon (often called Achilles tendon) attaches at the posterior surface of the calcaneus.
   - The **cuboid** articulates with the calcaneus and proximal ends of of metatarsals IV and V.
   - The **navicular** articulates with the talus and the proximal articular surfaces of the cuneiform bones.
   - **Medial, intermediate** and **lateral cuneiform** bones articulate with the proximal surfaces of metatarsals I–III respectively.

From *Human Anatomy*, Ninth Edition, by Frederic H. Martini, Robert B. Tallitsch, and Judi L. Nath (2018), reproduced by permission of Pearson Education.

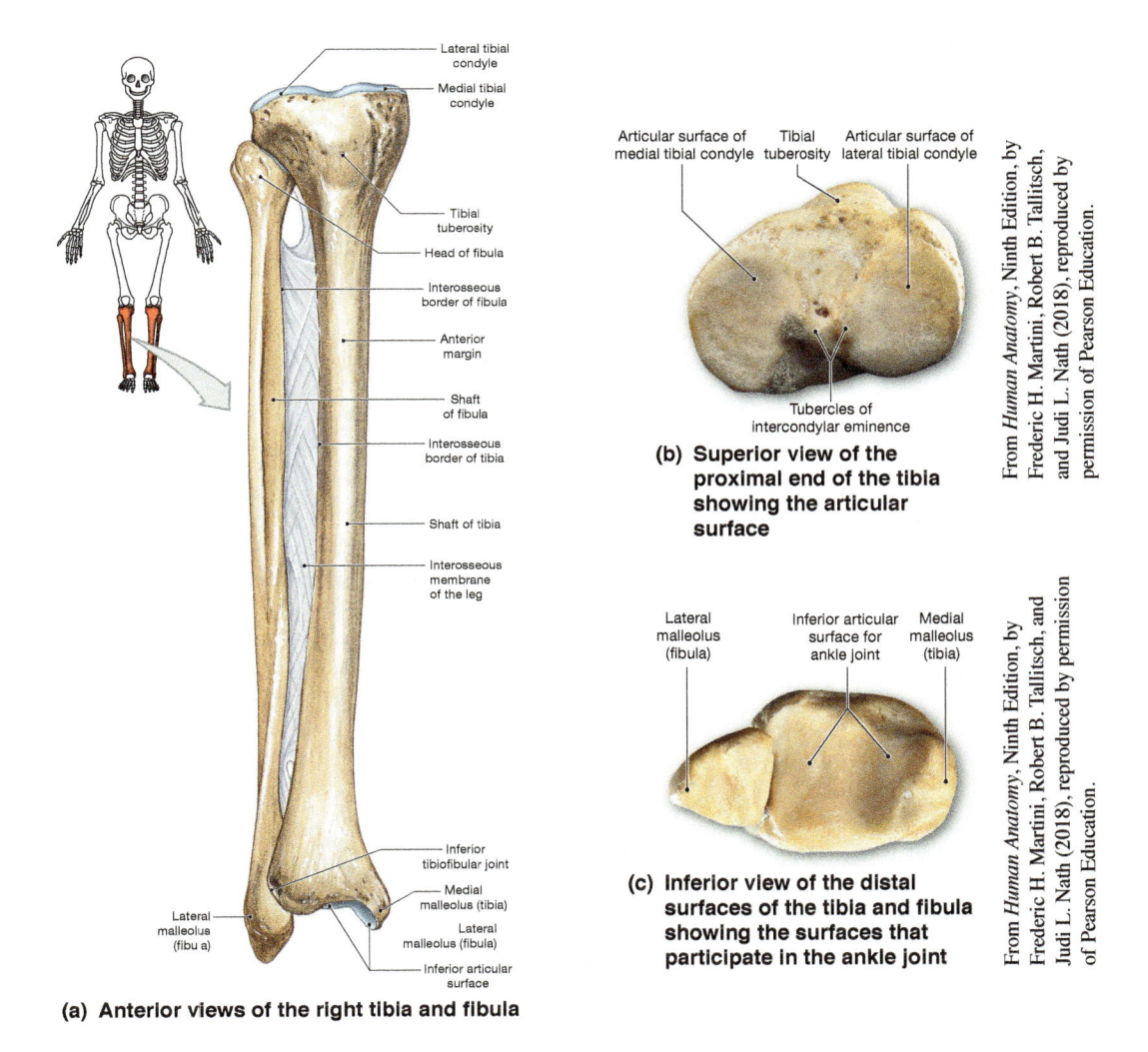

Figure 2.19 **Anterior view of the right Tibia and Fibula.**

2. The five **metatarsal bones** articulate with the cuneiform bones and the cuboid. The metatarsals are numbered I–V, beginning with the great toe (hallux).

3. Fourteen **phalanges** comprise the toes. Each of the four lateral toes has three phalanges: proximal, middle and distal.

4. The **hallux** (great toe) has only two phalanges: a proximal and distal phalanx.

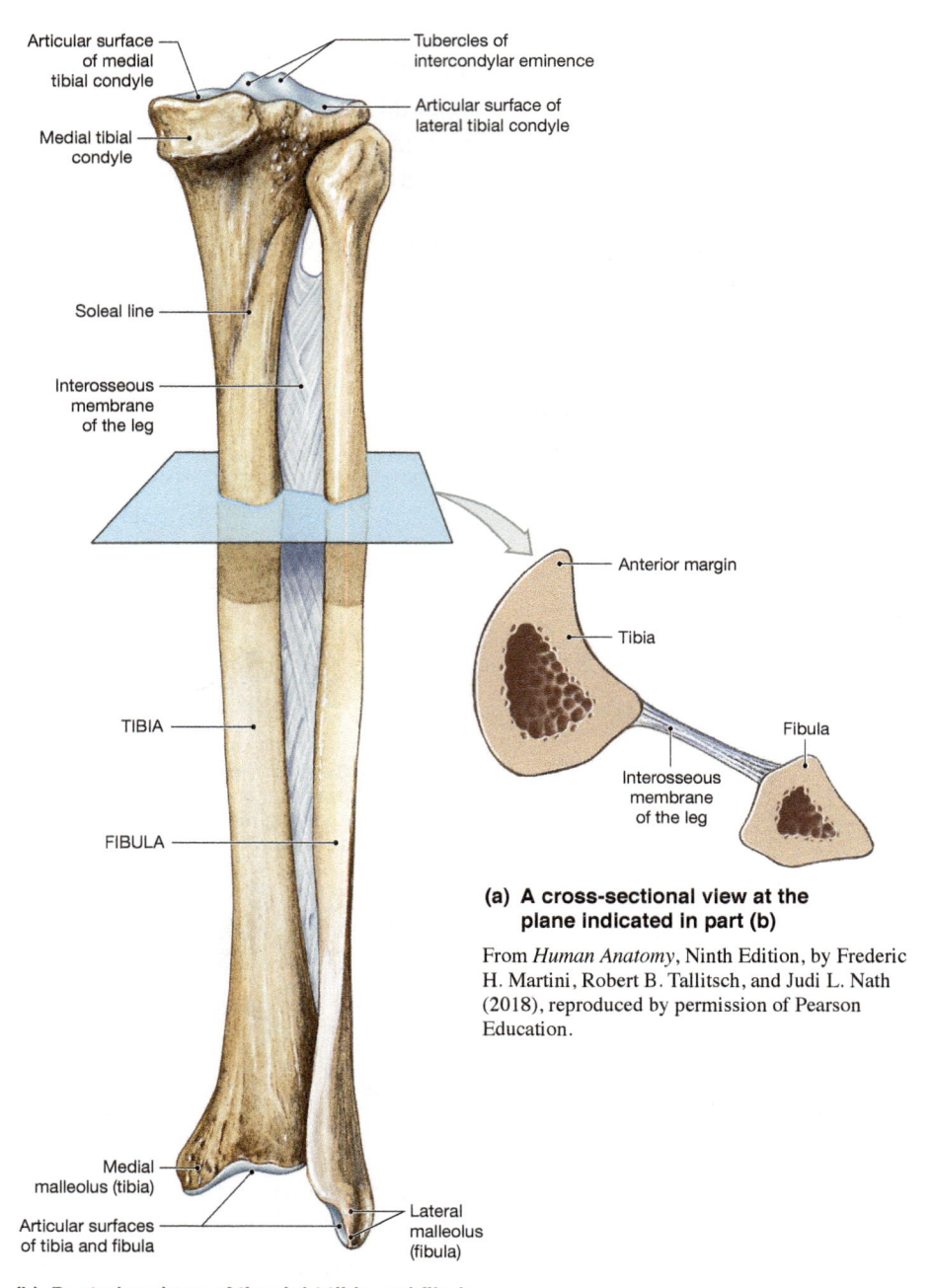

(a) A cross-sectional view at the plane indicated in part (b)

From *Human Anatomy*, Ninth Edition, by Frederic H. Martini, Robert B. Tallitsch, and Judi L. Nath (2018), reproduced by permission of Pearson Education.

(b) Posterior views of the right tibia and fibula

From *Human Anatomy*, Ninth Edition, by Frederic H. Martini, Robert B. Tallitsch, and Judi L. Nath (2018), reproduced by permission of Pearson Education.

Figure 2.20 **Posterior view of the Right Tibia and Fibula.**

From *Human Anatomy*, Ninth Edition, by Frederic H. Martini, Robert B. Tallitsch, and Judi L. Nath (2018), reproduced by permission of Pearson Education.

From *Human Anatomy*, Ninth Edition, by Frederic H. Martini, Robert B. Tallitsch, and Judi L. Nath (2018), reproduced by permission of Pearson Education.

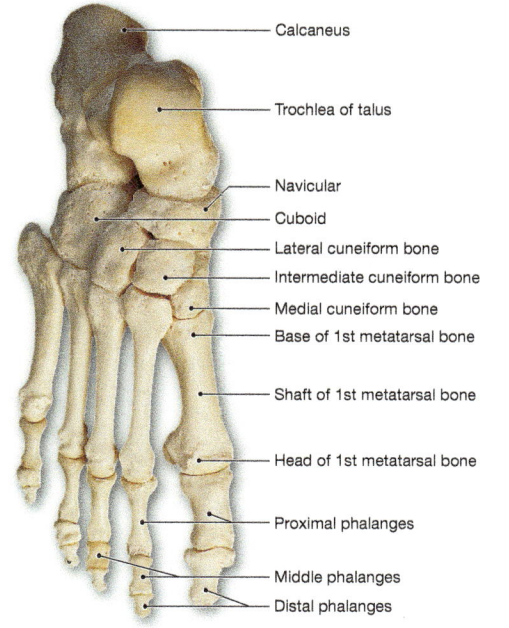

(a) Superior view of the bones of the right foot.

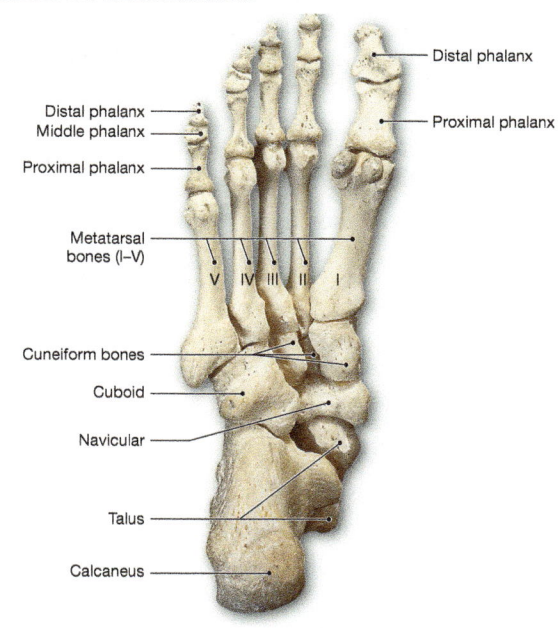

(b) Inferior (plantar) view

Figure 2.21a Superior and Inferior Views of Right Foot.

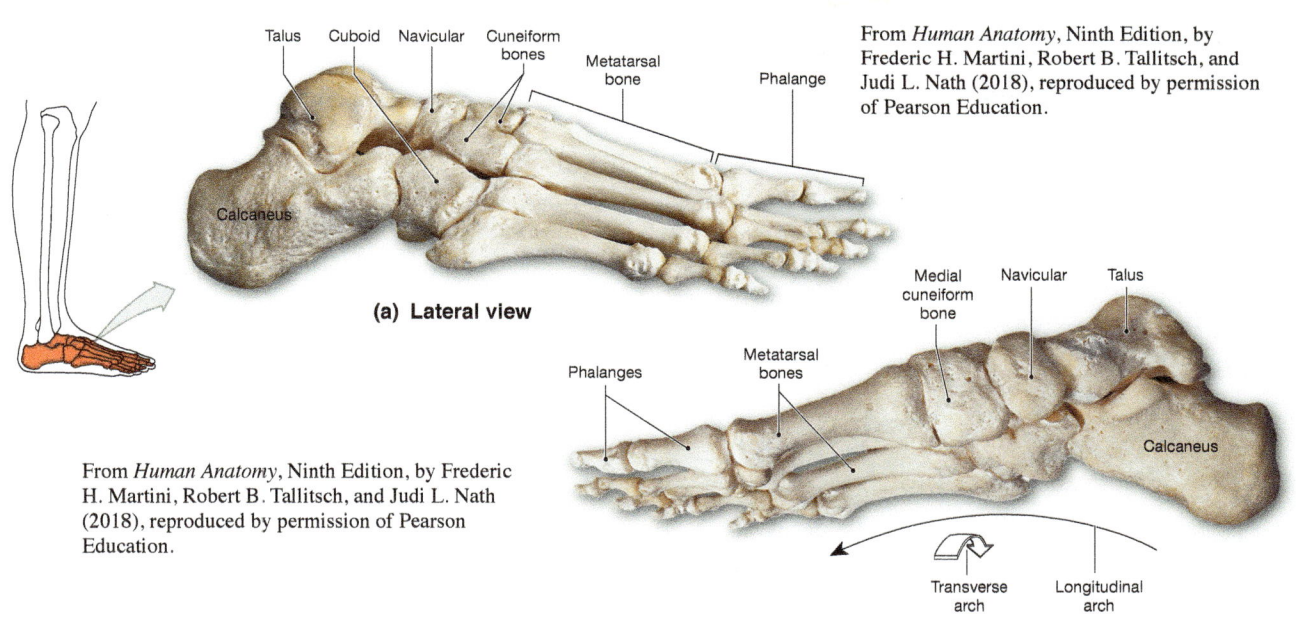

(a) Lateral view

From *Human Anatomy*, Ninth Edition, by Frederic H. Martini, Robert B. Tallitsch, and Judi L. Nath (2018), reproduced by permission of Pearson Education.

From *Human Anatomy*, Ninth Edition, by Frederic H. Martini, Robert B. Tallitsch, and Judi L. Nath (2018), reproduced by permission of Pearson Education.

(b) Medial view showing the relative positions of the tarsal bones and the orientation of the transverse and longitudinal arches

Figure 2.21b Lateral and Medial Views of the Right Foot.

CHAPTER TWO *The Skeletal System: Axial & Appendicular Divisions*

III. JOINTS

JOINTS: FUNCTIONAL CLASSIFICATION

List an example of each functional classification of joints.

1. **Synarthroses** (immovable) _____
2. **Amphiarthroses** (slightly movable) _____
3. **Diarthroses** (freely movable) _____

Synovial joints are diarthroses that are distinguished by having the following associated structures:

- Synovial membrane
- Synovial cavity
- Articular cartilage
- Fibrous capsule
- Ligaments that strengthen the capsule and may be found inside the joint as well.
- Tendons, which provide attachments of muscles.

JOINTS: SUBTYPES OF SYNOVIAL JOINTS

List an example of each type of joint listed below.

1. **Ball-and-socket** _shoulder_
2. **Hinge** _knee_
3. **Pivot** _elbow_
4. **Gliding (Plane) joint** _____
5. **Ellipsoid joint** _____
6. **Saddle** _____

Table 2.1: Structural Classification of Joints

Functional Category	Type	Description
Synarthrosis (No Movement)		
At synarthroses, bony edges are close together and sometimes interlock. They allow no movement	Suture	Joints between bones of the skull. Edges of bones are interlocking.
	Gomphosis	Joint between a tooth and bone of alveolus in maxilla or mandible. Teeth anchored to bone by a periodontal ligament.
	Synchondrosis	Connection between two bones or parts of bones composed of hyaline cartilage; first costal cartilage, cartilaginous pad between the epiphysis and metaphysis of a growing bone.
	Synostosis	Complete bony fusion between two bones.
Amphiarthrosis (Little Movement)		
Amphiarthroses permit limited motion and it is usually passive (i.e., not actively caused by voluntary motion). Bones may be connected by ligaments or cartilage	Syndesmosis	Two bones connected by a ligament.
	Symphysis	Two bones connected by a fibrocartilaginous pad, such as an intervertebral disc or symphysis pubis
Diarthrosis (Free Movement)		
Diarthroses allow active motion by voluntary muscles.	Synovial	Joints that permit a wide range of motion. Most mobile joints are synovial joints.

Study and Review Questions – The Skeletal System

CHAPTER TWO

Answers to these questions are found in Chapter Two of this guide.

1. What structures pass through the optic canals of the sphenoid bone? _Optic nerves_
2. What structure of the sphenoid bone houses the **pituitary gland**? _sella turcica_
3. Name the porous region of the **ethmoid bone**. _cribriform plate_
    b. What structures pass through this porous region? _olfactory nerves_
4. What structure of the temporal bone helps form the **temporomandibular joint**? _mandibular fossa_
5. List two identifying characteristics of cervical vertebrae 3-7.
The spinous process is short & points directly posteriorly & _the vertebrae foramen is large & generally triangular_
6. With what structure of the coxal bone does the head of the femur articulate? _acetebulum_
7. With what structure of the scapula does the clavicle articulate? _acromium process_
8. Match the term in **column A** with the correct bone in **column B**. Write the letter or letters of your answer in the blank by the appropriate term in column A. Some bones may be used more than once.

Column A	Column B
_d_ Glenoid cavity	A. Ulna
_c_ Lesser tubercle	B. Radius
_a, b_ Styloid process	C. Humerus
_a_ Olecranon	D. Scapula
_c_ Deltoid tuberosity	

9. Match the term in **column A** with the correct bone in **column B**. Write the letter or letters of your answer in the blank by the appropriate term in column A. Some bones may be used more than once.

Column A	Column B
_c_ Greater trochanter	A. Fibula
_c, d_ Medial condyle	B. Calcaneus
_a_ Lateral malleolus	C. Femur
_c_ Linea aspera	D. Tibia
_c_ Gluteal tuberosity	

EXERCISES IN HUMAN ANATOMY

10. List two distinguishing characteristics of a thoracic vertebra.
    The spinous processes are & the vertebral foramen is circular
    large & point inferiorly
11. With what structures of a thoracic vertebra does a rib articulate?
    demifacets of the body & transverse processes

12. List the tarsal bones that articulate with the metatarsals.
    medial, intermediate lateral, & cuboid.
    cuneiforms

13. Which suture separates the frontal bone from the two parietal bones? coronal.

14. Match the term in **column A** with the bone in **column B**.

    Column A   **Column B**
    _d_ Foramen magnum   A. Sphenoid
    _b_ Frontal process   B. Maxilla
    _c_ Mastoid process   C. Temporal
    _a_ Greater wings   D. Occipital
    _b_ Sinus
    _a_ Sella turcica

15. __Fontanels__ begin as membranous "soft spots" of an infant's skull.

THREE
Histology

I. BODY LANGUAGE

The terms listed in this **Body Language** section are roots of words. The definitions of these terms will help you comprehend the meaning of words containing these prefixes or suffixes.

1. **Blast**—Bud or sprout. A fibroblast is the cell that forms new collagen fibers.
2. **Chondro**—Cartilage. *Chondrocytes* are cartilage cells.
3. **Clast**—Break. An osteoclast breaks down bone tissue.
4. **Cyte**—Cell. Osteocytes are mature bone cells.
5. **Derma**—Skin. *Dermis* is the layer of tissue beneath the epidermis.
6. **Endo**—Inside. Endothelial cells are the inner lining of blood vessels.
7. **Epi**—Upon. Epidermis is superficial to the dermis.
8. **Exo**—Outside. Exocrine glands discharge their secretions through a duct.
9. **Kerato**—Hard and horn-like. *Keratinized* stratified squamous epithelium is tough and hard.
10. **Lemma**—Husk. The plasmalemma is the membrane that contains the cell.
11. **Lipo**—Fat.
12. **Melano**—Black. *Melanin* is the skin pigment, found in the stratum germinativum that contributes to skin color.
13. **Osteo**—Bone. *Osteocytes* are mature bone cells.
14. **Peri**—Around. Periosteum is the connective tissue around bones.
15. **Pilo**—Hair. The *arrector pili* muscle is a small muscle attached to the hair follicle.
16. **Sarco**—Flesh. Sarcolemma is the cell membrane of a muscle cell.
17. **Sebo**—*Sebum* is an oily substance secreted by sebaceous glands.
18. **Sudo**—Sweat.

II. OVERVIEW OF BASIC TISSUE TYPES

A **tissue** is a group of similar cells that work with each other to perform the same basic function. The four basic tissue types are **epithelial**, **connective**, **muscle** and **nervous**. Each tissue type has subtypes that have specific functions. An **organ** is a group of tissues that works in close relationship to perform specialized functions. Organs have specific functions and distinguishable shapes.

Study all the tissue types described in this section using illustrations and photomicrographs. *You are responsible for identifying each tissue, knowing its functions and its locations in the body.*

III. EPITHELIAL TISSUE

Epithelial tissue performs different functions based on its location in the body. Epithelial tissue covers body surfaces, lines body cavities, and forms glands. (Figs. 3.1–3.7).

Epithelial tissue is also classified by the shapes of cells and organization into layers. The cells of epithelia may be flat (**squamous**), square (**cuboidal**), or tall and thin (**columnar**). Epithelial tissue is further classified as **simple** or **stratified**. "Simple" epithelial tissues are one cell layer thick and stratified tissues are two or more layers thick. Epithelial tissues are attached to the underlying connective tissue by a **basement membrane**. Epithelial tissues have polarity, meaning that cells (or layers of cells) have distinct surfaces. The surface attached to the basement membrane is the **basal surface**. The surface that contacts the external surface of the body, or the lumen of a body cavity is the **apical surface**. The surface that contacts cells to the side is the **lateral surface**.

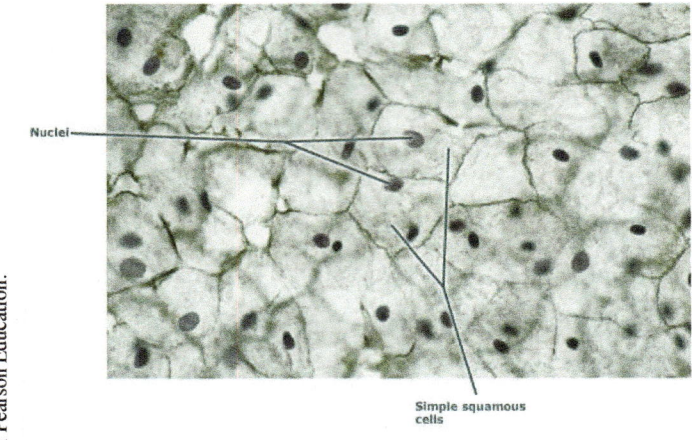

Figure 3.1

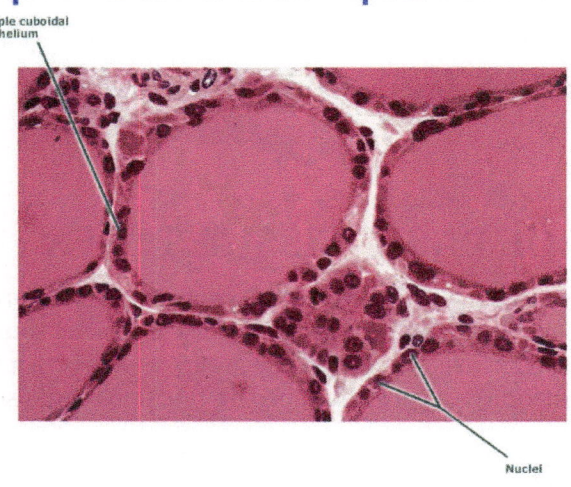

Figure 3.2

Simple Columnar Epithelial Tissue

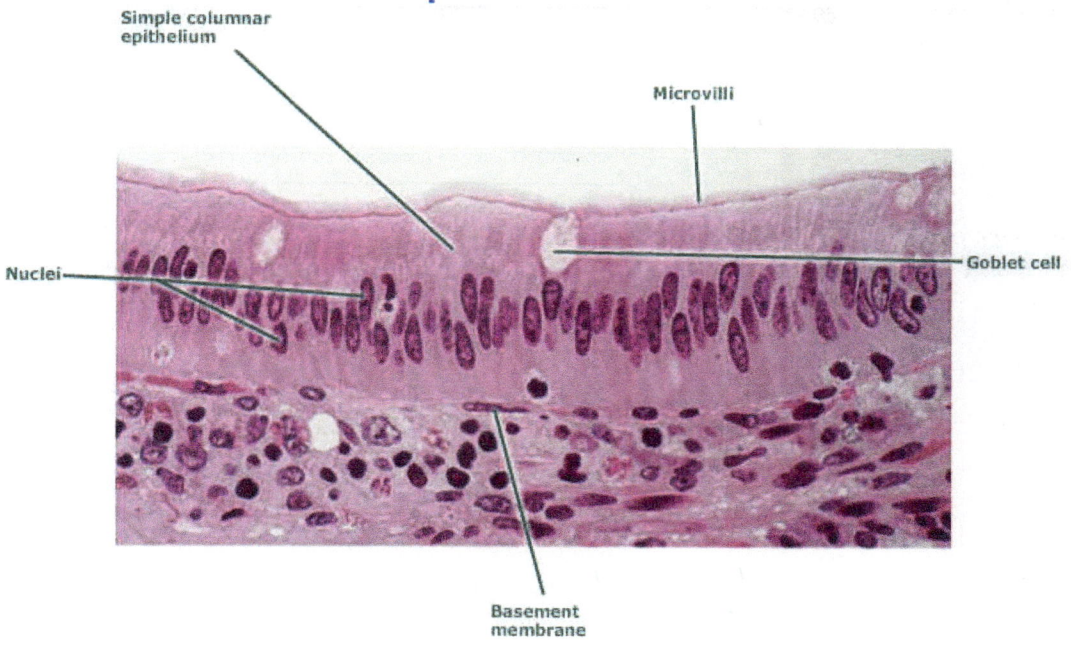

Figure 3.3

Pseudostratified Ciliated Columnar Epithelial Tissue

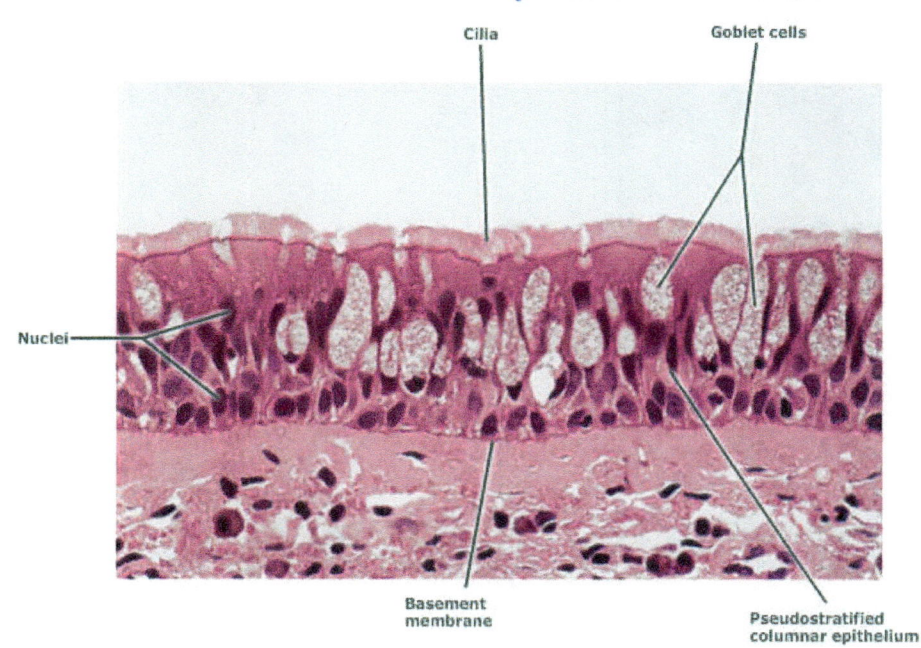

Figure 3.4

CHAPTER THREE *Histology* 47

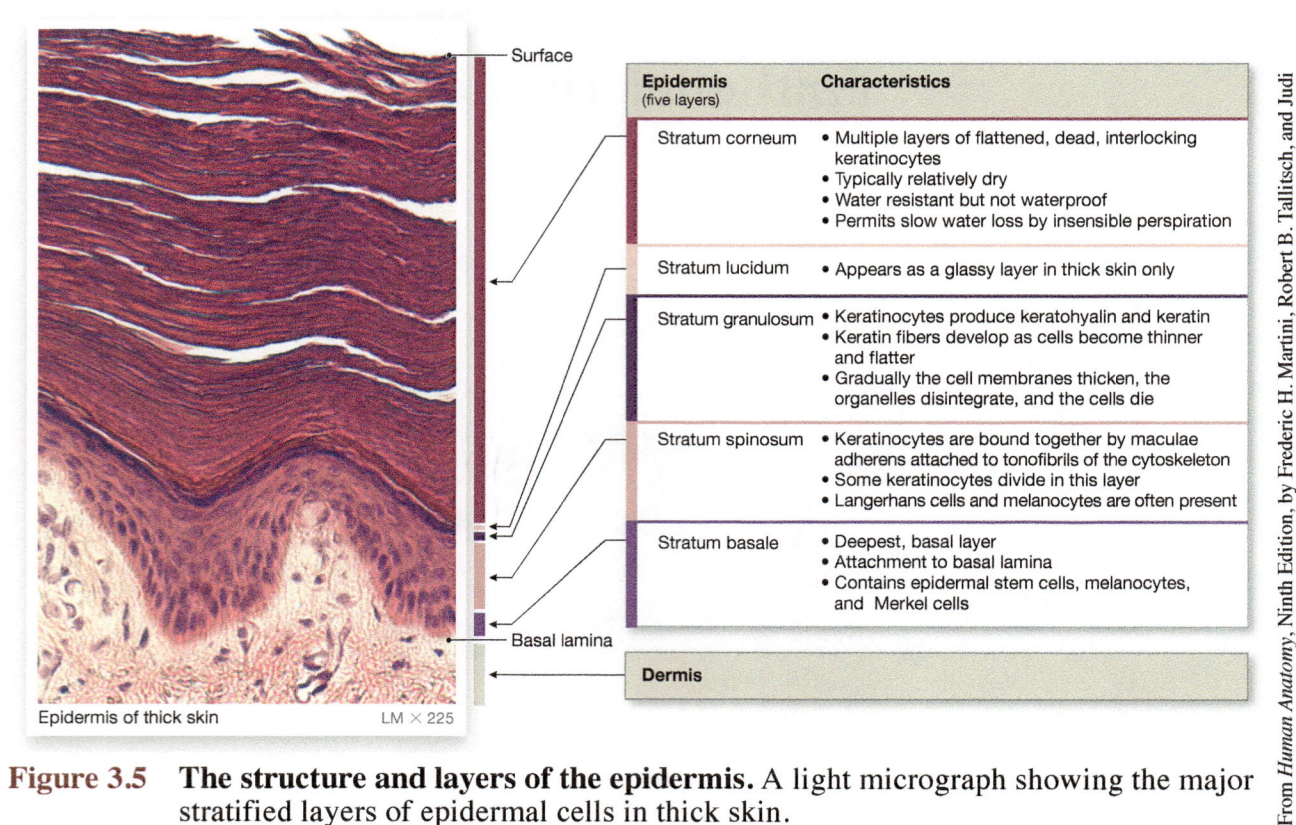

Epidermis (five layers)	Characteristics
Stratum corneum	• Multiple layers of flattened, dead, interlocking keratinocytes • Typically relatively dry • Water resistant but not waterproof • Permits slow water loss by insensible perspiration
Stratum lucidum	• Appears as a glassy layer in thick skin only
Stratum granulosum	• Keratinocytes produce keratohyalin and keratin • Keratin fibers develop as cells become thinner and flatter • Gradually the cell membranes thicken, the organelles disintegrate, and the cells die
Stratum spinosum	• Keratinocytes are bound together by maculae adherens attached to tonofibrils of the cytoskeleton • Some keratinocytes divide in this layer • Langerhans cells and melanocytes are often present
Stratum basale	• Deepest, basal layer • Attachment to basal lamina • Contains epidermal stem cells, melanocytes, and Merkel cells

Figure 3.5 **The structure and layers of the epidermis.** A light micrograph showing the major stratified layers of epidermal cells in thick skin.

Transitional Epithelium

LOCATIONS: Urinary bladder; renal pelvis; ureters

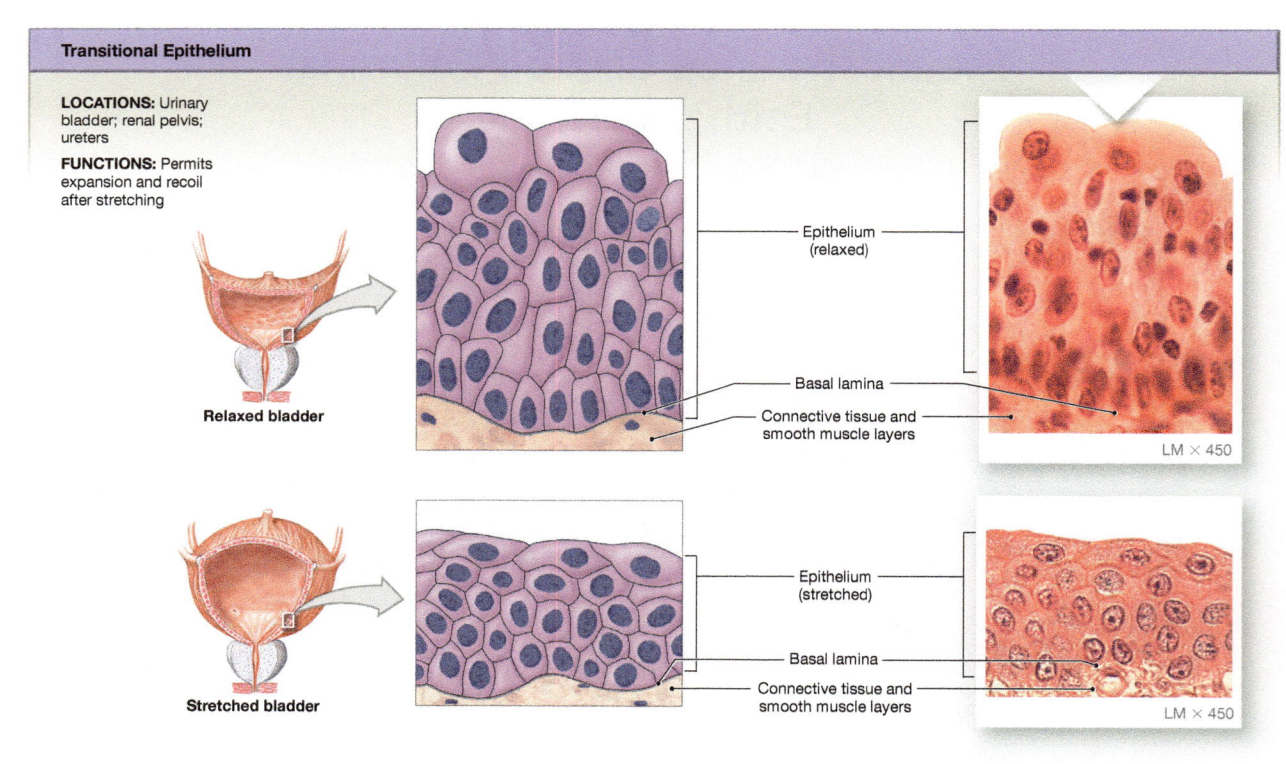

FUNCTIONS: Permits expansion and recoil after stretching

Figure 3.6 **Transitional epithelium.** A sectional view of the transitional epithelium lining the urinary bladder. The cells from an empty bladder are in the relaxed state, while those lining a full urinary bladder show the effects of stretching on the arrangement of cells in the epithelium.

Complete Introductory Human Anatomy Lab Guide

Glandular Epithelium
(Pancreatic Tissue)

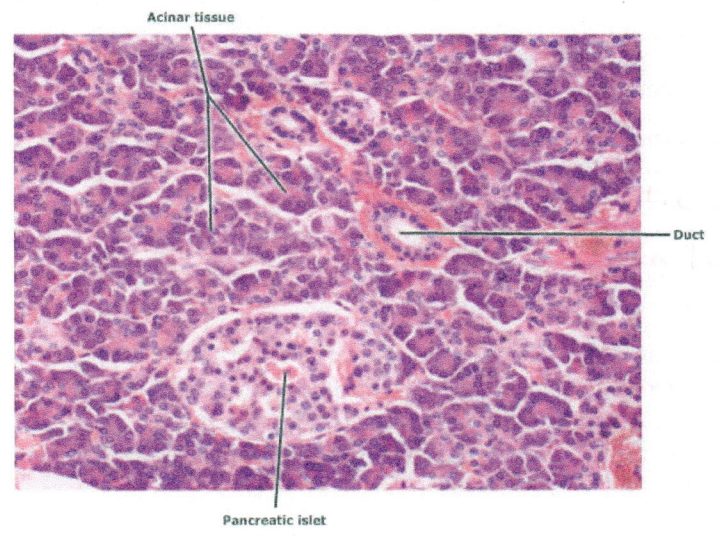

Figure 3.7

From Practice Anatomy Lab 3.0, First Edition, by Ruth Heisler et al. (2012), reproduced by permission of Pearson Education.

1. **Simple squamous epithelium** consists of a single layer of flat cells, joined closely with a minimum of intercellular material. Cells are mononucleate and have a "fried egg" shape (Fig. 3.1).

    Locations: Simple squamous epithelium is found in alveolar sacs in the lungs, the glomerular capsule (Bowman's capsule) of the kidney and in the endothelium of the heart and blood vessels. Capillary walls consist of a layer of simple squamous epithelial tissue.

    Functions: gas exchange (between capillaries & alveoli), absorption, secretion and filtration

2. **Simple cuboidal epithelium** is a single layer of cube-shaped cells. The nucleus of simple cuboidal epithelial tissue is large and centrally located. Cube-shaped cells line the lumen of the kidney tubule, for example (Fig. 3.2).

    Locations: kidney tubules, lining the ducts of glands and the external layer of the ovary and thyroid follicles.

    Functions: secretion and absorption

3. **Simple cuboidal epithelium** (higher magnification): The **basement membrane** is the surface by which epithelial cells are attached to underlying tissue, and is distinct in this magnification. Observe that, whether cuboidal cells are viewed in cross-section or longitudinal section, they appear cube-shaped.

4. **Simple columnar epithelial tissue:** Simple columnar epithelial cells are single-layered tall, rectangular cells with their nuclei located near the basement membrane (Fig. 3.3).

    The epithelial lining of the small intestine is composed of simple columnar epithelium. This slide shows a cross section through a portion of the small intestines. **Microvilli** are apical surface features of simple columnar epithelial tissue that increase surface area for absorption, particularly in the small intestines.

Also, note the **goblet cells** found among the columnar cells. Goblet cells secrete a slimy protein called **mucin** that, when mixed with water, forms mucus.

    Locations: Simple columnar epithelial tissue forms the mucous lining of the gastrointestinal tract from the stomach to anus, but is particularly distinct in the mucosal layer of the small intestine.

    Functions: secretion and absorption

5. **Simple columnar epithelium** (higher magnification): Observe slides or photomicrographs showing a section of a **villus** in the small intestines. Villi are multicellular structures that increase the surface area of the lining of the intestine. Microvilli are folds of the plasmalemma of the cell to increase the surface area of an individual cell. Microvilli are subcellular structures. Note the microvilli along the apical surface of the columnar epithelial cells. **Microvilli** and **villi** increase the surface area for absorption (Fig. 3.3).

6. **Stratified squamous epithelium:** This tissue is formed from numerous layers of flattened cells. True squamous-shaped cells are located at the apical surface (free surface). Cells are more cube-shaped near the basement membrane. The two types of stratified squamous epithelium are **keratinized** and **non-keratinized**. Stratified squamous epithelium is tolerant of abrasion and so is found in places that are subject to physical wear.

    Locations: The **keratinized** type of stratified squamous epithelium forms the epidermis, while **non-keratinized** stratified squamous epithelium lines moist surfaces such as the mouth, esophagus and vagina.

    Function: protection

7. **Pseudostratified ciliated columnar epithelial tissue** is named such because, though all cells are attached to the basement membrane, not all cells reach the free surface. Varied cell length gives the tissue the appearance of being many-layered, but it is actually only one layer thick (Fig. 3.5). Other characteristics of Pseudostratified ciliated columnar epithelium include **cilia** and **goblet cells**. Cilia are extensions of individual cells that are capable of active motion. They consist of an array of microtubules covered with plasmalemma.

    Note that nuclei of the Pseudostratified ciliated columnar epithelium are located at different levels in each cell: a characteristic that further contributes to the "stratified" appearance. **Lamina propria** is a type of loose connective tissue binding the epithelial layer to deeper structures.

    Locations: Pseudostratified ciliated columnar epithelium is found lining the lumen of the **trachea** and **primary bronchi**. It can also be found lining the ducts of glands and parts of the male reproductive tract.

    Functions: secretion, protection and movement of mucus by cilia

8. **Transitional epithelium** is a type of stratified epithelium that is specialized to tolerate stretching. It forms the lining of the urinary bladder and is subject to stretching (distention) as the bladder fills and empties. Cells of the superficial layer are called **dome cells** because of their rounded apical surfaces (Fig. 3.6). They become flattened when the bladder is distended.

    Locations: forms the lining of the renal pelvis, ureter and urinary bladder

    Function: stretching and recoiling

9. **Glandular epithelium is specialized to produce secretions:** This example is of **pancreatic glandular epithelium.** The group of light-colored cells in the center is a **pancreatic islet** (Islet of Langerhans) (Fig. 3.7).

- **Pancreatic islets** have endocrine functions and secrete both **insulin** and **glucagon**.
- The surrounding dark-colored cells are **acinar cells**. Acinar cells secrete digestive enzymes into ducts that eventually unite to form the pancreatic duct.

Many glands are formed from epithelium. Locate additional examples of glandular epithelium.

IV. CONNECTIVE TISSUE

Connective tissue is the most abundant tissue type in the body. It is characterized by three components:

1. specialized cells
2. extracellular protein fibers
3. extracellular fluid known as the ground substance.

It **binds, protects** and **supports** organs and forms the framework of the body and is never found on an exposed body surface. Connective tissues are classified into three major types:

1. connective tissue proper
2. supporting connective tissue, and
3. fluid connective tissue.

Connective Tissue Proper

Connective tissue proper is characterized by having multiple cell types, a variety of extracellular fibers and a thick fluid ground substance. Subtypes are based on the relative proportions of the components and types of cells and fibers. Connective tissue proper is subdivided into Loose and Dense Connective Tissues. (Figs. 3.8–3.14)

Areolar Connective Tissue

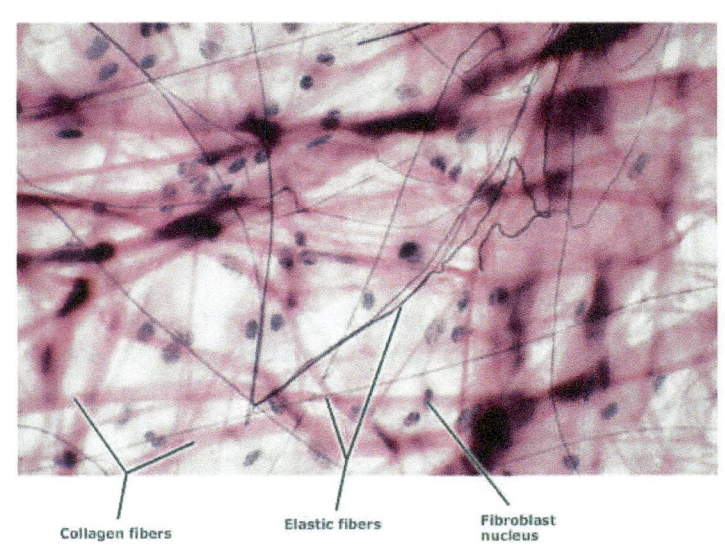

Figure 3.8

Adipose Connective Tissue

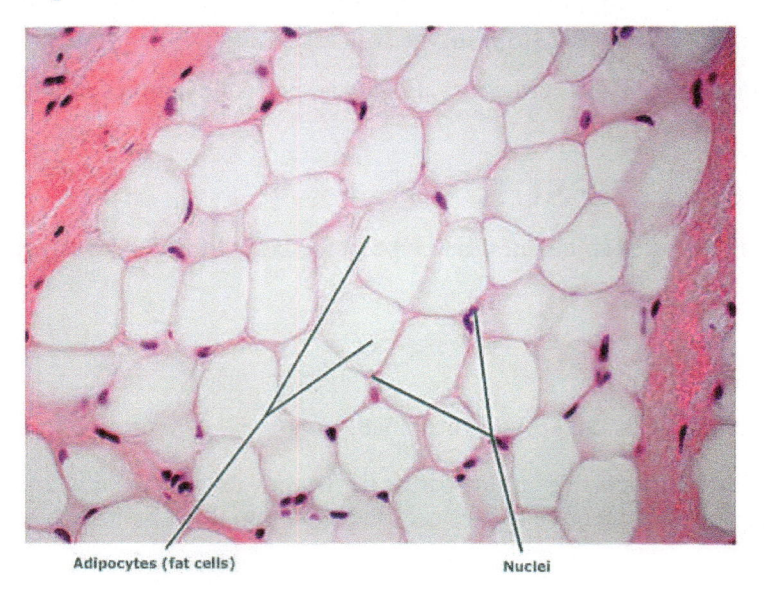

Figure 3.9

Loose Connective Tissue

1. **Areolar connective tissue** forms a network around organs, muscles, blood vessels and nerves. Look for the following structures:

    - Areolar connective tissue is found in the dermis of the skin (described below) and in the connective tissue deep to the dermis. It forms the foundation of mucous membranes as **lamina propria**.
    - Areolar connective tissue contains **elastic fibers, reticular fibers** and **collagen fibers.**
    - Pink-stained fibers are **collagen fibers**.
    - The thin, dark fibers are **elastic fibers**.
    - **Reticular fibers** are too fine to see in this illustration.
    - Locate **nuclei of fibroblasts** (dark ovals).
    - **Fibroblasts** produce extracellular fibers & ground substance.
    - Extracellular **matrix** is made up of the fibers and ground substance.

    Locations: Areolar connective tissue is found surrounding organs and in the superficial fascia (connective tissue between skin and muscles).

    Function: binding and support

2. **Areolar connective tissue** (higher magnification): locate elastic fibers, collagen fibers and nuclei of fibroblasts. Reticular fibers may be seen as a spider web-like network (Fig. 3.8).

3. **Adipose connective tissue** is characterized by having a high proportion of **adipocytes** that store lipids (fats) bound together in a basement membrane. (Fig. 3.9)

    The cytoplasm and nuclei in adipose cells are pressed against the side of the cell to make room for fatty deposits. Most of the volume of the adipose cell is taken up with fat.

Locations: Adipose connective tissue is located in numerous regions of the body including the subcutaneous layer. Adipose connective tissue also surrounds and protects major organs and it is found in the medullary cavity of long bones.

Functions: storage of fats as energy, support, protection, shock absorption and insulation

Dense Connective Tissue

Dense connective tissues have a greater proportion of fibers and relatively little ground substance. The most common cells are fibroblasts.

(Figs. 3.10–3.12)

4. **Dense irregular connective tissue** is composed almost entirely of irregularly arranged collagen fibers. The irregular arrangement allows for stress to be applied in several directions.

    Location: Dense irregular connective tissue is located in the **dermis (reticular layer), periosteum of bones, membrane capsules** around various organs and **joint capsules.**

    Function: Dense irregular connective tissue provides strength and resistance to stress.

5. **Dense regular connective tissue:**

    a. **Collagen fibers** have a wavy, parallel arrangement. Parallel collagen fibers provide great tensile strength (resisting stretching).
    b. Observe the nuclei of fibroblasts between the collagen fibers. These nuclei appear as small, dark specks within the collagen fibers.

    Location: Dense regular connective tissue is located in tendons and ligaments.

    Function: Dense regular connective tissue provides strong connection between bone and muscles or bone and bone.

Dense Irregular Connective Tissue

LOCATIONS: Capsules of visceral organs; periostea and perichondria; nerve and muscle sheaths; dermis

FUNCTIONS: Provides strength to resist forces applied from many directions; helps prevent overexpansion of organs such as the urinary bladder

Collagen fiber bundles

LM × 111

From *Human Anatomy*, Ninth Edition, by Frederic H. Martini, Robert B. Tallitsch, and Judi L. Nath (2018), reproduced by permission of Pearson Education.

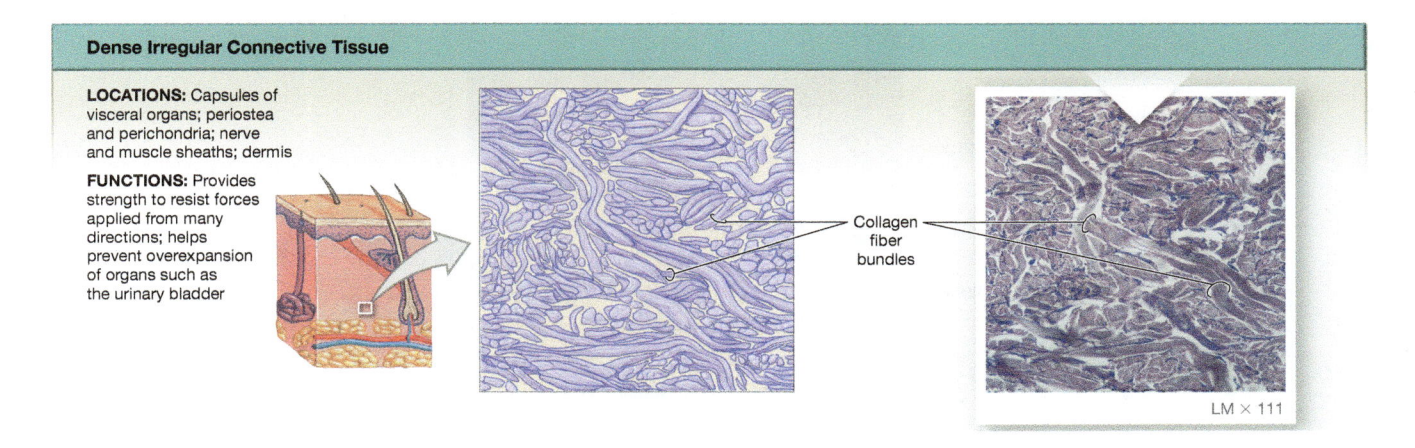

Figure 3.10 **Deep Dermis.** The deep portion of the dermis of the skin consists of a thick layer of interwoven collagen fibers oriented in various directions.

Elastic Tissue

LOCATIONS: Between vertebrae of the spinal column (ligamentum flavum and ligamentum nuchae); ligaments supporting penis; ligaments supporting transitional epithelia; in blood vessel walls

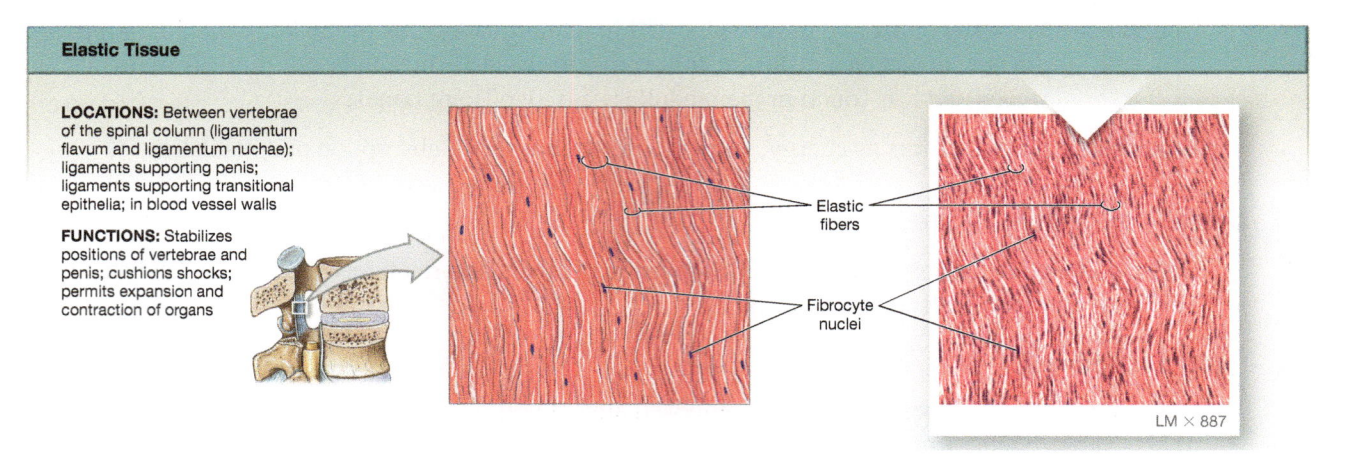

FUNCTIONS: Stabilizes positions of vertebrae and penis; cushions shocks; permits expansion and contraction of organs

Figure 3.11 Elastic Ligament. Elastic ligaments extend between the vertebrae of the spinal column. The bundles of elastic fibers are fatter than the collagen fiber bundles of a tendon or typical ligament.

From *Human Anatomy*, Ninth Edition, by Frederic H. Martini, Robert B. Tallitsch, and Judi L. Nath (2018), reproduced by permission of Pearson Education.

6. **Elastic connective tissue:** Microscopically, elastic fibers appear as darkly stained lines. Fibers of the protein elastin comprise the primary type of fibers in elastic connective tissue.

   Location: Elastic connective tissue is found in the walls of the aorta and large arteries. Elastic tissue is also present in the yellow ligaments of the vertebral column.

   Function: Elastic fibers in arteries help regulate blood pressure, and in other regions, allow stretching of various organs.

From *Human Anatomy*, Ninth Edition, by Frederic H. Martini, Robert B. Tallitsch, and Judi L. Nath (2018), reproduced by permission of Pearson Education.

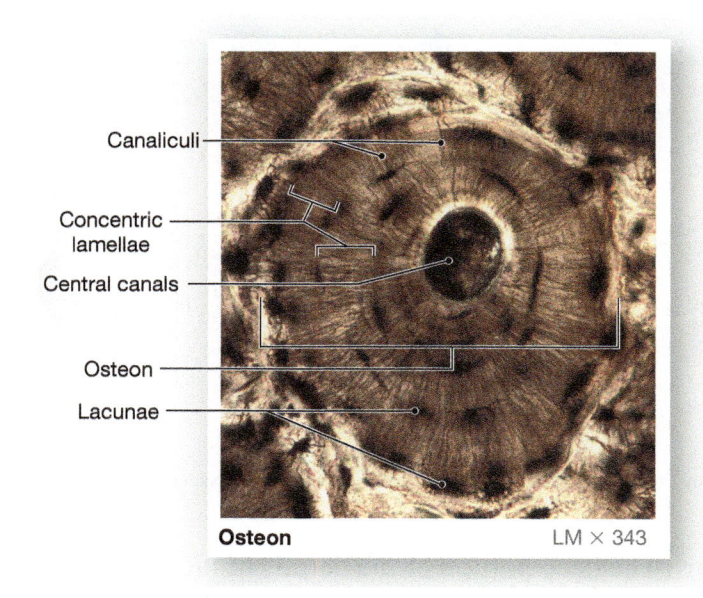

Figure 3.12   A single osteon at higher magnification.

7. **Elastic connective tissue** (higher magnification): shown again in the walls of the aorta. Observe the network of darkly stained elastic fibers. Elastic fibers are abundant in the walls of arteries.

Supporting and Fluid Connective Tissues

(Figs. 3.13–3.14)

8. **Bone connective tissue** (low power): Several **osteons** (Haversian systems) can be studied simultaneously at a lower magnification. Each osteon is made up of a central canal, lamellae, canaliculi and lacunae (Figs. 3.12 and 3.13).

From *Human Anatomy*, Ninth Edition, by Frederic H. Martini, Robert B. Tallitsch, and Judi L. Nath (2018), reproduced by permission of Pearson Education.

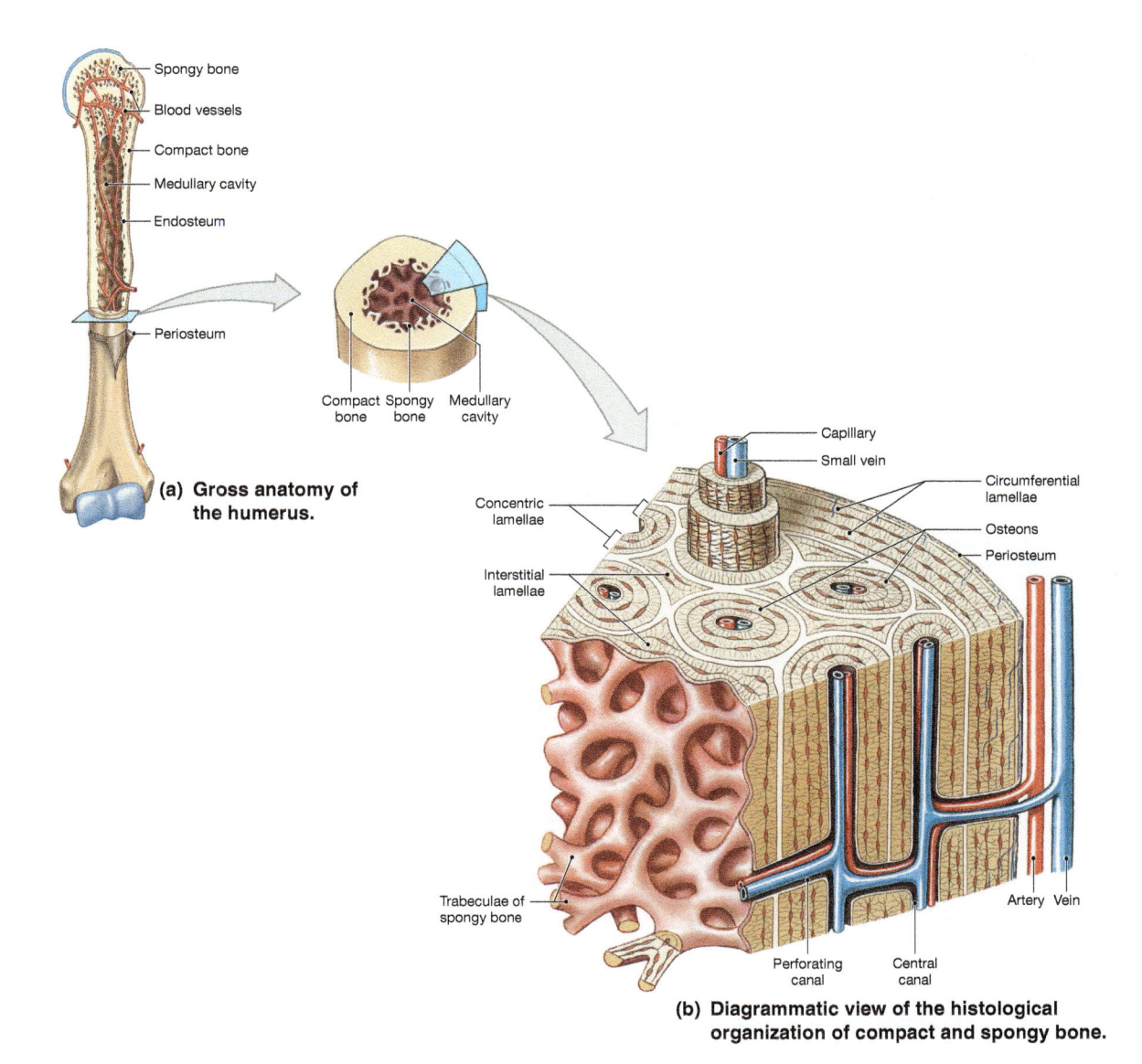

Figure 3.13 **The Internal Organization in Representative Bones.** The structural relationship of compact and spongy bone in representative bones.

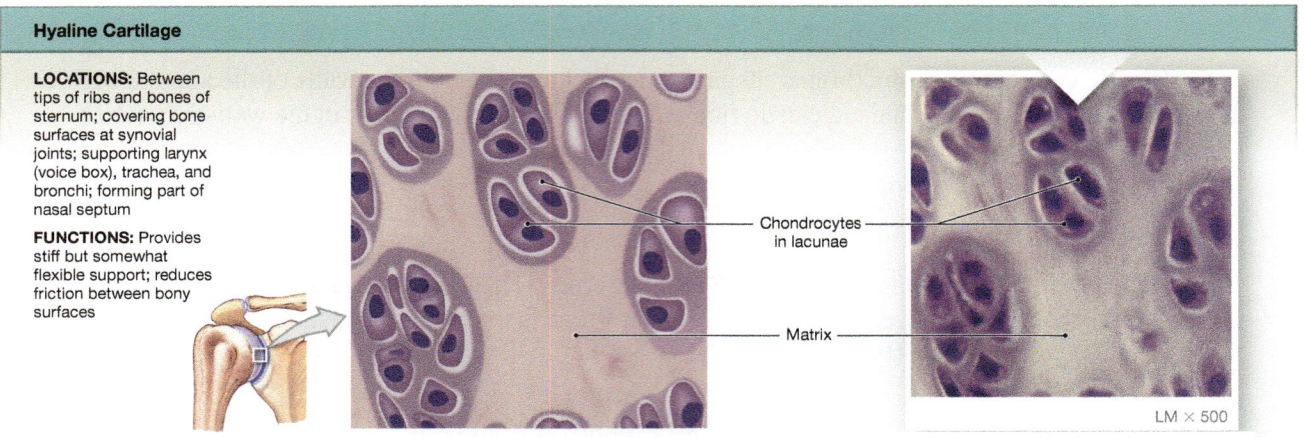

Hyaline Cartilage

LOCATIONS: Between tips of ribs and bones of sternum; covering bone surfaces at synovial joints; supporting larynx (voice box), trachea, and bronchi; forming part of nasal septum

FUNCTIONS: Provides stiff but somewhat flexible support; reduces friction between bony surfaces

— Chondrocytes in lacunae
— Matrix

LM × 500

(a) Hyaline cartilage. Note the translucent matrix and the absence of prominent fibers.

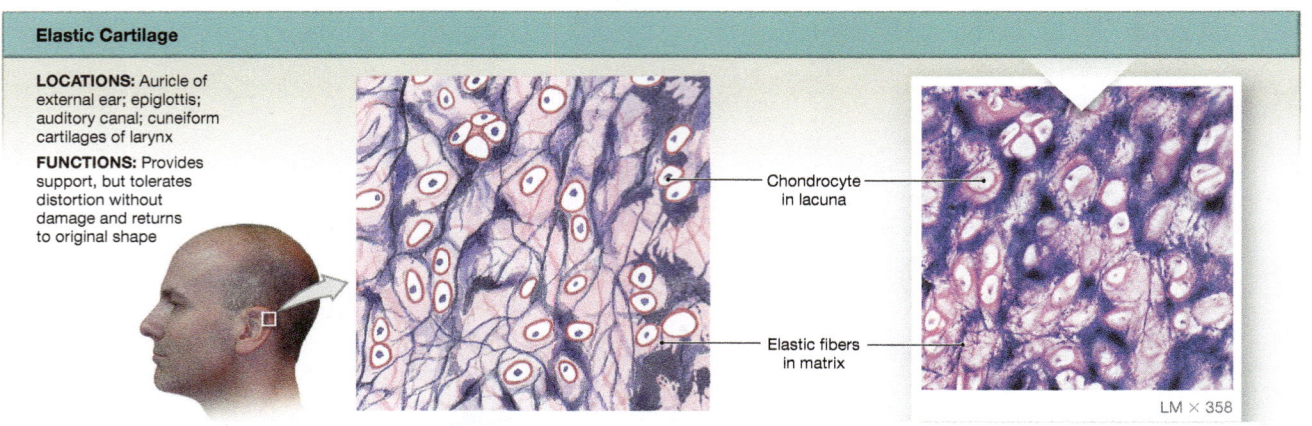

Elastic Cartilage

LOCATIONS: Auricle of external ear; epiglottis; auditory canal; cuneiform cartilages of larynx

FUNCTIONS: Provides support, but tolerates distortion without damage and returns to original shape

— Chondrocyte in lacuna
— Elastic fibers in matrix

LM × 358

(b) Elastic cartilage. The closely packed elastic fibers are visible between the chondrocytes.

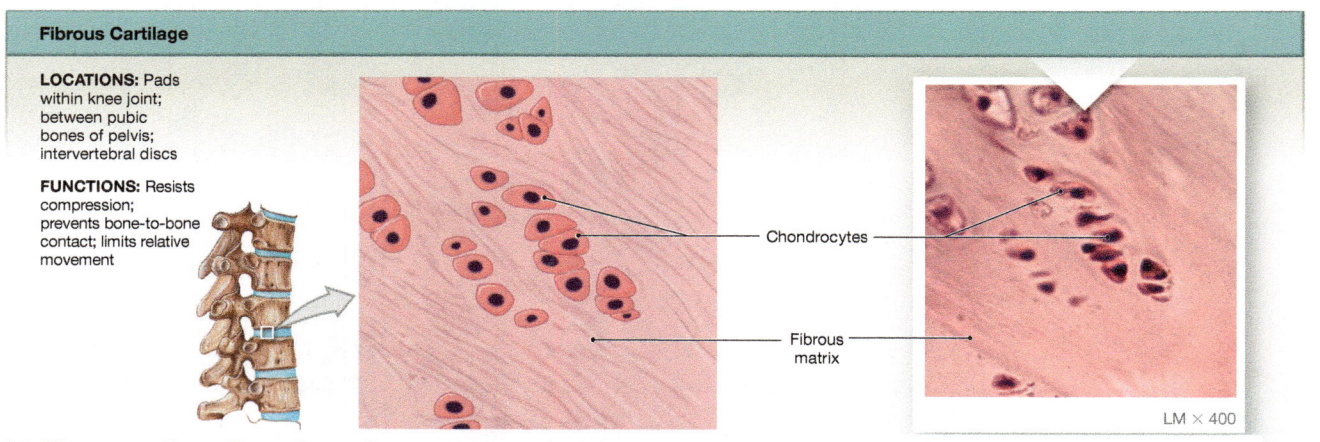

Fibrous Cartilage

LOCATIONS: Pads within knee joint; between pubic bones of pelvis; intervertebral discs

FUNCTIONS: Resists compression; prevents bone-to-bone contact; limits relative movement

— Chondrocytes
— Fibrous matrix

LM × 400

(c) Fibrous cartilage. The collagen fibers are extremely dense, and the chondrocytes are relatively far apart.

From *Human Anatomy*, Ninth Edition, by Frederic H. Martini, Robert B. Tallitsch, and Judi L. Nath (2018), reproduced by permission of Pearson Education.

Figure 3.14 Histology of the Three Types of Cartilage. Cartilage is a supporting connective tissue with a firm, gelatinous matrix.

Functions of **bone** include the following:

- It provides the rigid framework of the body and supports internal organs.
- Bones serve as sites for muscle attachment.
- It contains many blood vessels, collagen fibers and calcium salts.
- Bone stores minerals such as calcium, phosphorous and magnesium that are needed in physiological processes.
- It also stores the cells that produce blood cells in the red marrow.

9. **Bone connective tissue** (higher magnification): Structures found in an osteon are distinguishable at higher magnification (400x) (Fig. 3.12).

    - The **central canal** (Haversian canal) is the dark, central portion of each osteon containing an artery, vein and nerve. Blood vessels within each central canal supply materials to and remove wastes from the osteocytes (mature bone cells).
    - **Lamellae** are formed by calcified bone arranged in concentric circles around the Haversian canal.
    - **Lacunae** containing **osteocytes** (mature bone cells) appear as dark spots between lamellae. Osteocytes cannot be distinguished inside these lacunae.
    - **Canaliculi** connect the central canal to lacunae and lacunae to each other. They seem to radiate outward from the central canal.

10. **Hyaline cartilage connective tissue** is found in the trachea. Double-celled lacunae are characteristic of hyaline cartilage. Chondrocytes are found in the lacunae. Hyaline cartilage is avascular and contains collagen fibers that are very fine; they are not usually visible as fibers, giving the matrix its gel-like appearance. Locate the following structures within hyaline cartilage connective tissue (Fig. 3.14).

    - **Chondrocytes** (cartilage cells) can be seen in each lacuna.
    - **Lacunae** may contain one or several cells, but double-celled lacunae are typical of hyaline cartilage connective tissue. The walls of the lacunae stain slightly darker than the surrounding tissue.
    - **Matrix** is the substance between lacunae.

    Locations: **Hyaline cartilage** is located in the fetal skeleton, articular surfaces of long bones and "c"–shaped rings of the trachea. Hyaline cartilage connective tissue also makes up epiphyseal plates of bones in growing children, the tip of the nose and part of the larynx.

    Functions: Hyaline cartilage functions to support various structures and its smooth surface reduces friction between ends of bones at joints.

11. **Elastic Cartilage Connective Tissue** is characterized by having chondrocytes in lacunae with closely packed elastic fibers in a gel-like matrix. Locate the following structures within elastic cartilage connective tissue (Fig. 3.14).

    Locations: Elastic cartilage is located in the external ear and auditory canal, and epiglottic cartilages.

    Functions: Tolerates distortion and returns to original shape.

12. **Fibrous Cartilage Connective Tissue** has prominent collagen fibers visible in micrographs between lacunae. Locate the following structures within elastic cartilage connective tissue (Fig. 3.15).

    - Chondrocytes
    - Lacunae
    - Elastic fibers: fine, darkly staining fibers in the matrix

    Locations: Menisci of knee, intervertebral discs, pubic symphysis.

    Functions: Tolerates compression; fibers resist tension and limit distortion (Fig. 3.15). Locate the following structures within elastic cartilage connective tissue (Fig. 3.15).

    - Chondrocytes
    - Lacunae
    - Collagen fibers: wavy, lightly staining fibers in the matrix

13. **Blood connective tissue:** This is a scanning electron micrograph of **erythrocytes** (red blood cells). **Blood** is considered a type of connective tissue because it consists of cells in an intercellular matrix. It carries oxygen and nutrients throughout the body and is composed of both formed elements (cells and cellular fragments) and plasma. (Fig. 3.15)

    - **Erythrocytes** are the most numerous cell types in this slide. Red blood cells are non-nucleated.
    - **Leukocytes**, also called white blood cells, are cells of the immune system. They have prominent nuclei. There are five types of leucocytes (Fig. 3.15)
    Neutrophils—large phagocytic cells with irregular nuclei and neutrally staining granules in the cytoplasm.
    Eosinophils—cells with a bilobed nucleus and acidic staining granules; they are attracted to antigens.

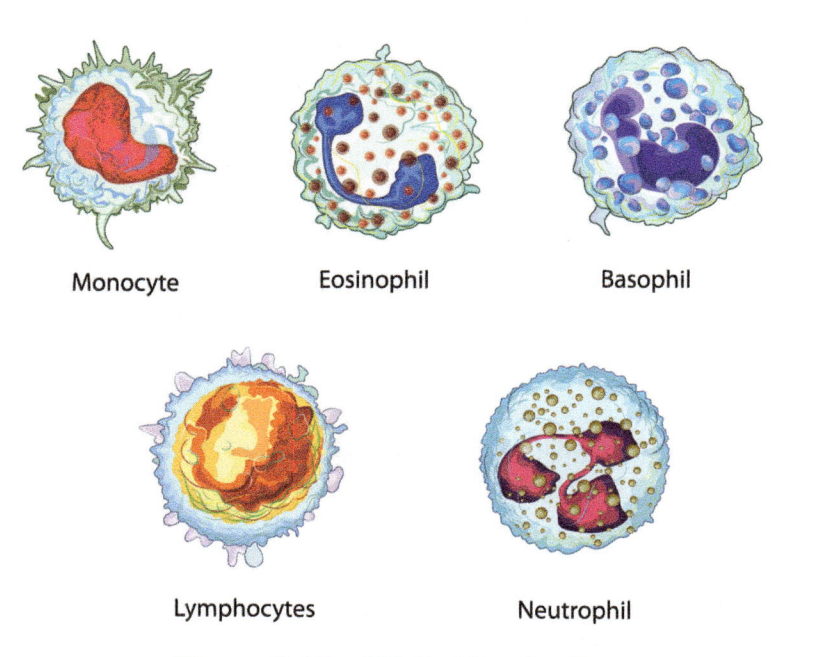

Figure 3.15 White blood cells.

Basophils—cells have cytoplasmic granules that stain with basic dyes. They release histamine into damaged tissues.

Monocytes—the largest leucocytes with large nuclei and agranular cytoplasm. They are phagocytic.

Lymphocytes—small cells, but have relatively large nuclei. They are responsible for immunity to specific pathogens.

- **Platelets** initiate blood clotting. Platelets are not cells, but rather are fragments of the cytoplasm of megakaryocytes found in the bone marrow.

V. MUSCLE TISSUE

Skeletal muscles perform voluntary movement, support organs and are connected to bones either by directly attaching to the periosteum, or by tendons. Skeletal muscle fibers, which are the cells of muscles, contain numerous **myofibrils**, which shorten when the cells contract. Muscle cells are bound together in groups called fascicles. Fascicles are surrounded by connective tissue. Numerous fascicles make up each whole muscle. (Figs. 3.16–3.18)

1. **Skeletal muscle**: Observe the following characteristics of skeletal muscle tissue. Observe muscle cells in longitudinal section and in cross-section (Fig. 3.16a, b).

    - Skeletal muscle cells are **striated** and **multinucleate**. A cell with multiple nuclei is called a syncytium.
    - **Nuclei** are located at the periphery of the skeletal muscle cells.
    - Skeletal muscle cells are long and cylindrical.
    - Striations appearing on skeletal muscle tissue cells result from the alternating bands of actin and myosin.
    - Skeletal muscle functions in movement, posture and heat production.

2. **Skeletal muscles:** Myofibrils are arranged parallel to each other from one end of the cell to the other. There are many **myofibrils** in each muscle cell (Fig 3.16a).

3. **Cross-section of skeletal muscle tissue:** Locate the fascicles, muscle cells (fibers) and myofibrils in cross-section. (Figs. 3.16a,b)

    - A muscle is composed of several **fascicles**.
    - In turn, each fascicle is composed of many **muscle cells** (muscle fibers)
    - One muscle cell (muscle fiber) is made up of many **myofibrils**.
    - Small dots inside each muscle cell are the cross-sections of myofibrils.
    - Skeletal muscle cells are multinucleate.
    - Note the peripherally located nuclei (dots between muscle cells).

Cardiac muscle tissue is found exclusively in the heart. Cardiac muscle tissue is striated, but involuntary. The cells of cardiac muscle tissue are branched and mononucleate.

1. **Cardiac muscle tissue:**

    Cardiac muscle tissue is **striated** similar to skeletal muscle but is **involuntary** like smooth muscle. Unique characteristics of cardiac muscle tissue include **branched cells** and **intercalated discs**. Cardiac muscle tissue also has a single, centrally located nucleus. (Fig. 3.17)

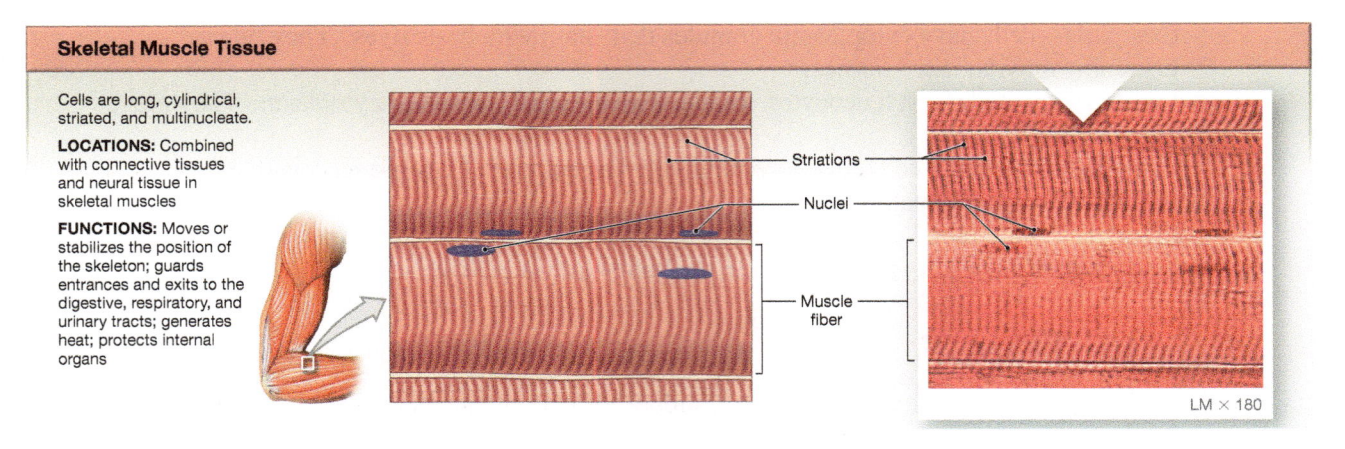

Skeletal Muscle Tissue

Cells are long, cylindrical, striated, and multinucleate.

LOCATIONS: Combined with connective tissues and neural tissue in skeletal muscles

FUNCTIONS: Moves or stabilizes the position of the skeleton; guards entrances and exits to the digestive, respiratory, and urinary tracts; generates heat; protects internal organs

Labels: Striations, Nuclei, Muscle fiber — LM × 180

From *Human Anatomy*, Ninth Edition, by Frederic H. Martini, Robert B. Tallitsch, and Judi L. Nath (2018), reproduced by permission of Pearson Education.

Figure 3.16 **Skeletal Muscle Fibers.** Note the large fiber size, prominent banding pattern, multiple nuclei, and unbranched arrangement.

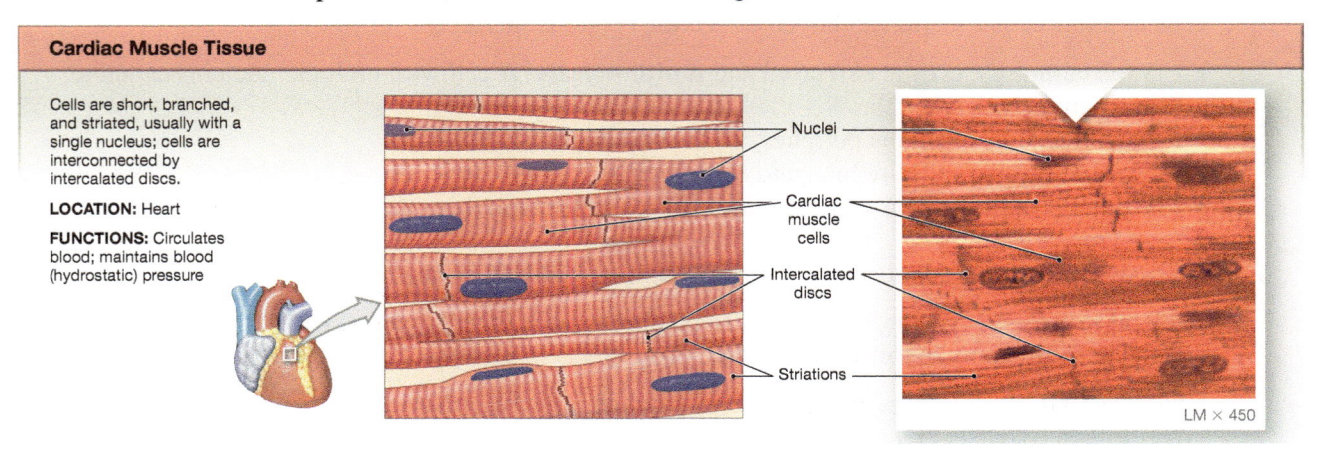

Cardiac Muscle Tissue

Cells are short, branched, and striated, usually with a single nucleus; cells are interconnected by intercalated discs.

LOCATION: Heart

FUNCTIONS: Circulates blood; maintains blood (hydrostatic) pressure

Labels: Nuclei, Cardiac muscle cells, Intercalated discs, Striations — LM × 450

From *Human Anatomy*, Ninth Edition, by Frederic H. Martini, Robert B. Tallitsch, and Judi L. Nath (2018), reproduced by permission of Pearson Education.

Figure 3.17 **Cardiac Muscle Cells.** Cardiac muscle cells are smaller than skeletal muscle cells, are branched, and have single nuclei.

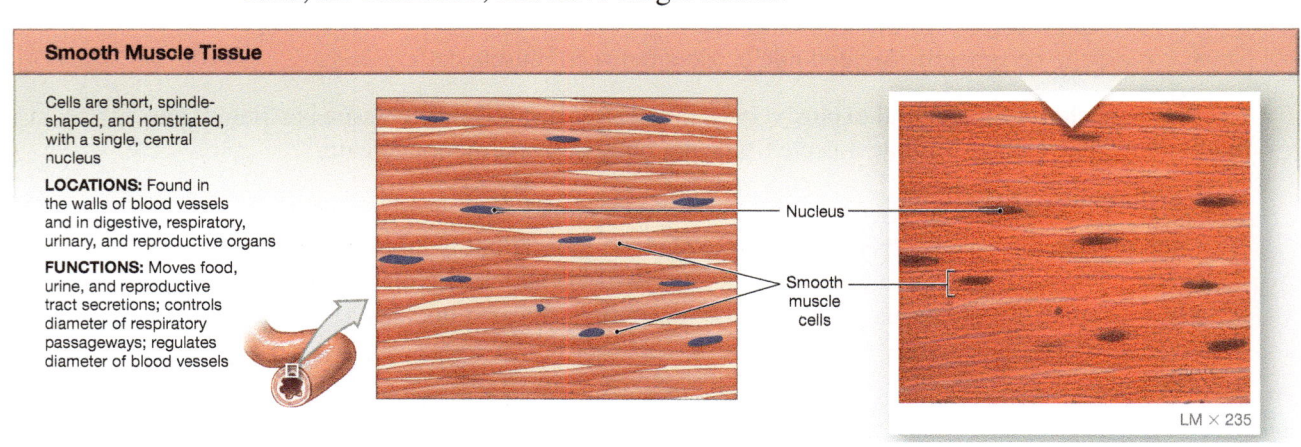

Smooth Muscle Tissue

Cells are short, spindle-shaped, and nonstriated, with a single, central nucleus

LOCATIONS: Found in the walls of blood vessels and in digestive, respiratory, urinary, and reproductive organs

FUNCTIONS: Moves food, urine, and reproductive tract secretions; controls diameter of respiratory passageways; regulates diameter of blood vessels

Labels: Nucleus, Smooth muscle cells — LM × 235

Figure 3.18 **Smooth Muscle Cells.** Smooth muscle cells are small and spindle shaped, with a central nucleus. They do not branch, and there are no striations.

Complete Introductory Human Anatomy Lab Guide

Location: Cardiac muscle tissue is located exclusively in the heart.

Functions: Cardiac muscle tissue's function is to pump blood to all parts of the body and sustain blood pressure.

2. **Cardiac muscle tissue** (higher magnification): Locate examples of **intercalated discs** and **branching cells**.

From *Human Anatomy*, Ninth Edition, by Frederic H. Martini, Robert B. Tallitsch, and Judi L. Nath (2018), reproduced by permission of Pearson Education.

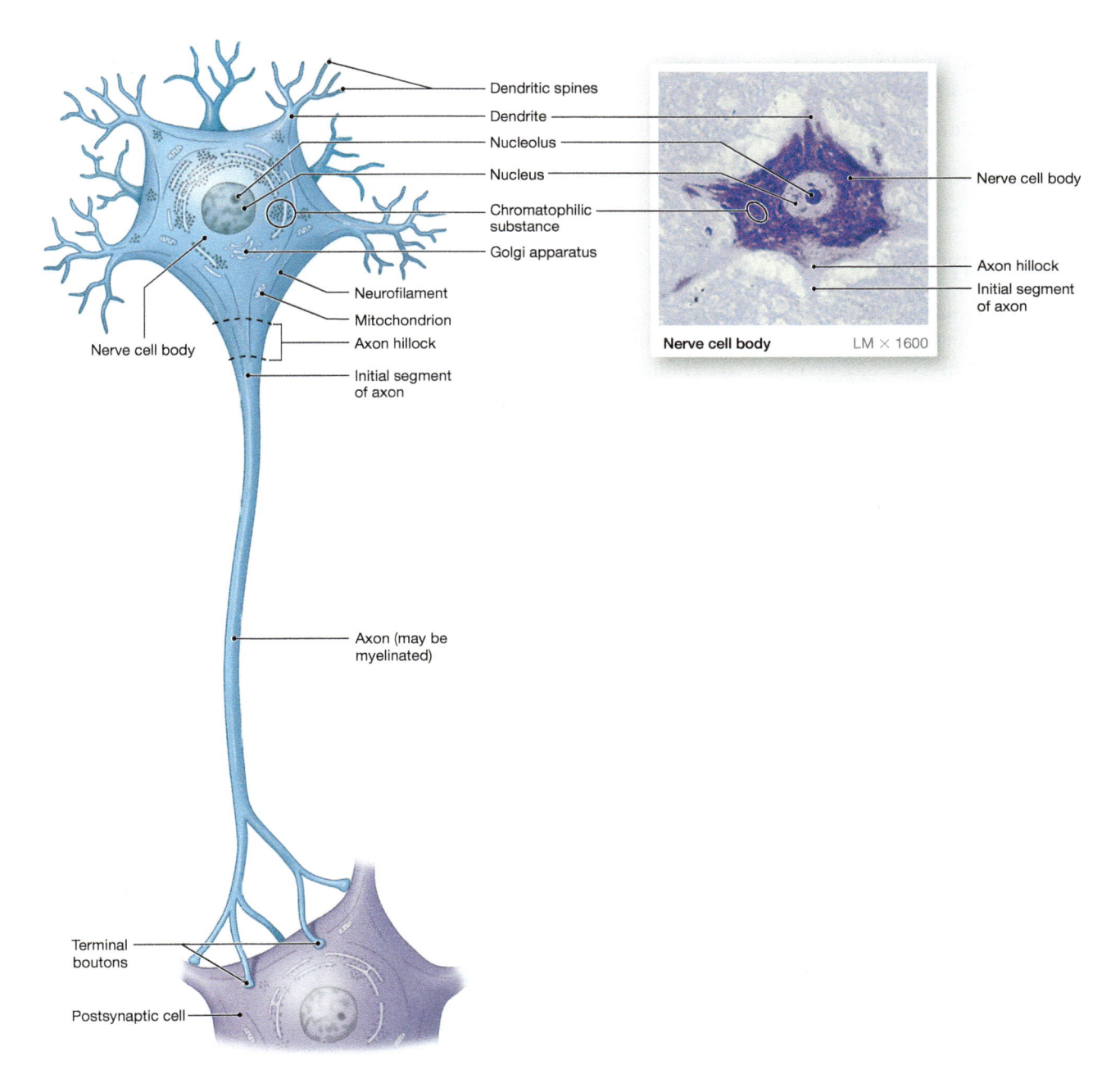

Figure 3.19   **Multipolar neuron.**

CHAPTER THREE   *Histology*

Smooth Muscle Tissue

1. **Smooth muscle tissue:**

    Smooth muscle cells are spindle-shaped, have a single, centrally-located nucleus and lack striations. Smooth muscle cells are mononucleate. Smooth muscle is also involuntary muscle tissue (Fig. 3.18).

    Locations: Smooth muscle is located in the walls of hollow (visceral) organs such as blood vessels, stomach walls, intestinal walls and urinary bladder.

    In most locations, smooth muscle is composed of two layers, the **circular muscularis** and **longitudinal muscularis**.

    Function: Smooth muscle's functions include moving food through gastrointestinal tract, regulation of the diameter of blood vessels and bronchioles, and moving urine through the urinary tract.

VI. NERVOUS TISSUE

Two major cell types make up nervous tissue, **neurons** and **neuroglial cells**. **Neurons** are conductive cells that exhibit sensitivity to stimulation, convert stimuli to impulses and conduct impulses to other neurons. Neurons are involved in initiation and transmission of nerve impulses.

Neuroglial cells are the supporting cells of the nervous system. Functions of neuroglial cells include support, protection (blood-brain barrier) and production of myelin sheath. (See Chapter 6 for more information.)

2. **Neurons:**
    - A neuron consists of a cell body, also known as the **soma**, that contains the nucleus, nucleolus and cytoplasm.
    - Cell processes extend from the soma.
    - This type of neuron has one axon and many dendrites, and is therefore called **multipolar**.
    - The axon is connected to the soma by the axon hillock.

VII. THE INTEGUMENT

Examine images of structures within and near the skin. Using photomicrographs and anatomical models locate and identify the following structures found within the skin. (Figures 3.20a–d)

- **Sudoriferous glands** are highly coiled glands that secrete sweat through ducts.
- **Sebaceous glands** are located near hair follicles and secrete oil into hair follicles.
- **Hair follicles** are found in thin skin. Epidermis surrounds the outer surface of the follicle.

1. **Thin skin:** Observe the epidermis and underlying dermis.
    - Epidermis is composed of stratified squamous epithelial tissue.
    - The dermis has two layers. The more superficial papillary layer is composed loose areloar tissue; the deeper reticular layer is composed of dense irregular connective tissue.

Section of thick skin

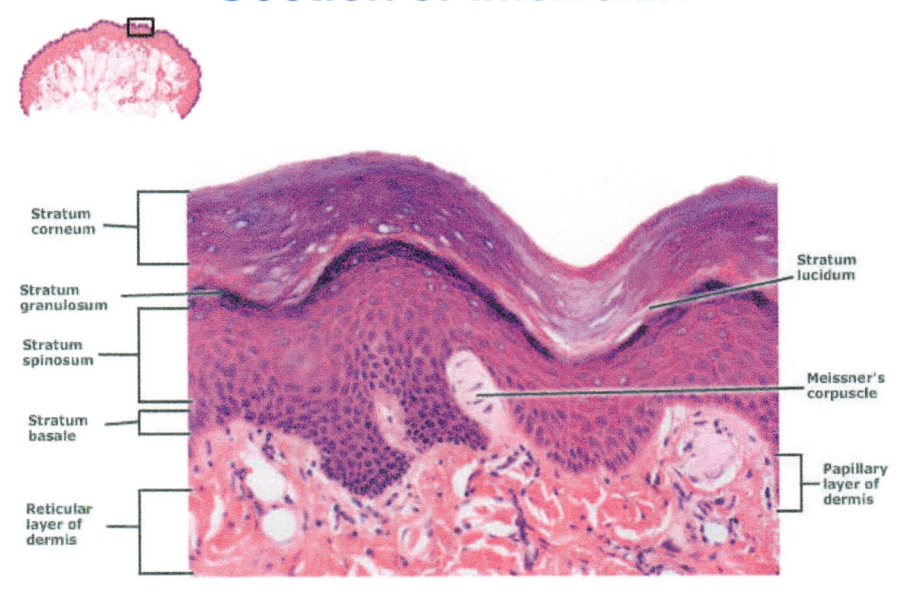

Figure 3.20a Section of thick skin.

Meissner Corpuscles in Thick Skin

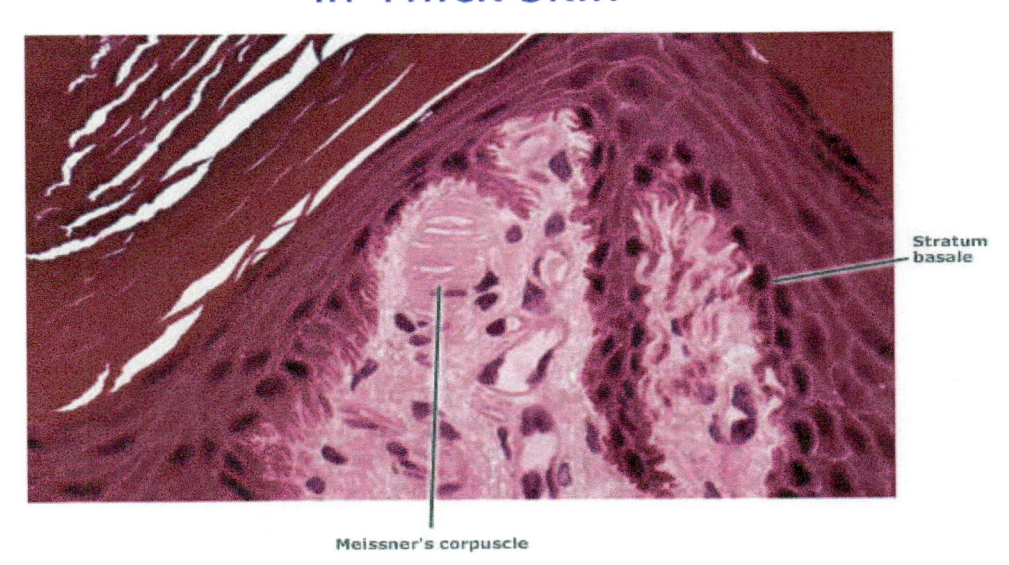

Figure 3.20b

CHAPTER THREE   *Histology*

Pacinian Corpuscles

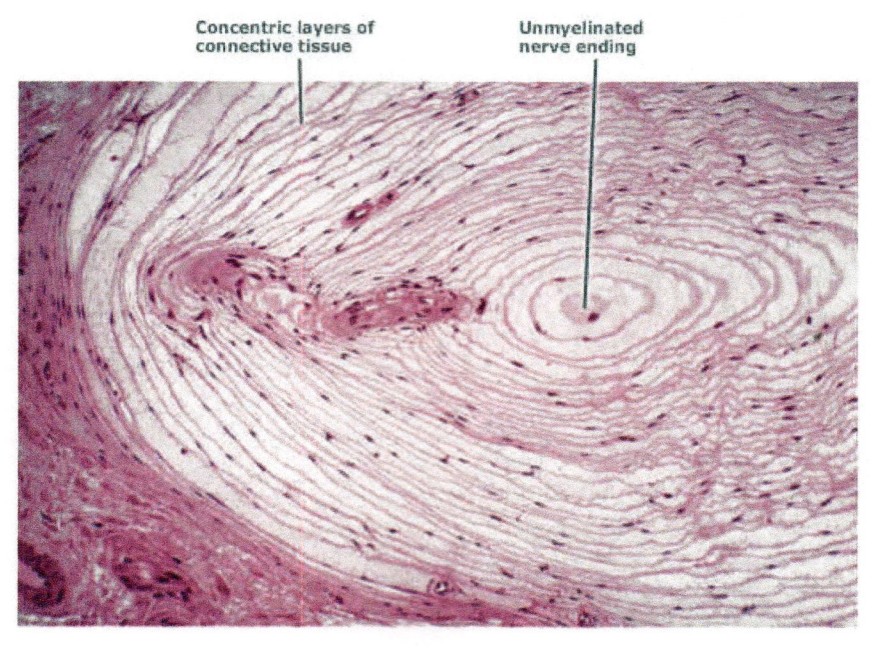

Figure 3.20c

Hair Follicle, Sebaceous Gland & Arrector Pili Muscle

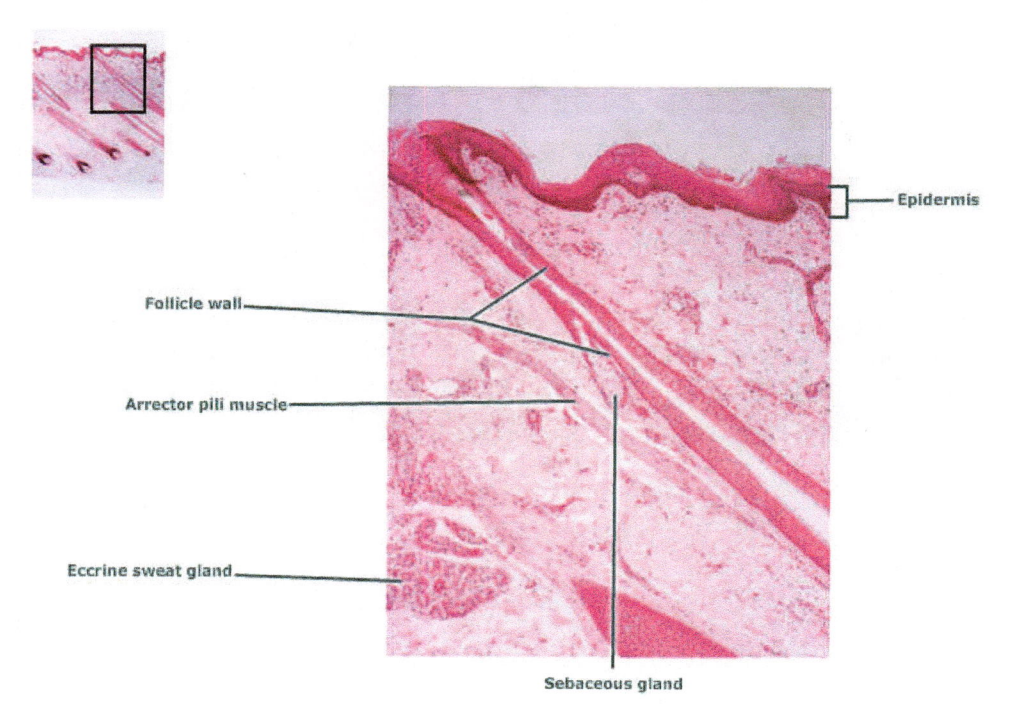

Figure 3.20d

Complete Introductory Human Anatomy Lab Guide

- Note the hair in the hair follicle (Fig 3.20d). Hair follicles are only located with "thin" skin. Note that the stratum basale of the epidermis extends deeply into the dermis surrounding the hair follicle.
- **Sebaceous glands** secrete sebum into hair follicles.

2. **Thick skin:** Five layers of epidermis are distinguishable.
    - **Stratum germinativum** (stratum basale) is the deepest layer of the epidermis and site of mitotic division. Cells known as **melanocytes** are located in the stratum germinativum. Melanocytes are responsible for producing the pigment granules, which contain melanin. **Skin color** is determined in part by the activity of melanocytes. (Fig. 3.20c)
        - **Melanin** is a brownish pigment, which, based on the amount secreted, causes the skin to be darker or lighter. Melanocytes are present in relatively the same number in all individuals. Active melanocytes secrete melanin, which causes the skin to become darker.
    - **Stratum spinosum** has a spiny appearance due to the desmosomes joining the cells to each other.
    - **Stratum granulosum**—Keratin gives this layer its granular appearance.
    - **Stratum lucidum** is a narrow, clear layer and is not present in thin skin.
    - **Stratum corneum** is the thickest, most superficial layer and is continually sloughed off and replaced.

3. **Thick skin:**
    - Note the thick **stratum corneum** and the absence of hair follicles.
    - **Meissner corpuscles** are found in the dermal papillae. These corpuscles function in discriminating touch (light touch). (Fig. 3.20a)

4. **Tactile corpuscle (Meissner's corpuscle):** Locate the oval-shaped Meissner's corpuscles within the dermal papillae.
    - **Skin receptors**—Examine two of the types of skin receptor using photomicrographs and the skin model.
    - **Tactile corpuscles (Meissner's corpuscles)** are for discriminating touch and **Lamellated corpuscles (Pacinian corpuscles)** function to detect pressure.

5. **Lamellated corpuscle (Pacinian corpuscle):** Pacinian corpuscles are found deep in the dermis. Pacinian corpuscles function in deep touch (pressure). (Fig. 3.20b)

6. **Hair follicle with sebaceous gland and arrector pili muscle:**
    - **Sebaceous glands** secrete sebum (an oily substance) and usually open into a hair follicle.
    - The **arrector pili muscle** is attached to the dermal papillae and to connective tissue surrounding the hair follicle. Arrector pili muscles cause the hair to become erect (goose bumps). (Fig. 3.20d)

7. **Sudoriferous** (sweat) **glands**: This slide shows sweat glands in thick skin. Sweat glands are highly coiled tubular structures. The duct of the sweat gland carries water, salts and wastes such as urea and uric acid to the surface of the skin. Sweat glands thus have **excretory** as well as **thermoregulatory** functions.

VIII. MEMBRANES

Membranes are thin sheets of epithelial tissue and an underlying layer of connective tissue, which cover organs or line body cavities. The two categories of membrane are **epithelial** and **fibrous membranes**.

1. **Epithelial membranes** are subdivided into **mucous** and **serous** membranes.
   - **Mucous membranes** line the digestive, respiratory, urinary and reproductive tracts. Mucous membranes open to the exterior of the body.
   - **Serous membranes** line the thoracic and abdominal cavities and other closed cavities.

2. **Fibrous membranes** cover organs and bones.
   - **Superficial fascia** is made up of areolar connective tissue. It lies directly under the skin between skin and muscles.
   - **Deep fascia** is dense irregular connective tissue that covers muscles and divides groups of muscles into compartments.
   - **Periosteum** is a dense irregular connective tissue covering that surrounds the diaphyses of bone.
   - **Synovial membranes** line joint cavities.

FOUR

Selected Muscles of the Appendicular & Axial Skeleton

Materials

Prone and supine human donor bodies and anatomical models
Latex gloves and wooden probes

In this section of the course we will begin using human donor bodies. Students are reminded that these bodies are the remains of people who chose to make a selfless and generous donation after their death. Furthermore, hundreds of hours were invested in the preparation of these dissections for your benefit. These dissections can be used for several years if they are kept moist and covered when not in use. Please help us get the maximum benefit from these invaluable donations.

Like most introductory courses in anatomy, this course is organized by organ systems. However, the study of muscles, particularly in the limbs is more efficient if we learn the nerves that innervate them and the blood supply at the same time. Muscles are best organized by compartments, as these are groups of muscles of similar position on a limb. In most cases all the muscles in a compartment are innervated by a single nerve, and only one or two arteries supply blood to all the muscles of a compartment. This chapter on the musculature will include the nerves and arteries that serve the limbs and all of these structures should be learned along with the muscles.

I. BODY LANGUAGE

Your study of human muscles will entail an in-depth examination of many of the muscles of the human body. You will learn the **origin, insertion, action,** and **nerve innervation** of *all* the muscles in this chapter. You will use prosected human donor bodies, anatomical models or images to examine these muscles.

Each muscle has an origin and an insertion. **Origin** usually refers to the more proximal attached end of the muscle. The **insertion** of a muscle is the attached end that is more distal or lateral and crosses the joint where the primary movement takes place.

Muscles work in coordination with each other to permit voluntary and purposeful movement. As one muscle contracts another relaxes. **Agonists** (prime movers) are muscles that initiate a particular movement. The **antagonist** is a muscle that contracts to return a body part to its original position, making a movement opposite to that of the agonist. **Synergists** are muscles that assist the agonist.

Muscles can be named for their **shape, size, fiber arrangement, location** or **action.** For example, the deltoid is named for its shape and the rectus femoris is named for its fiber arrangement. Many muscles are named for more than one attribute.

The muscle table accompanying each muscle group provides you with a precise and simplified format for learning about each muscle. Use these tables while working with the prosected donor body, anatomical models or illustrations.

Vocabulary for Muscles

1. **Agonist**—(prime mover) is a muscle that initiates a particular movement.
2. **Antagonist**—is a muscle that contracts to return a body part to its original position, making a movement opposite to that of the agonist.
3. **Fixator**—simultaneous contraction of an agonist and antagonist to hold a proximal joint in place to allow motion at a distal joint.
4. **Insertion**—is the attached end of a muscle that is more distal or lateral and is at the joint where the primary movement takes place.
5. **Origin**—refers to the more proximal attached end of the muscle.
6. **Ligament**—A tough band of connective tissue that connects a bone to another bone.
7. **Synergist**—a muscle that assists the agonist.
8. **Tendon**—A tough band of connective tissue that connects muscle to bone or muscle to muscle, often serving as the part of a muscle that attaches to its origin or insertion.
9. **Aponeurosis**—A broad and flattened tendon in the form of a sheet.

Vocabulary for Movements

To understand muscle function you must know the definitions of movements. Be able to demonstrate all of these motions with your study partners.

- **Flexion** – a movement that reduces the angle between articulating elements.
- **Extension** – the opposite; movement that increases the angle between elements.
- **Abduction** – a movement away from the longitudinal axis of the body.
- **Adduction** – the opposite; a movement toward the longitudinal axis of the body.
- **Rotation** –
  - Medial, rotates the anterior aspect of the limb toward the ventral body surface
  - Lateral, rotates the anterior surface of the limb away from the ventral aspect of the body
- **Circumduction** – rotation of a limb in a circular arc about its long axis.

Some movements apply only to particular body parts.
- **Pronation & supination** – rotation of the hand between the palm-down and palm-up positions.
- **Dorsiflexion** – extension of the foot at the ankle.
- **Plantarflexion** – flexion of the foot as in pointing the toes.
- **Eversion** – lateral or outward rotation of the foot.
- **Inversion** – medial or inward rotation of the foot.
- **Elevation and depression** – with respect to the shoulders or mandible.
- **Protraction and retraction** of the jaw.
- **Rotation and lateral flexion** of the head or torso.

II. MUSCLES OF THE UPPER LIMB

Muscles That Move the Pectoral Girdle

1. The **pectoralis minor** is a small triangle-shaped muscle of the anterior chest, located deep to the pectoralis major. (Fig. 4.1)
2. The **serratus anterior** is a muscle with a "saw-toothed" border arising from the ribs posterolateral and inferior to the pectoralis major. (Fig. 4.1)

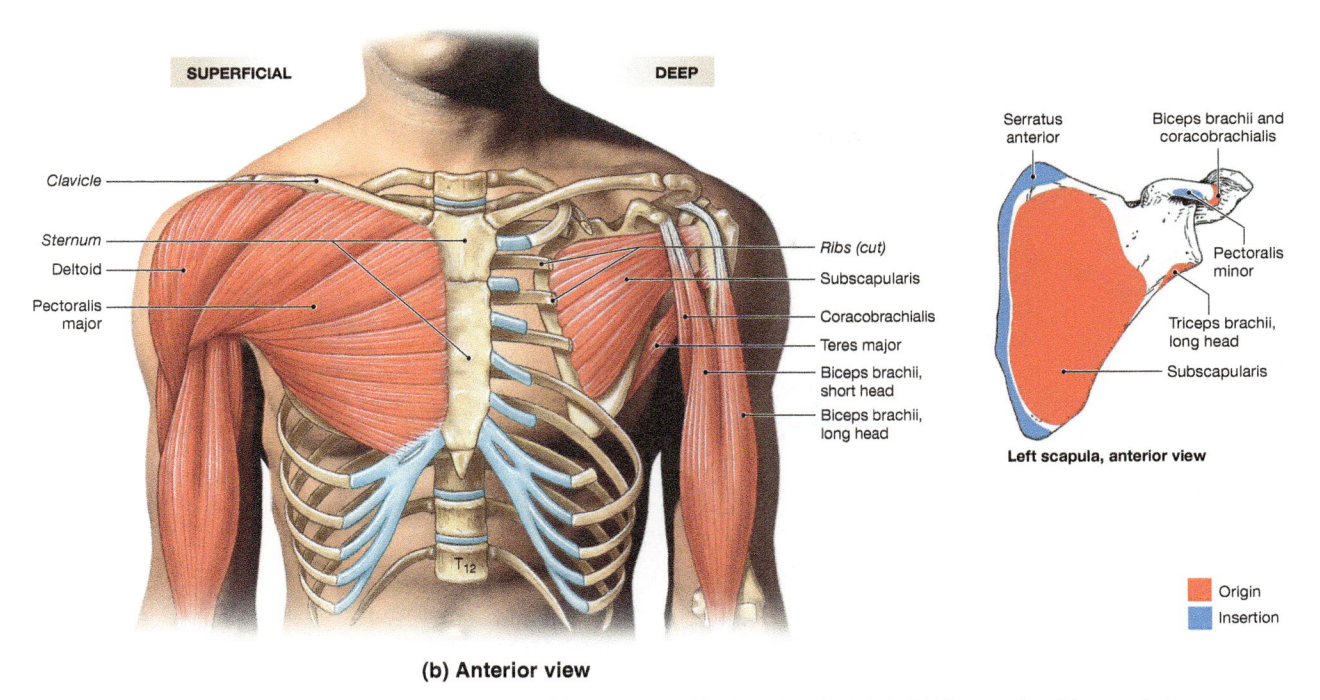

(b) Anterior view

From *Human Anatomy*, Ninth Edition, by Frederic H. Martini, Robert B. Tallitsch, and Judi L. Nath (2018), reproduced by permission of Pearson Education.

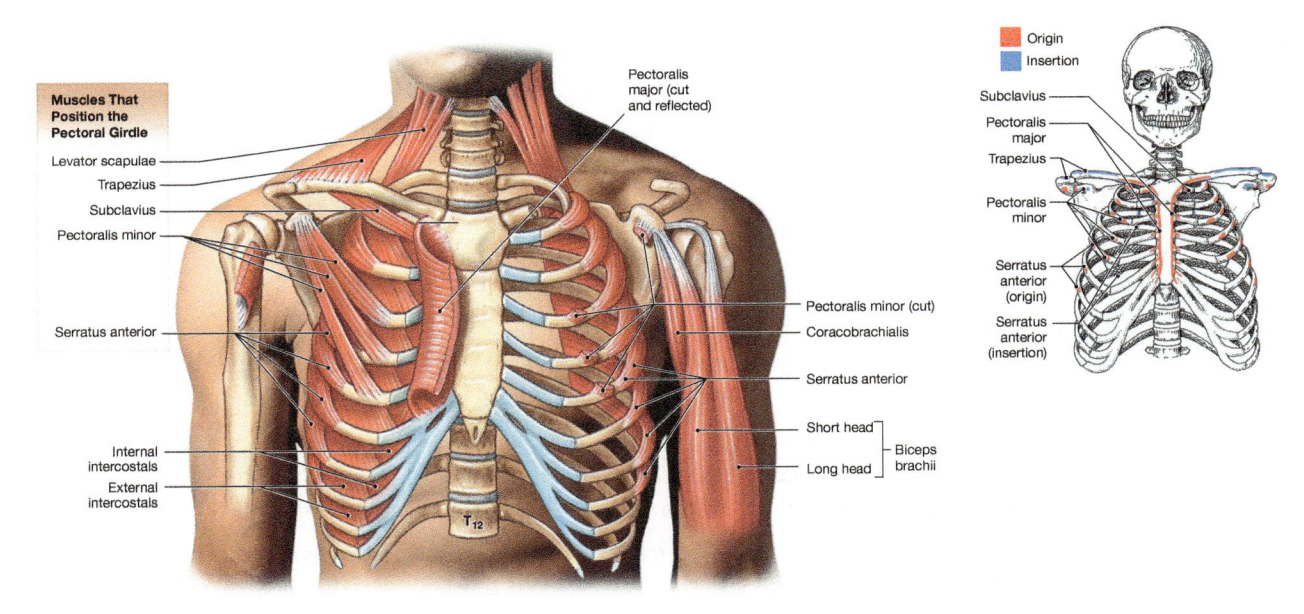

(a) **Muscles That Position the Pectoral Girdle, Part II.** Anterior view showing superficial muscles and deep muscles of the pectoral girdle. Selected origins and insertions are detailed.

From *Human Anatomy*, Ninth Edition, by Frederic H. Martini, Robert B. Tallitsch, and Judi L. Nath (2018), reproduced by permission of Pearson Education.

Figure 4.1 Muscles That Move the Arm *(continued)*

CHAPTER FOUR   *Selected Muscles of the Appendicular & Axial Skeleton*

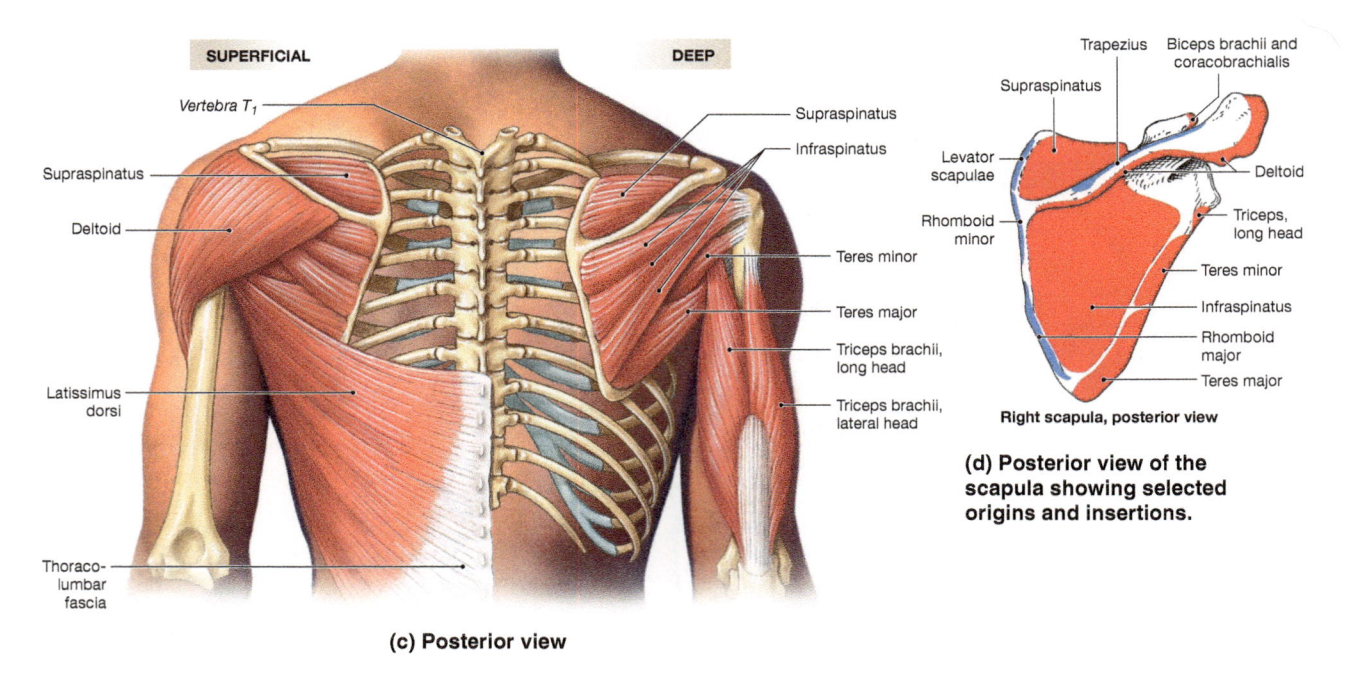

(c) Posterior view

(d) Posterior view of the scapula showing selected origins and insertions.

From *Human Anatomy*, Ninth Edition, by Frederic H. Martini, Robert B. Tallitsch, and Judi L. Nath (2018), reproduced by permission of Pearson Education.

Figure 4.1   Muscles That Move the Arm

Figure 4.1 Superficial muscles of the anterior and posterior thorax and shoulder acting on the scapula and arm. (a) Anterior view. The superficial muscles, which cause arm movements, are shown at the left. These muscles have been removed at the right to show the muscles that stabilize or move the pectoral girdle. (b) Posterior view. The superficial muscles of the back are shown for the left side of the body, but are removed at the right to reveal the deeper muscles acting on the scapula and the rotator cuff muscles that help move the shoulder joint.

3. The **trapezius** is a large, superficial muscle located on the posterior neck and upper back. The trapezius covers many of the deeper muscles of the neck and back (Fig. 4.2). Trapezius is named for its trapezoid shape.

4. The **levator scapulae** is a strap-shaped muscle lying deep to the trapezius. Levator scapulae can be seen attached to the superior border of the scapula.

5. The **rhomboid major** is located deep to the trapezius and attaches to the medial border (vertebral border) of the scapula and also to the spinous processes of thoracic vertebrae (Fig. 4.2). The rhomboids are named for their rhomboid-like shape.

6. The **rhomboid minor** is located superior to the rhomboid major. The rhomboid minor has attachments to the vertebrae and the medial (vertebral) border of the scapula.

MUSCLES THAT MOVE THE ARM

1. The **pectoralis major** is the large triangle-shaped muscle occupying most of the superficial, anterior chest (Fig. 4.1).

2. The **deltoid** caps the shoulder and should be studied on both the supine and prone body.

3. The **latissimus dorsi** is the large superficial muscle that occupies most of the mid and lower back. The latissimus dorsi forms part of the posterior portion of the axilla (armpit).
4. The **teres major** is located along the inferolateral border of the scapula superior to the latissimus dorsi. The teres major enters the posterior arm and inserts at the intertubercular groove of the humerus.
5. The **coracobrachialis** arises from the coracoid process and inserts on the humerus. It is a flexor of the humerus.

Rotator Cuff—the following four muscles of the shoulder make up the rotator cuff

6. The **supraspinatus** lies deep to the trapezius and is located **above** the spine of the scapula. It inserts into the greater tubercle. It is the muscle that is most frequently involved in a rotator cuff injury. (Fig. 4.2).
7. The **infraspinatus** lies deep to the trapezius and is located **below** the spine of the scapula. (Fig. 4.2)
8. The **teres minor** is located just superior to the teres major and then inserts at the greater tubercle of the humerus. The tendon of the long head of the triceps brachii passes between the teres minor and teres major.
9. The **subscapularis** is located in the subscapular fossa on the anterior surface of the scapula. It inserts on the lesser tubercle. Its primary action is medial rotation of the arm.

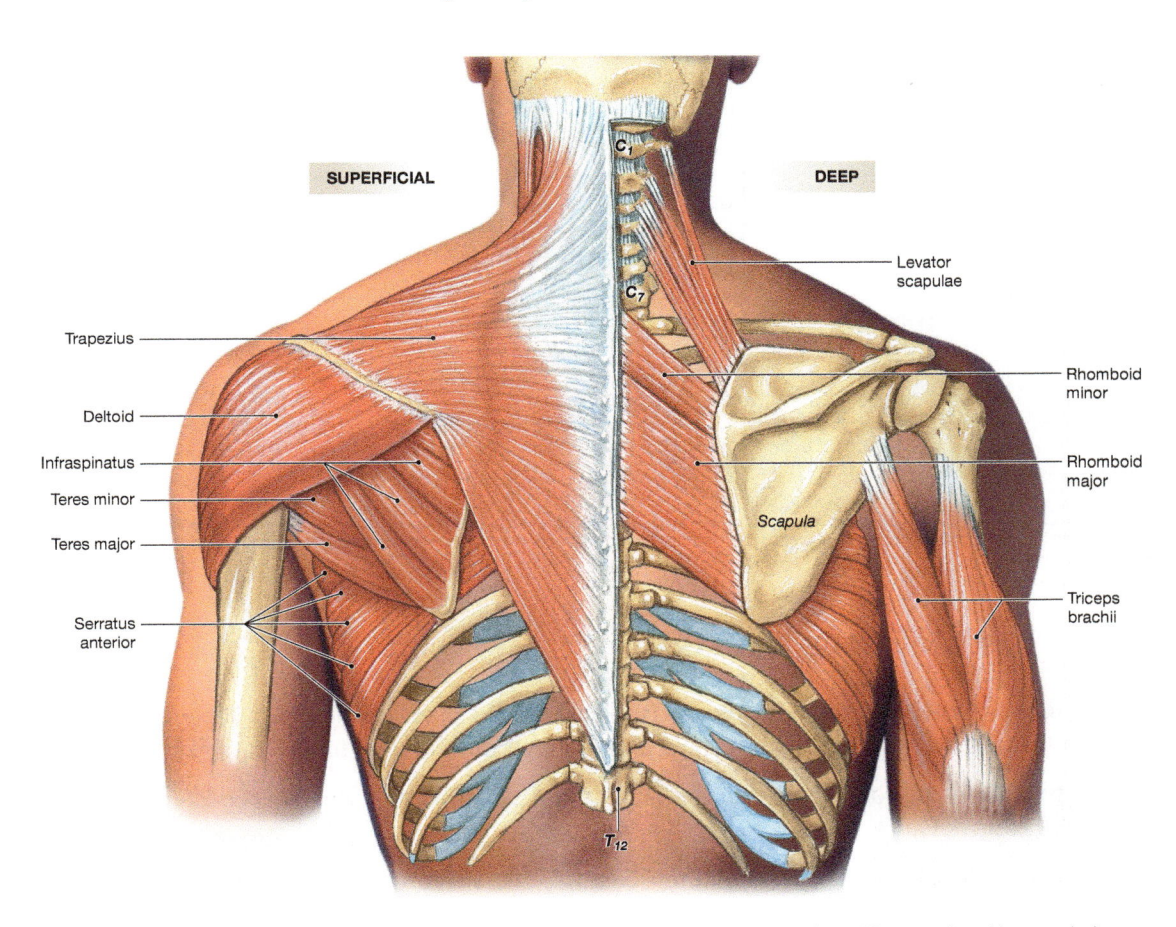

From *Human Anatomy*, Ninth Edition, by Frederic H. Martini, Robert B. Tallitsch, and Judi L. Nath (2018), reproduced by permission of Pearson Education.

Figure 4.2 Muscles of the Back & Shoulder

Figure 4.2 Posterior view. Muscles that move the scapula attach mainly to its vertebral border, superior angle and spine.

MUSCLE TABLE 1: MUSCLES THAT POSITION THE PECTORAL GIRDLE

Muscle	Origin	Insertion	Action	Innervation
Muscles of the Anterior Thorax and Shoulder				
Pectoralis minor	Anterior surfaces of ribs 3–5	Coracoid process of the scapula	Depresses & moves scapula anteriorly; elevates ribs 3 – 5 in forced inspiration when scapula is stationary	Medial pectoral nerve
Serratus anterior	Anterior margins of ribs 1–9	Anterior surface of vertebral border & inferior angle of scapula	Protracts and rotates scapula upward & laterally, so glenoid cavity moves superiorly	Long thoracic nerve
Muscles of the Posterior Thorax and Shoulder				
Trapezius	Occipital bone, ligamentum nuchae & spines of thoracic vertebrae	Clavicle, acromion process and spine of scapula	Elevates clavicle; retracts, elevates and depresses scapula; rotates scapula upward; extends neck when shoulder is fixed	Cranial nerve XI
Levator scapulae	Transverse processes of C1–C4	Superior angle, vertebral border of the scapula	Elevates scapula	Dorsal scapular nerve & cervical nerves 3–5
Rhomboid major	Spinous processes of T2–T5	Vertebral border of the scapula from spine to inferior angle	Retraction and downward rotation of scapula	Dorsal scapular nerve
Rhomboid minor	Spinous processes of C7–T1	Vertebral border of the scapula	Retraction and downward rotation of scapula	Dorsal scapular nerve

MUSCLES THAT MOVE THE FOREARM

1. The **biceps brachii** has two heads and is located on the anterior surface of the arm. Both origins of the biceps brachii are on the scapula and it inserts at the radial tuberosity (Figs. 4.1 and 4.3).

2. The **brachialis** lies deep to the biceps brachii, but a portion of it can be seen lateral to the biceps brachii (Fig. 4.1).

3. The **brachioradialis** is a superficial muscle of the lateral forearm. The brachioradialis passes over the anterior forearm and inserts just above the styloid process of the radius. This muscle inserts on the anterior surface of the forearm, and therefore it flexes the forearm.

4. The **triceps brachii** has three points of origin and is most easily viewed and studied on the prone body. The triceps brachii forms most surface of the posterior arm (Fig. 4.2). The three heads of the triceps have a common insertion at the olecranon process of the ulna.

Muscle Table 2: Muscles that Move the Arm

Muscle	Origin	Insertion	Action	Innervation
Muscles on Anterior – Chest and Shoulder				
Pectoralis major	Inferior and medial region of clavicle, sternum & costal cartilage of ribs 2 - 6	Greater tubercle and lateral lip of intertubercular sulcus of the humerus	Flexes, adducts & rotates arm medially at the shoulder	Medial & lateral pectoral nerves
Deltoid	Lateral clavicle, acromion and spine of scapula	Deltoid tuberosity of the humerus	*Entire deltoid:* abduction of shoulder; *anterior deltoid:* flexion and medial rotation of humerus; *posterior deltoid:* extension and lateral rotation of humerus	Axillary nerve
Muscles on Posterior – Back and Shoulder				
Latissimus dorsi	Spines of inferior thoracic and all lumbar and sacral vertebrae; thoracolumbar fascia & lower 4 ribs	Intertubercular sulcus of the humerus	Extends, adducts & rotates arm medially at the shoulder	Thoracodorsal nerve
Teres major	Inferior angle of the scapula	Medial lip of Intertubercular sulcus of the humerus	Extends, adducts & rotates arm medially at the shoulder	Lower subscapular nerve
Muscles on Posterior – Rotator Cuff Muscles				
Supraspinatus	Supraspinous fossa	Greater tubercle of the humerus	Assists deltoid in abducting arm	Suprascapular nerve
Infraspinatus	Infraspinous fossa	Greater tubercle of the humerus	Adducts arm & rotates arm laterally	Suprascapular nerve
Teres minor	Lateral border of the scapula	Greater tubercle of the humerus	Extends, adducts & rotates arm laterally at the shoulder	Axillary nerve
Subscapularis	Subscapular fossa	Lesser tubercle of the humerus	Rotates arm medially at the shoulder	Upper and lower Subscapular nerves

Chapter Four   *Selected Muscles of the Appendicular & Axial Skeleton*

Muscle Table 3: Muscles that Move the Forearm

Muscle	Origin	Insertion	Action	Innervation
Muscles of the Anterior Compartment of the Arm and Forearm				
Coracobrachialis	Coracoid process of scapula	Shaft of humerus, medially	Adduction and flexion at shoulder	Musculocutaneous nerve
Biceps brachii • Long head	Supraglenoid tubercle of scapula	Radial tuberosity	Flexes arm; flexes & supinates forearm	Musculocutaneous nerve
• Short head	coracoid process of scapula	Radial tuberosity	Flexes arm; flexes & supinates forearm	Musculocutaneous nerve
Brachialis	Distal half of the anterior surface of humerus	Ulnar tuberosity and coronoid process	Flexes forearm at the elbow	Musculocutaneous & radial nerves
Muscles of the Posterior Compartment of the Arm and Forearm				
Brachioradialis*	Superior to lateral epicondyle of humerus	Lateral side of styloid process of radius	Flexes forearm at the elbow	Radial nerve
Triceps brachii • Long head	Infraglenoid tubercle of scapula	Olecranon of ulna	Extension at elbow and extension and adduction at shoulder	Radial nerve
• Lateral head	Superior, lateral border of humerus superior to radial groove	Olecranon of ulna	Extension at elbow	Radial nerve
• Medial head	Posterior surface of humerus, inferior to radial groove	Olecranon of ulna	Extension at elbow	Radial nerve

*Though the brachioradialis is a flexor of the forearm, it is located in the posterior compartment of the forearm (lateral compartment, if further subdivided).

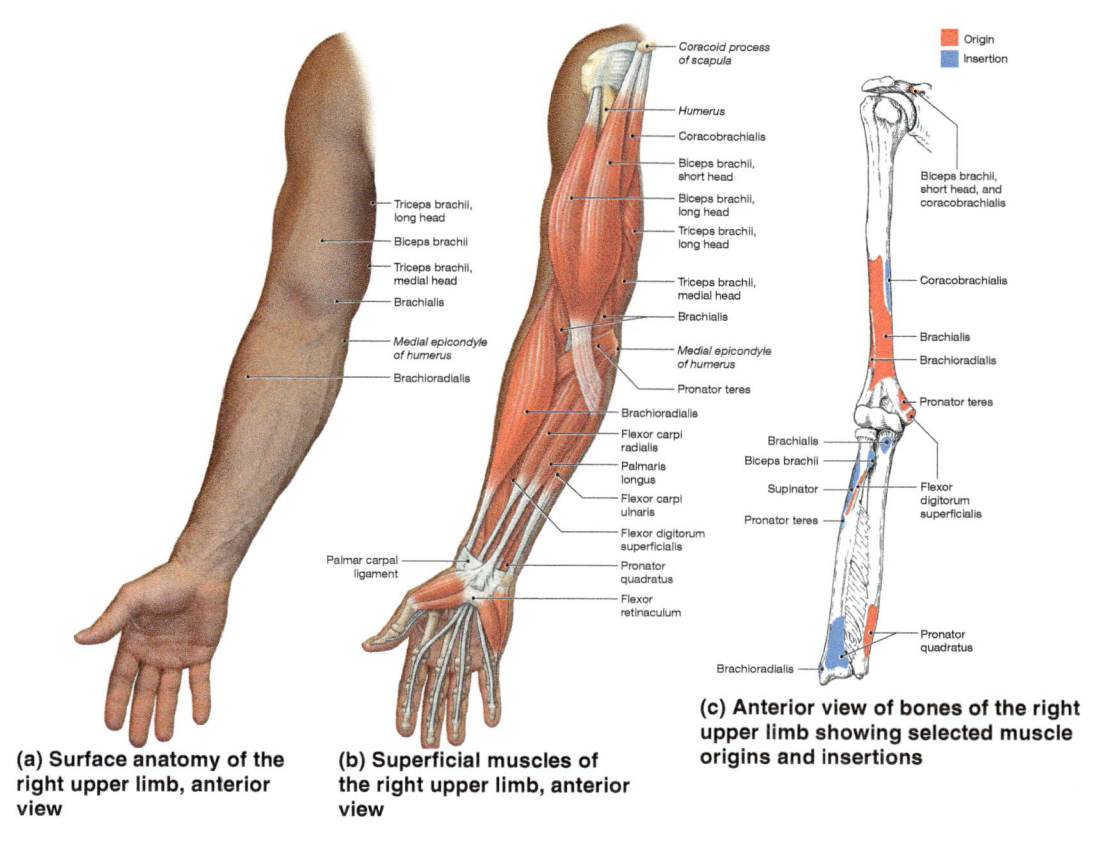

(a) Surface anatomy of the right upper limb, anterior view

(b) Superficial muscles of the right upper limb, anterior view

(c) Anterior view of bones of the right upper limb showing selected muscle origins and insertions

From *Human Anatomy*, Ninth Edition, by Frederic H. Martini, Robert B. Tallitsch, and Judi L. Nath (2018), reproduced by permission of Pearson Education.

Figure 4.3 Muscles That Move the Forearm and Hand, Part I

Muscles That Move the Wrist, Hand & Fingers

Superficial Anterior Forearm Muscles

The **flexor carpi radialis, flexor carpi ulnaris** and **palmaris longus** are located on the anterior surface of the forearm, adjacent to the brachioradialis (Fig. 4.3).

The **pronator teres** is another anterior forearm muscle located between the brachioradialis and flexor carpi radialis. The pronator teres **pronates** the forearm (Fig. 4.3).

A band of fascia called the **flexor retinaculum** secures tendons of the anterior forearm muscles at the wrist (Fig. 4.3).

Superficial Posterior Forearm Muscles

The **extensor carpi radialis longus, extensor carpi radialis brevis** and **extensor carpi ulnaris** and **extensor digitorum** are located on the posterior forearm. The extensor carpi radialis longus is next to the brachioradialis. The **extensor digitorum** is adjacent to the extensor carpi ulnaris (Fig. 4.4).

Tendons of the posterior forearm muscles are held in place by the **extensor retinaculum** (Fig. 4.4).

Chapter Four   *Selected Muscles of the Appendicular & Axial Skeleton*

(a) Surface anatomy of the right upper limb, posterior view

(b) A diagrammatic view of a dissection of the superficial muscles

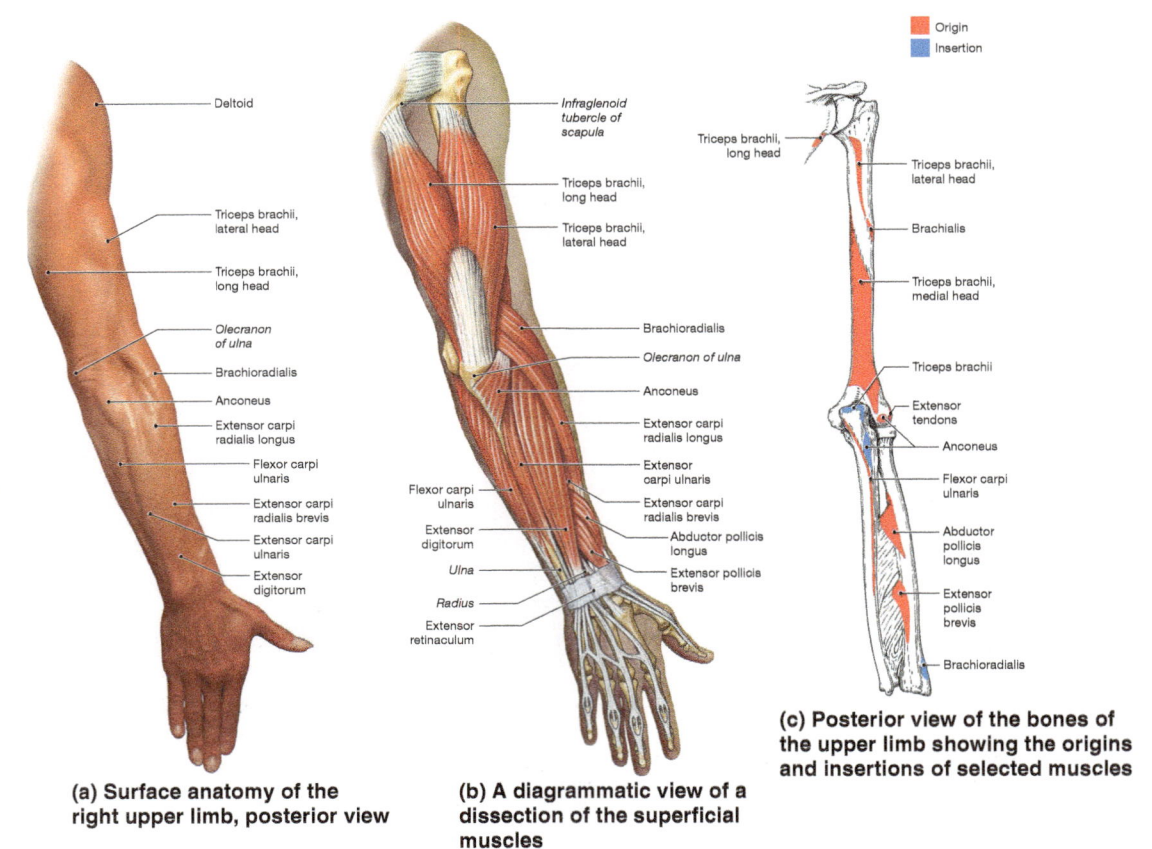

(c) Posterior view of the bones of the upper limb showing the origins and insertions of selected muscles

From *Human Anatomy*, Ninth Edition by Frederic H. Martini, Michael J. Timmons, and Robert B. Tallitsch

Figure 4.4 Muscles That Move the Forearm and Hand, Part II

Muscle Table 4:
Muscles that Move the Wrist, Hand & Fingers

Muscle	Origin	Insertion	Action	Nerve Supply
Anterior Forearm • Flexor carpi radialis, • Flexor carpi ulnaris, • Palmaris longus, • Flexor digitorum superficialis	Medial epicondyle of humerus	Carpals & phalanges	Flex and deviate wrist to radial side (abduction)	Median nerve (radialis and palmaris longus) Ulnar nerve (flexor carpi ulnaris)
			Flex and deviate wrist to ulnar side (adduction)	
			Flex wrist	
			Flex digits	
Posterior Forearm • Extensor carpi radialis longus, and brevis, • Extensor carpi ulnaris, • Extensor digitorum	Distal humerus and lateral epicondyle of humerus	Carpals & phalanges	Extend & deviate wrist to radial side	Radial nerve
			Extend and deviate wrist to ulnar side.	
			Extend digits	

Complete Introductory Human Anatomy Lab Guide

III. MUSCLES OF THE SPINE & NECK

Muscles of the Anterior and Lateral Neck

1. **Sternocleidomastoid** is an anatomical landmark dividing the anterior and posterior triangles of the neck. It extends from the sternum and clavicle to the mastoid process of the temporal bone. When the sternocleidomastoid on one side contracts, its action is lateral rotation of the head and neck to the opposite side. When both sternocleidomastoid muscles contract, their action is neck flexion.

2. **Scalene muscles** are small, flat muscles that insert on the first two ribs. Their actions include aiding inspiration and neck flexion.

MUSCLE TABLE 5: MUSCLES OF THE NECK AND VERTEBRAL COLUMN

Muscle	Origin	Insertion	Action	Innervation
Muscles of the Anterior and Lateral Neck				
Sternocleidomastoid	Medial clavicle and manubrium	Mastoid process of the temporal bone; superior nuchal line of occipital bone	Flexes neck when both sides contract; laterally flexes neck toward opposite side when one side contracts	CN XI
-Anterior scalene	Transverse processes of C3 – C6	Superior surface of first rib	Raises ribs and flexes neck; one side bends neck and rotates to *opposite* side	Cervical spinal nerves
-Middle scalene	Transverse processes of atlas and C3 – C7	Superior surface of first rib	Raises ribs and flexes neck; one side bends neck and rotates to *same* side	Cervical spinal nerves
-Posterior scalene	Transverse processes of C4 – C6	Superior surface of second rib	Raises ribs and flexes neck; one side bends neck and rotates to *same* side	Cervical spinal nerves
Muscles of the Posterior Vertebral Column				
Splenius capitis	Spinous processes and nuchal ligament of lower cervical & upper thoracic vertebrae	Mastoid process of temporal bone; transverse processes of upper cervical vertebrae	Extends & rotates the neck	Dorsal rami of cervical spinal nerves
Erector Spinae (formed from three major subdivisions noted below)				
• Iliocostalis group	Ribs 6–12; Iliac crest and sacral crest	Ribs and transverse processes of vertebrae	Extension and rotation of vertebral column.	Dorsal rami of spinal nerves
• Longissimus group	Transverse processes of vertebrae	Mastoid process of temporal bone; transverse processes of vertebrae	Extension and rotation of vertebral column; Rotation and lateral flexion of neck	Dorsal rami of spinal nerves

(Continued)

Muscle Table 5: Muscles of the Neck and Vertebral Column (Continued)

Muscle	Origin	Insertion	Action	Innervation
Muscles of the Posterior Vertebral Column				
• Spinalis group	Spines of lower thoracic and upper lumbar vertebrae	Spinous process of superior thoracic vertebrae	Extends neck and vertebral column	Dorsal rami of spinal nerves
Quadratus lumborum	Iliac crest; lumbar fascia, iliolumbar ligament	Rib 12 and transverse processes of lumbar vertebrae	Acting together: extends lumbar spine, unilaterally, elevates pelvic girdle.	Ventral rami of thoracic and lumbar spinal nerves

Muscles of the Posterior Neck and Spine

1. **Erector spinae** are a group of overlapping muscles of the axial skeleton, located adjacent to the spinal column. These muscles are arranged in three subdivisions from medial to lateral: the **spinalis, longissimus,** and **iliocostalis**.

2. **Splenius capitis** is a muscle of the posterior neck. The splenius capitis lies deep to the superior region of the trapezius muscle.

3. **Quadratus lumborum** is a large muscle forming the posterior abdominal wall in the lumbar region. Contracting alone, a single quadratus lumborum flexes the vertebral column laterally and elevates the pelvic girdle on that side.

IV. BLOOD SUPPLY TO THE UPPER LIMB & TORSO

Arterial Supply to the Upper Limb & Torso

Identify the specified arteries in the upper limb of the donor body. Branches of the **subclavian artery**, **axillary artery** and **brachial artery** are the main arteries supplying the arm. Branches of the **radial artery** and **ulnar artery** supply the forearm and hand. (Fig. 4.5.)

1. The **subclavian artery** and its branches supply the muscles and tissues of the shoulder proximally.

2. The **axillary artery** is the direct continuation of the subclavian artery lateral to the clavicle. Its branches supply the muscles of the shoulder and the anterior, posterior and lateral body walls.

3. The **brachial artery** continues from the axillary artery lateral to the pectoralis minor. With the deep brachial artery it supplies the muscles and tissues of the arm. On the anterior surface of the elbow the brachial artery branches to form the radial and ulnar arteries.

4. The **radial artery** runs down the radial side of the forearm. Its pulsations can be felt at the wrist and it is commonly used to monitor the pulse. It continues into the hand as the deep palmar arch with a connection to the superficial palmar arch.

5. The **ulnar artery** runs parallel to the radial artery on the ulnar side of the forearm. It continues into the hand as the superficial palmar arch.

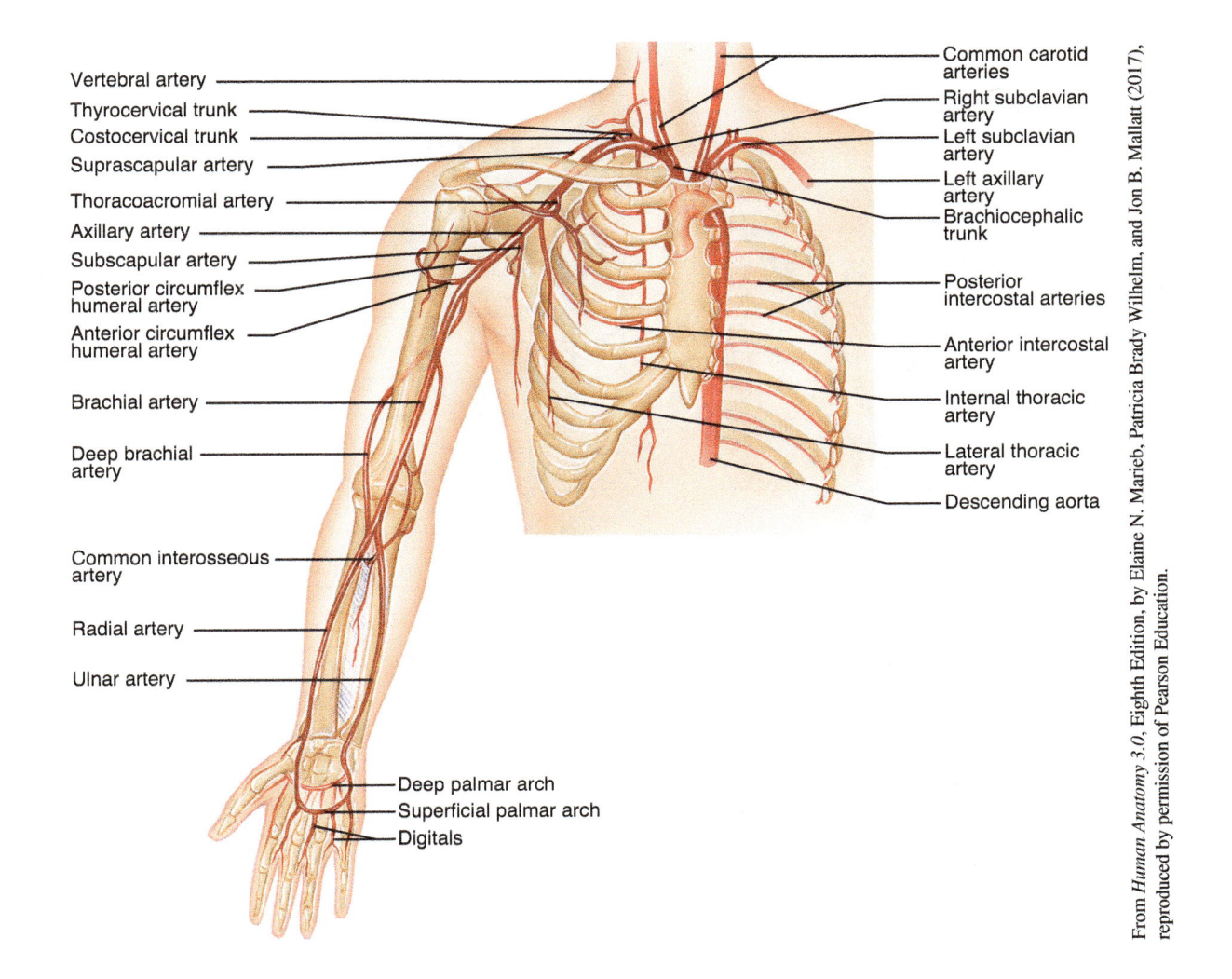

Figure 4.5 Arteries of the Right Upper Limb and Thorax

VEINS OF THE UPPER LIMB & TORSO

The venous drainage of the upper extremity follows the reverse pattern of the arteries. The radial and **ulnar veins** drain into the **brachial vein**. The brachial vein becomes the **axillary vein** in the armpit region. The axillary vein drains into the **subclavian vein**. Deep veins course parallel to the arteries of the same name.

SUPERFICIAL VEINS OF THE ARM

Superficial veins do not have a corresponding artery and are often visible through the skin. These veins drain the subcutaneous tissue into the deeper veins. Identify the superficial veins in the upper limb of the donor body, illustrations, or on your lab partners. (Fig. 4.6).

1. The **cephalic vein** lies superficially and laterally on the arm. The cephalic vein drains into the axillary vein between the deltoid muscle and pectoralis major.

2. The **basilic vein** lies medially along the arm drains with the brachial vein to form the axillary vein.

3. The **median cubital vein** connects the cephalic vein with the basilic vein in the antecubital fossa. The median cubital vein is often used for withdrawal of blood samples.

CHAPTER FOUR   *Selected Muscles of the Appendicular & Axial Skeleton*

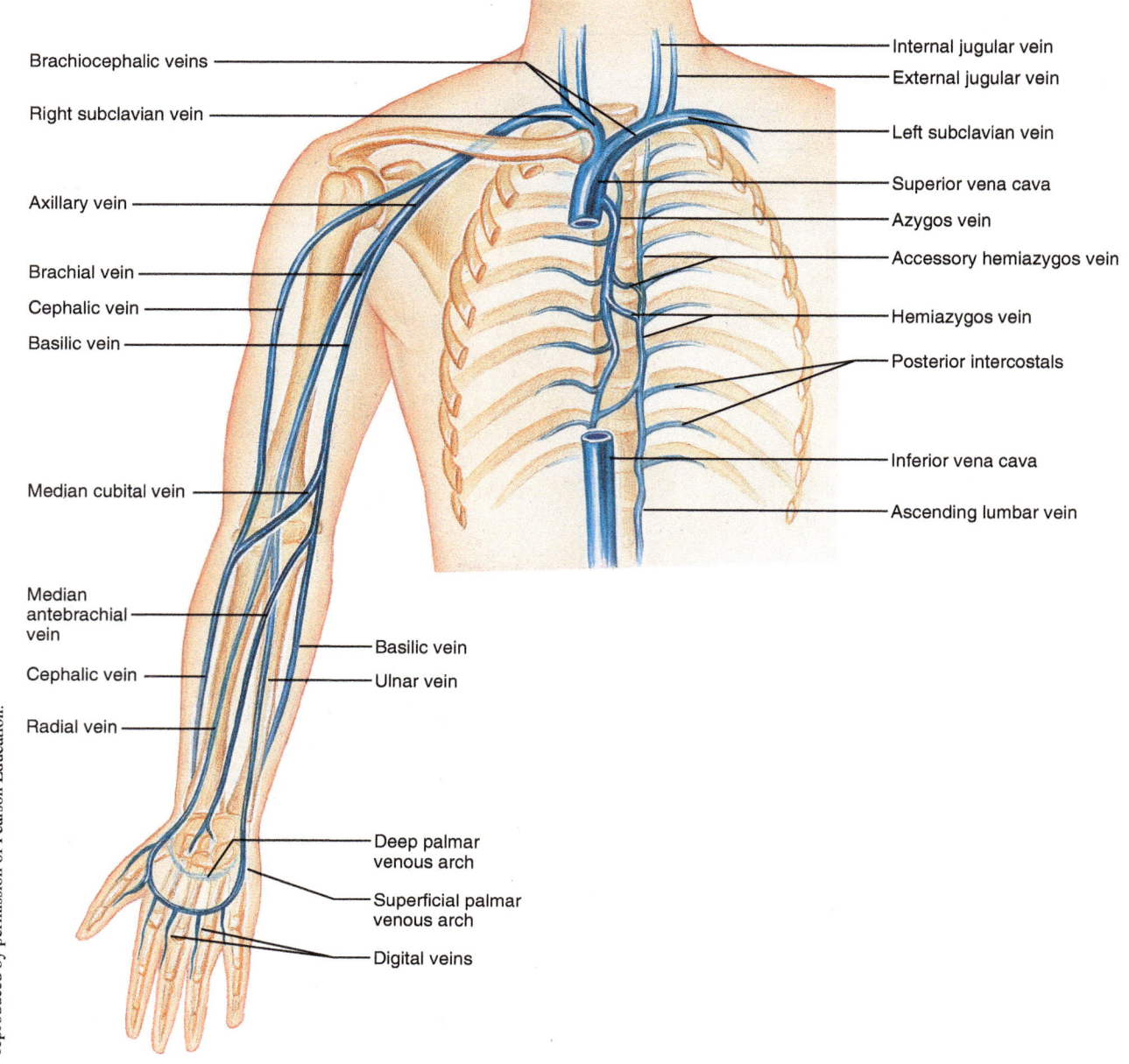

Figure 4.6 Veins of the Right Upper Limb and Shoulder

V. INNERVATION OF THE PECTORAL REGION & UPPER LIMB

Cervical Nerves

Cervical nerves arise from the ventral rami of spinal nerves C1–C4. Branches of cervical **nerves** supply the levator scapulae, scalene muscles and skin of the neck and shoulder.

The Brachial Plexus

The **brachial plexus** (Fig. 4.7) is a system of nerves originating from the ventral rami of cervical nerves 5–8 and thoracic nerve 1 (C5–C8 and T1). These nerves join to form the complex network of nerves that supply sensory and motor innervation to the shoulder and upper limb.

Nerves that contribute to the brachial plexus join together and divide in a complex pattern that distributes fibers from the spinal nerves to the final named nerves. To understand the brachial plexus, we divide it into five zones:

- **Roots** – the ventral rami of cervical nerves 5-8 and the first thoracic nerve are called the roots of the brachial plexus.
- **Trunks** – the roots combine to make three trunks; superior, middle and inferior.
- **Divisions** – each trunk splits to form an anterior and posterior division. Anterior division nerves typically go to the anterior side of the upper limb and posterior division to the opposite side.
- **Cords** – divisions from different trunks combine to make cords; lateral cord, posterior cord and medial cord.
- **Branches** – the five major nerves of the upper limb are branches from the cords; smaller branches come from other places on the brachial plexus.

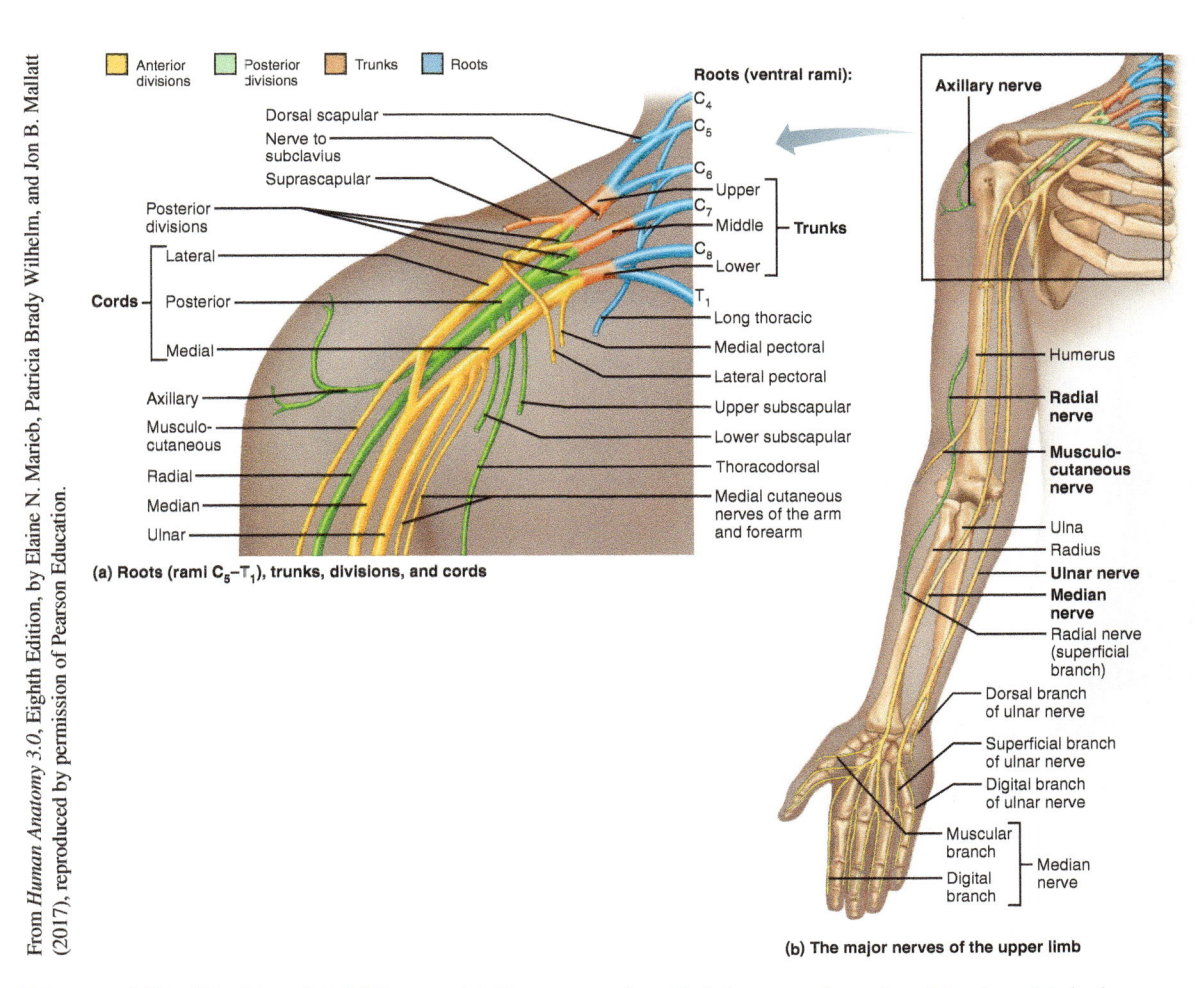

Figure 4.7 **The Brachial Plexus.** (a) Roots, trunks, divisions, and cords of the brachial plexus. (b) Distribution of the major peripheral nerves of the upper limb.

CHAPTER FOUR   *Selected Muscles of the Appendicular & Axial Skeleton*   81

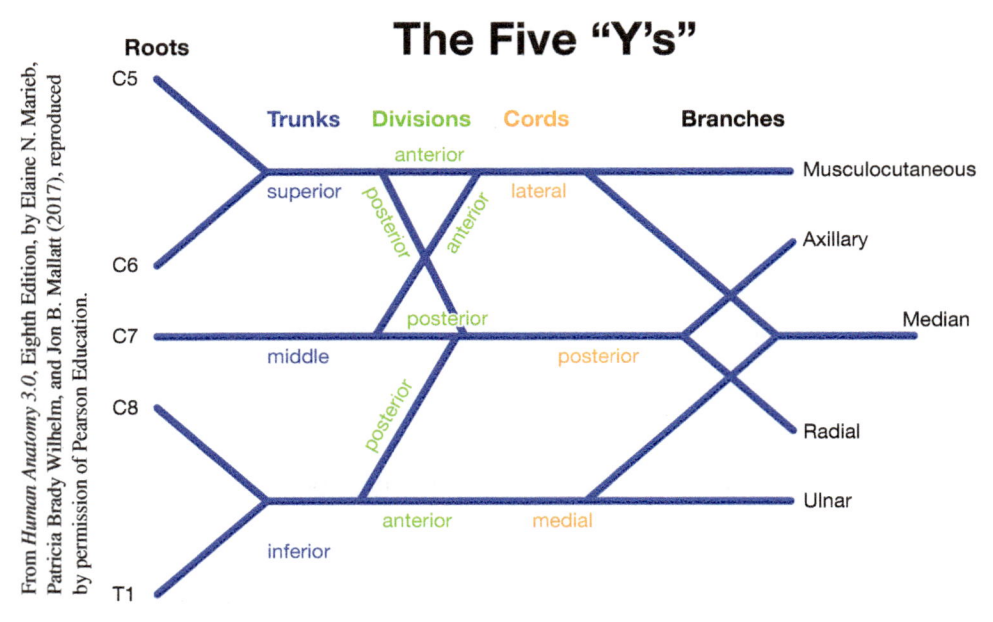

Figure 4.7c   **Schematic of Brachial Plexus**

1. Three large nerves arise from the **lateral** and **medial cords** of the brachial plexus. These three nerves form a characteristic "M" shape.

   - The **musculocutaneous** nerve is the most lateral limb of the "M ." It innervates the muscles of the flexor compartment of the arm.
   - The **ulnar nerve** is the most medial limb of the "M" and innervates one and one-half muscles of the anterior compartment of the forearm muscles and the hypothenar muscles of the hand.
   - The **median nerve** receives a contribution from both the lateral and medial cords, and forms the middle limb of the "M". It innervates most of the muscles of the anterior compartment of the forearm muscles and the thenar muscles of the hand.

2. The **axillary** and **radial** nerves arise from the posterior cord of the brachial plexus. These nerves form the two "arms" of a "Y ," with the posterior cord forming the stem.

   - The **axillary nerve** travels through the axilla and innervates the deltoid and teres minor muscles.
   - The **radial nerve** is a large nerve innervating all of the extensor muscles of the posterior compartment of the arm and forearm.

3. Other branches of the brachial plexus arise from ventral rami of cervical nerves 5–7 or branch directly from the lateral, medial or posterior cord. (Fig. 4.5)

   - The **long thoracic nerve** arises from branches of ventral rami of C5–C7 and innervates the serratus anterior muscle.
   - The **medial** and **lateral pectoral nerves** branch from the medial and lateral cords of the brachial plexus to innervate the pectoralis major and pectoralis minor muscles.
   - The **dorsal scapular nerve** branches from the ventral ramus of C5 and innervates the levator scapulae and the rhomboids major and minor muscles.
   - The **subscapular nerve** arises from the **posterior cord** and branches of lower cervical nerves. The subscapular nerve innervates the subscapularis and teres major muscle.
   - The **suprascapular nerve** branches from C5 and C6 to innervate the supraspinatus and infraspinatus.

VI. MUSCLES OF THE LOWER LIMB

MUSCLES THAT MOVE THE THIGH

The Gluteal Group

(Figs. 4.8 & 4.9a, 4.9c)

1. The **gluteus maximus** is a large, superficial muscle forming the majority of the buttock. It functions primarily in powerful extension of the thigh as in climbing stairs.

2. The **gluteus medius** lies deep to the gluteus maximus. A portion of the gluteus medius is visible superior to the gluteus maximus. The gluteus medius is "sandwiched" between the gluteus maximus and minimus.

3. The **gluteus minimus** covers a portion of the posterolateral surface of the ilium. It is the smallest of the gluteal muscles.

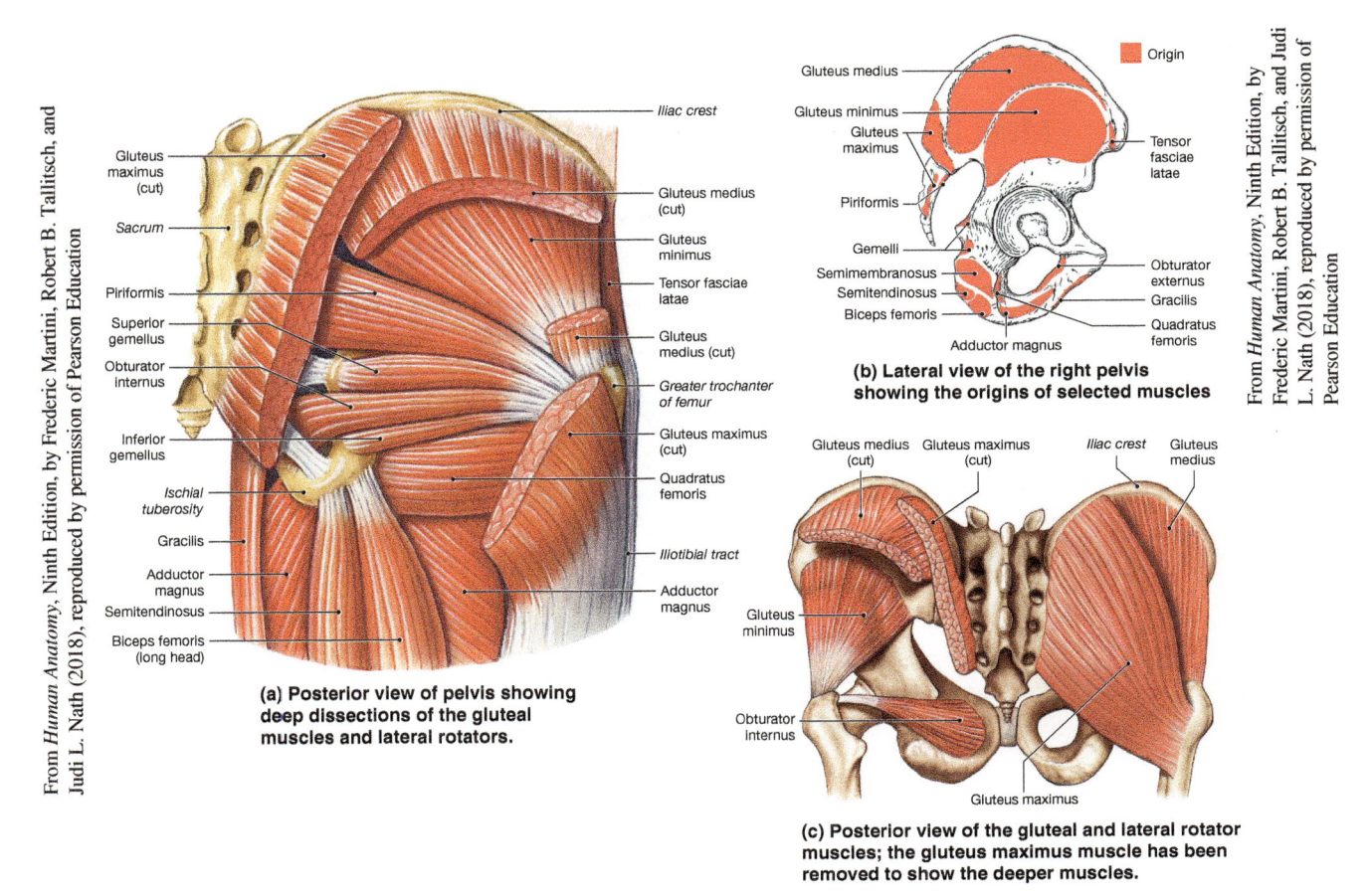

Figure 4.8 Muscles That Move the Thigh, Part I

Muscle Table 6: Muscles of the Posterior Hip
Muscles that flex, extend, abduct or rotate the thigh
The **ARTERIAL SUPPLY** for each muscle in this table are branches from the internal iliac artery.

\multicolumn{5}{c}{The Gluteal Group}				
Muscle	**Origin**	**Insertion**	**Action**	**Innervation**
Gluteus maximus	Iliac crest; sacrum & coccyx	Iliotibial tract & gluteal tuberosity of femur	Extension and lateral rotation of thigh at the hip	Inferior gluteal nerve
Gluteus medius	Anterior iliac crest; Posterior surface of ilium	Greater trochanter of the femur	Abducts & rotates thigh medially at the hip joint	Superior gluteal nerve
Gluteus minimus	Posterior surface of ilium	Greater trochanter of the femur	Abducts & rotates thigh medially at the hip joint	Superior gluteal nerve

Muscle Table 7: Muscles of the Posterior Hip
Muscles that flex, extend, abduct or rotate the thigh
The **ARTERIAL SUPPLY** for each muscle in this table are branches from the internal iliac artery.

\multicolumn{5}{c}{Lateral Rotators of the Thigh}				
Muscle	**Origin**	**Insertion**	**Action**	**Innervation**
Piriformis	Anterior surface of sacrum	Greater trochanter of the femur	Abducts & rotates extended thigh laterally; abducts thigh if hip is flexed; stabilizer of hip joint	Sacral nerves 1 & 2 (S_1 and S_2)
Superior & inferior gemellus	Spine of ischium; ischial tuberosity	Greater trochanter of femur	Rotates extended thigh laterally	Superior - nerve to obturator internus and superior gemellus; Inferior - nerve to quadratus femoris and inferior gemellus.
Obturator internus	Medial side of obturator membrane	Intertrochanteric fossa	Rotates thigh laterally	Nerve to obturator internus and superior gemellus
Quadratus femoris	Lateral border of ischial tuberosity	Crest between greater and lesser trochanter of the femur	Rotates thigh laterally	Nerve to quadratus femoris and obturator internus.

Muscle Table 8: Muscles that Flex the Thigh

	Flexors of the Thigh			
Muscle	**Origin**	**Insertion**	**Action**	**Innervation**
Iliacus	Iliac fossa	Lesser trochanter of femur	Flexion at hip, lumbar intervertebral joints	femoral nerve
Psoas major	transverse processes lumbar vertebrae			lumbar plexus

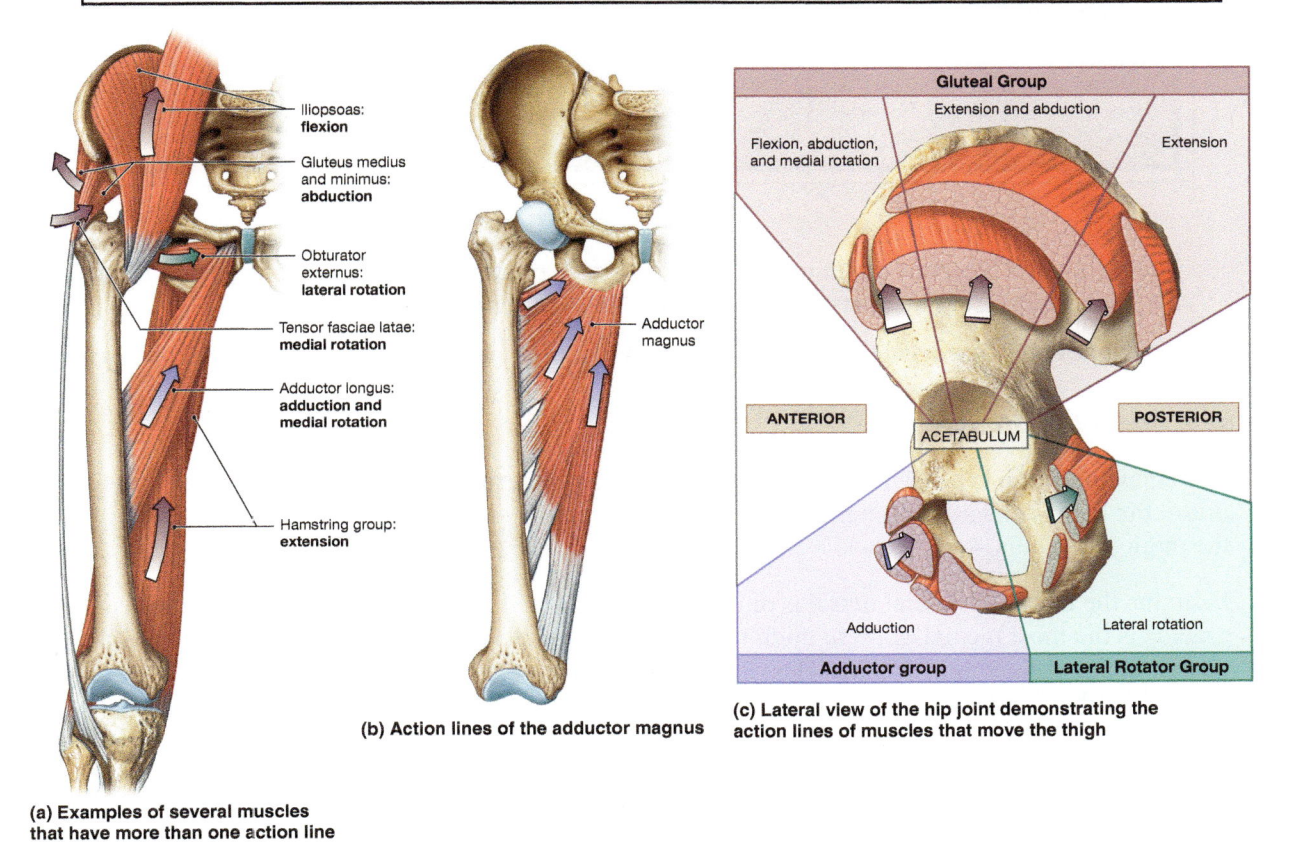

(b) Action lines of the adductor magnus

(c) Lateral view of the hip joint demonstrating the action lines of muscles that move the thigh

(a) Examples of several muscles that have more than one action line crossing the axis of the hip

From *Human Anatomy*, Ninth Edition, by Frederic Martini, Robert B. Tallitsch, and Judi L. Nath (2018), reproduced by permission of Pearson Education.

Figure 4.9a The Relationships between the Action Lines and the Axis of the Hip Joint

Lateral Rotators of the Thigh

(Fig. 4.8)

1. The **piriformis** is a lateral rotator of the thigh, inferior to the gluteus minimus. The sciatic nerve passes under the piriformis to enter the posterior thigh.

2. The **superior** and **inferior gemellus** are located deep to the gluteus maximus and inferior to the piriformis muscle.

CHAPTER FOUR   *Selected Muscles of the Appendicular & Axial Skeleton*

Muscle Table 9: Muscles of the Medial Compartment of the Thigh; Adductors of the thigh

Muscle	Origin	Insertion	Action	Innervation
Gracilis	Inferior rams of Pubic bone	Medial surface of body of the tibia	Adducts thigh at the hip joint; flexes leg at the knee	Obturator nerve
Adductor longus	Inferior rams of Pubic bone	Linea aspera of femur	Adducts, flexes & rotates thigh medially	Obturator nerve
Pectineus	Superior ramus of Pubic bone	Inferior to lesser trochanter of femur	Adducts & flexes thigh	Femoral nerve
Adductor magnus	Pubic bone & ischial tuberosity	Linea aspera of femur	Adducts, flexes & rotates thigh medially	Obturator & tibial division of sciatic nerve

3. The **obturator internus** arises on the internal surface of the pelvis and sends its tendon through the lesser sciatic foramen between the inferior and superior gemellus muscles.
4. The **quadratus femoris** lies deep to the gluteus maximus and originates at the ischial tuberosity.

The Adductor Group

The adductor group is a group of five muscles including the **gracilis, pectineus, adductor longus, adductor brevis** and **adductor magnus**. The primary action of this group of muscles is adducting the thigh (Figs. 4.9a, 4.9b).

Examine the more superficial muscles of this group: the gracilis, pectineus and adductor longus. The gracilis is the most medial of these thigh muscles. Muscles of this group are located in the medial compartment of the thigh. The muscles of this compartment are innervated by the obturator nerve (except for the pectineus - femoral n.)

1. The **gracilis** is a strap-shaped muscle located along the medial border of the thigh. The gracilis can be viewed in a supine or prone cadaver. In addition to adducting the thigh, the gracilis also flexes the leg at the knee joint.
2. The **adductor longus** is located just lateral to the gracilis.
3. The **pectineus** is superolateral to the gracilis.
4. The **adductor magnus** has several component parts. The posterior part of this muscle can be viewed between the gracilis and the semimembranous on the posterior thigh.

Muscles That Move the Leg

The Tensor Fasciae Latae

The tensor fasciae latae is located on the anterolateral aspect of the thigh and is enclosed within two layers of fascia lata, the deep muscular fascia of the thigh. It is unusual because it is not obviously a part of a muscular compartment. It is innervated by the superior gluteal nerve.

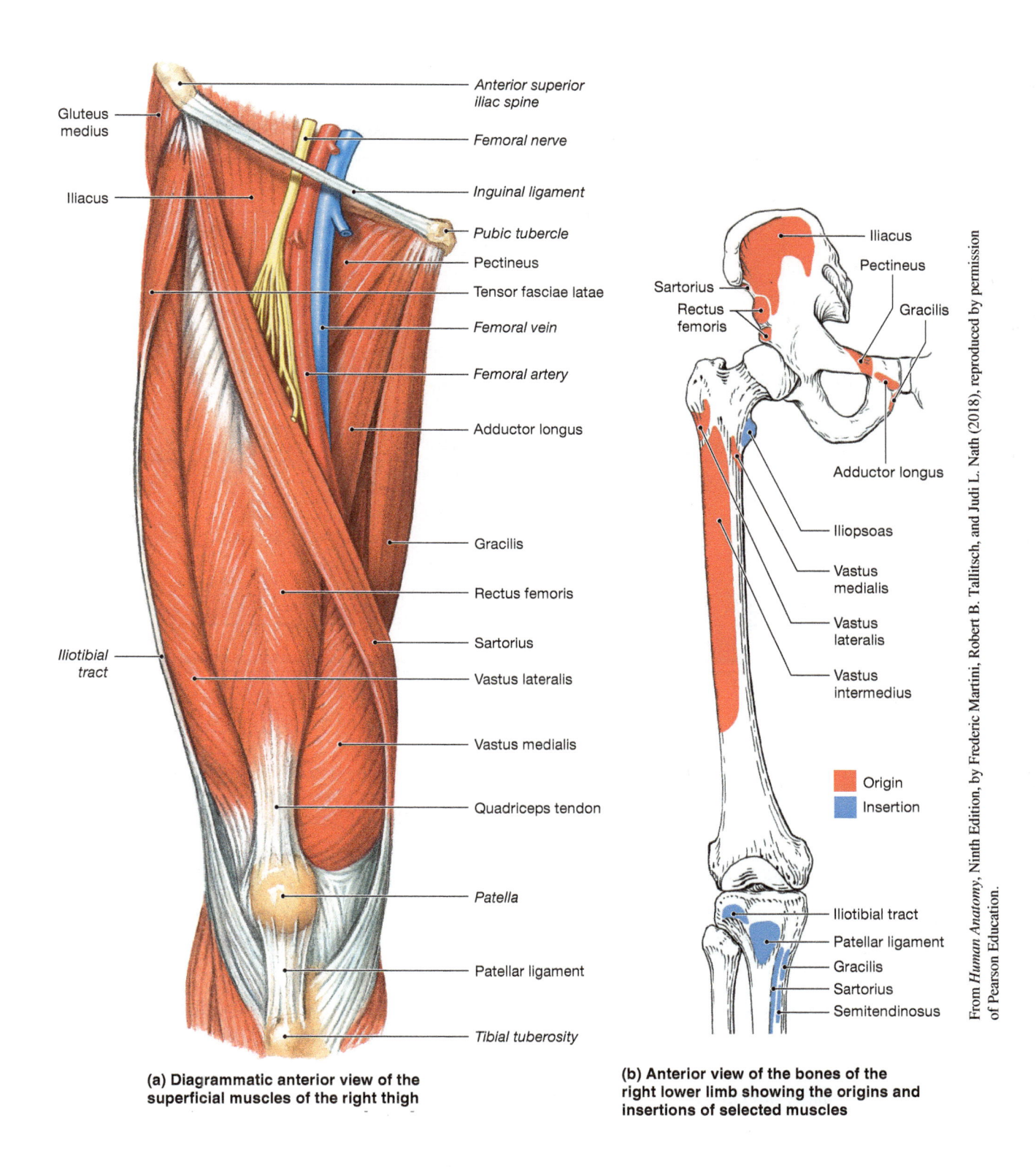

(a) Diagrammatic anterior view of the superficial muscles of the right thigh

(b) Anterior view of the bones of the right lower limb showing the origins and insertions of selected muscles

From *Human Anatomy*, Ninth Edition, by Frederic Martini, Robert B. Tallitsch, and Judi L. Nath (2018), reproduced by permission of Pearson Education.

Figure 4.9b Muscles That Move the Leg, Part I

CHAPTER FOUR   *Selected Muscles of the Appendicular & Axial Skeleton*   87

MUSCLE TABLE 10: MUSCLES OF THE ANTERIOR COMPARTMENT OF THE THIGH; MOVEMENTS AT THE THIGH AND LEG

The arterial supply of all muscles in the anterior compartment is branches of the femoral artery.

Muscle	Origin	Insertion	Action	Innervation
Tensor fasciae latae	Iliac crest and anterior superior iliac spine	Tibia by way of the iliotibial tract	Medial rotation at hip and abduction of the thigh; extension and lateral rotation at the knee	Superior gluteal nerve
Sartorius	Anterior superior iliac spine	Medial surface of body of the tibia near the tibial tuberosity	Flexes leg at the knee; Abducts and flexes thigh; rotates it laterally	Femoral nerve
Quadriceps femoris is formed from the following four muscles					
Rectus femoris	Anterior inferior iliac spine	**Common insertion:** Tibial tuberosity by way of the patella and patellar ligament	Flexes thigh; extends leg	Femoral nerve
Vastus lateralis	Femur anterior and inferior to greater trochanter; linea aspera of femur		Extends leg	Femoral nerve
Vastus medialis	Linea aspera of femur		Extends leg	Femoral nerve
Vastus intermedius	Anterolateral femoral shaft		Extends leg	Femoral nerve

The Sartorius

The **sartorius** is a long, strap-shaped muscle extending diagonally across the anterior thigh from the anterior superior iliac spine to the superior, medial surface of the tibia. It crosses both the hip and knee joints. The sartorius flexes and rotates the thigh laterally and flexes the leg at the knee joint.

The Quadriceps Femoris

The **Quadriceps femoris** is a group of four muscles that extend the leg at the knee joint. As a group, the quadriceps insert at the tibial tuberosity via the patella and the patellar ligament. The quadriceps femoris is formed from the following muscles. (Fig. 4.9b)

1. The **rectus femoris** is the large superficial muscle that lies along the anterior thigh. The rectus femoris crosses both the hip and knee joints. In addition to extending the leg, the rectus femoris also flexes the thigh.
2. The **vastus lateralis** lies laterally to the rectus femoris.
3. The **vastus medialis** lies medial to the rectus femoris.
4. The **vastus intermedius** lies deep to the rectus femoris between vastus lateralis and medius. The vastus intermedius is best studied by lifting the rectus femoris.

(a) Posterior view of superficial muscles of the right thigh

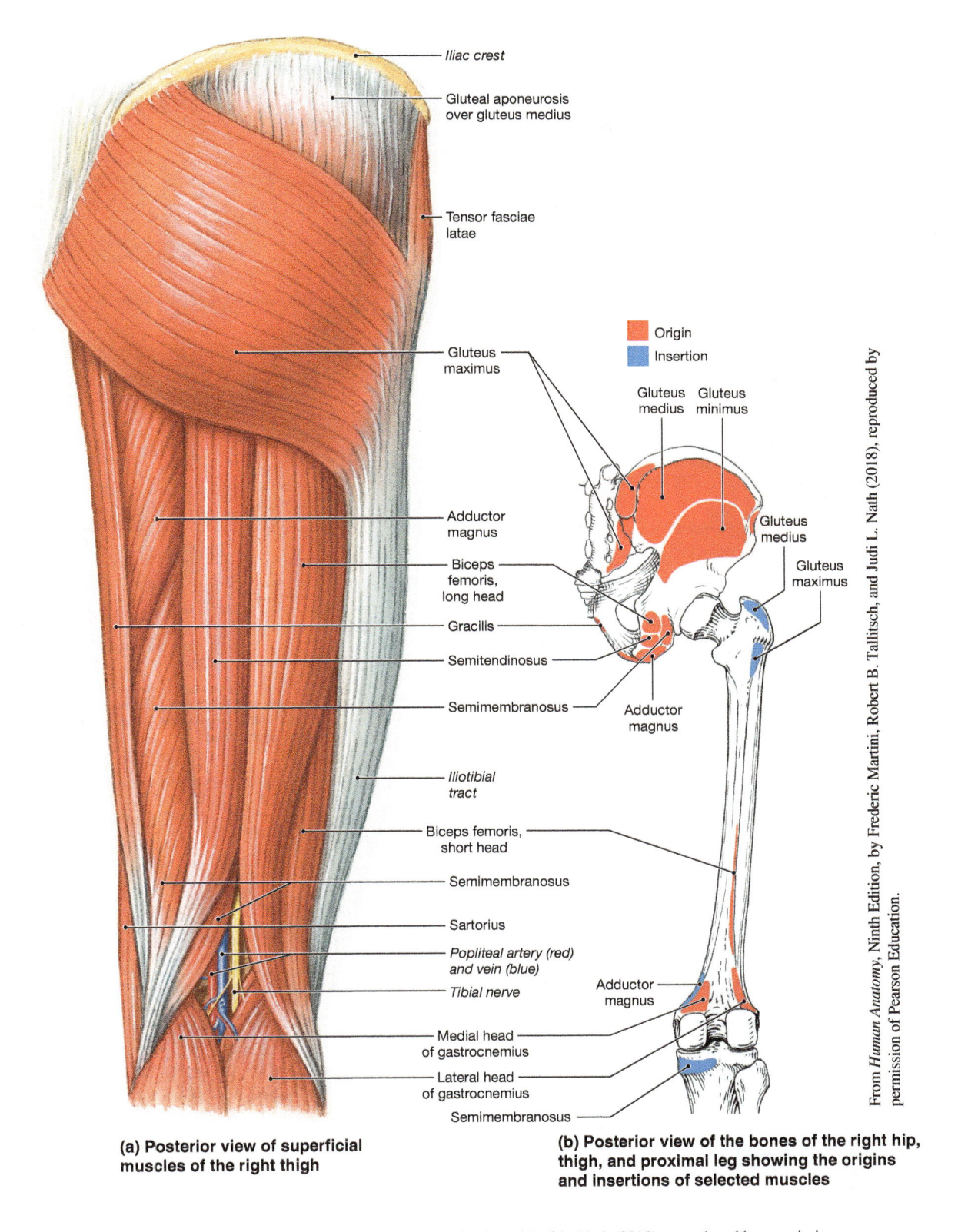

(b) Posterior view of the bones of the right hip, thigh, and proximal leg showing the origins and insertions of selected muscles

From *Human Anatomy*, Ninth Edition, by Frederic Martini, Robert B. Tallitsch, and Judi L. Nath (2018), reproduced by permission of Pearson Education.

Figure 4.9c   Muscles That Move the Leg, Part III *(Continued)*

CHAPTER FOUR   *Selected Muscles of the Appendicular & Axial Skeleton*   89

(c) Deep muscles of the posterior thigh

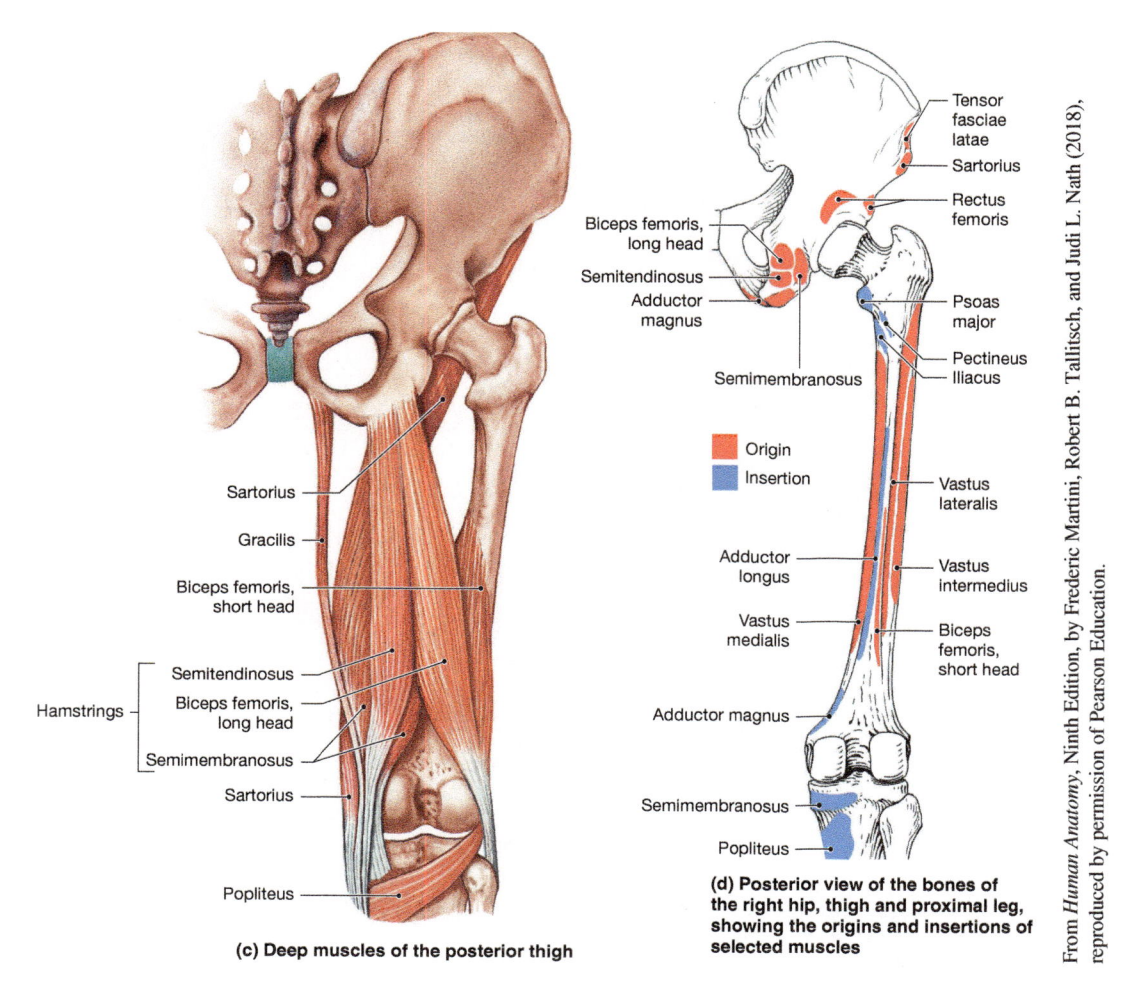

(d) Posterior view of the bones of the right hip, thigh and proximal leg, showing the origins and insertions of selected muscles

From *Human Anatomy*, Ninth Edition, by Frederic Martini, Robert B. Tallitsch, and Judi L. Nath (2018), reproduced by permission of Pearson Education.

Figure 4.9c   Muscles That Move the Leg, Part III

MUSCLE TABLE 11: MUSCLES OF THE POSTERIOR COMPARTMENT OF THE THIGH; THE HAMSTRING GROUP; FLEXORS OF THE LEG

Hamstring Group				
Muscle	**Origin**	**Insertion**	**Action**	**Innervation**
Biceps femoris • Long head • Short head	Ischial tuberosity; linea aspera of femur	Head of fibula	Extends thigh (long head); flexes leg	Tibial division of sciatic nerve (long head) and common fibular division (short head)
Semitendinosus	Ischial tuberosity	Medial surface of body of the tibia	Extends thigh; flexes leg	Tibial division of sciatic
Semimembranosus	Ischial tuberosity	Medial condyle of tibia	Extends thigh; flexes leg	Tibial division of sciatic nerve

The Hamstrings

Hamstrings occupy the posterior muscle compartment of the thigh and cross both the hip and knee joints. These muscles extend the thigh at the hip joint and flex the leg at the knee joint (Fig. 4.9c).

1. The **biceps femoris** is the most lateral of the hamstrings. The long head arises from the ischial tuberosity and the short head arises from the linea aspera of the femur. The two heads merge to insert on the head of the fibula.

2. The **semitendinosus** lies medial to the biceps femoris. Semitendinosus, as its name implies, has a long tendon of insertion.

3. The **semimembranosus** lies medial and deep to the semitendinosus. It originates from the ischial tuberosity by a broad flat tendon, hence the name semi**membranosus**.

MUSCLES THAT MOVE THE FOOT AT THE ANKLE JOINT

1. The **tibialis anterior** is the large, superficial muscle that lies along the lateral surface of the tibia on the anterior compartment of the leg (Figs. 4.10a, 4.10b).

MUSCLE TABLE 12: MUSCLES THAT MOVE THE FOOT AT THE ANKLE JOINT

Muscle	Origin	Insertion	Action	Innervation
Muscles of the Anterior Compartment of the Leg				
Tibialis anterior	Lateral condyle & diaphysis of tibia	First metatarsal & medial aspect of foot	Dorsiflexes & inverts the foot	Deep fibular nerve
Extensor digitorum longus	Proximal shaft of fibula; lateral condyle of tibia	Superior surface of phalanges 2–5	Extends toes 2–5; Dorsiflexes foot; prime mover of toe extension	Deep fibular nerve
Muscles of the Lateral Compartment of the Leg				
Fibularis longus	Proximal shaft of fibula; lateral condyle of tibia	1st metatarsal & medial cuneiform; 5th metatarsal	Plantar flexes & everts foot	Superficial fibular nerve
Fibularis brevis				
Muscles of the Posterior Compartment of the Leg				
Gastrocnemi-us	Lateral & medial condyles of femur	Calcaneus by way of the calcaneal tendon	Plantar flexion of foot	Tibial nerve
Soleus	Head & proximal shaft of the fibula; posteromedial surface of the tibia	Calcaneus by way of the calcaneal tendon	Plantar flexion of foot	Tibial nerve
Plantaris	Posterior femur	Long tendon into calcaneus	Flexion of knee and plantar flexion of foot	Tibial nerve

CHAPTER FOUR   *Selected Muscles of the Appendicular & Axial Skeleton*

(a) Anterior views showing superficial and deep muscles of the right leg

(b) Anterior view of the bones of the right leg showing the origins and insertions of selected muscles

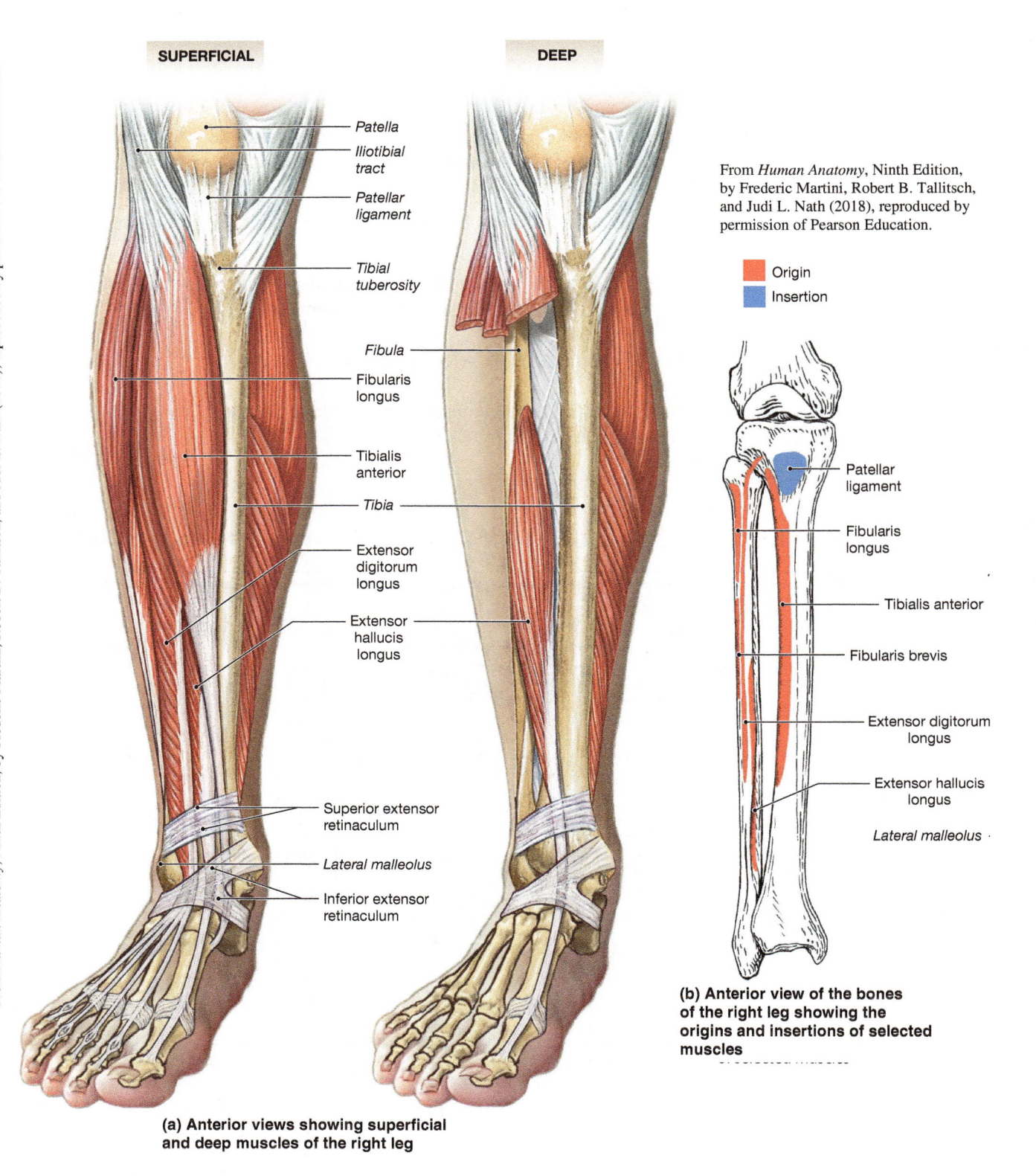

From *Human Anatomy*, Ninth Edition by Frederic H. Martini, Michael J. Timmons, and Robert B. Tallitsch

Figure 4.10a   Extrinsic Muscles That Move the Foot and Toes, Part III

Complete Introductory Human Anatomy Lab Guide

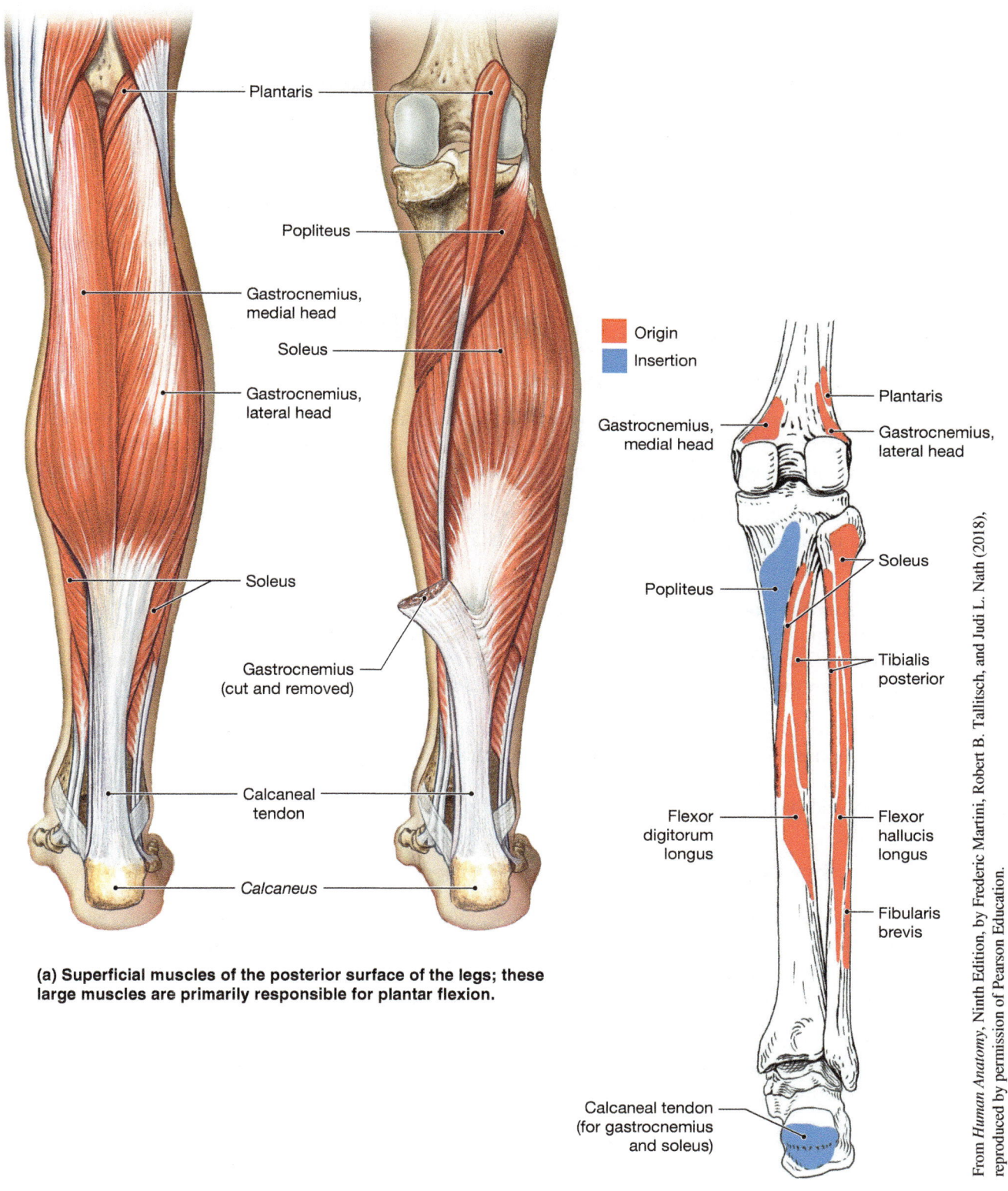

(a) Superficial muscles of the posterior surface of the legs; these large muscles are primarily responsible for plantar flexion.

(b) A posterior view of the bones of the right leg and foot showing the origins and insertions of selected muscles.

From *Human Anatomy*, Ninth Edition, by Frederic Martini, Robert B. Tallitsch, and Judi L. Nath (2018), reproduced by permission of Pearson Education.

Figure 4.10b Extrinsic Muscles That Move the Foot and Toes, Part I

CHAPTER FOUR   *Selected Muscles of the Appendicular & Axial Skeleton*

2. The **gastrocnemius** is the large, two-headed muscle of the posterior compartment of the leg. It crosses both the knee and ankle joints.

3. The **soleus** is deep to the gastrocnemius. The soleus and gastrocnemius insert together at the calcaneal tendon.

4. The **fibularis longus** is located lateral to the tibialis anterior, over the fibula. The fibularis brevis and longus are the two muscles of the lateral compartment of the leg.

5. The **extensor digitorum longus** is located lateral to the inferior portion of the tibialis anterior.

6. The plantaris is a small muscle attached to a very long tendon that inserts at the calcaneus.

VII. BLOOD SUPPLY OF THE LOWER EXTREMITIES

Arterial Supply to the Lower Extremity

The arterial supply to the lower extremities originates from the **descending abdominal aorta**. The descending abdominal aorta divides in the pelvic region into the **common iliac arteries** which branch into the **external iliac** and **internal iliac arteries**.

The external iliac arteries become the **femoral arteries** in the thigh and the femoral arteries continue as the **popliteal arteries** in the popliteal fossa. Branches of each of the femoral and internal iliac arteries supply the muscles of the lower extremity.

The **internal iliac** arteries branch into the **superior** and **inferior gluteal arteries**. The superior and inferior gluteal arteries supply the gluteal muscles. The **obturator artery** is another branch of the internal iliac artery that passes through the obturator canal. The obturator artery along with branches of the femoral artery supplies the adductors of the thigh.

Branches of the **femoral artery** supply most muscles of the thigh, including the quadriceps group. The popliteal artery is a continuation of the femoral artery. Branches of the popliteal artery supply the posterior and lateral compartments of the leg. The **deep femoral artery** branches from the femoral artery and supplies blood to the hamstring group.

Venous Return from the Lower Extremity

The venous drainage of the lower extremity follows the reverse pattern of the arteries. The **popliteal vein** drains into the **femoral vein**. The femoral vein becomes the **external iliac vein** inside the body cavity. The junction of the **external iliac** and **internal iliac veins** forms the **common iliac vein**. The common iliac vein then drains into the **inferior vena cava**.

Superficial veins drain subcutaneous tissues of the thigh and leg. Note the **great saphenous vein** that courses along the medial thigh and leg. The great saphenous vein drains into the femoral vein. The **small saphenous vein** is located on the posterior leg and drains into the popliteal vein.

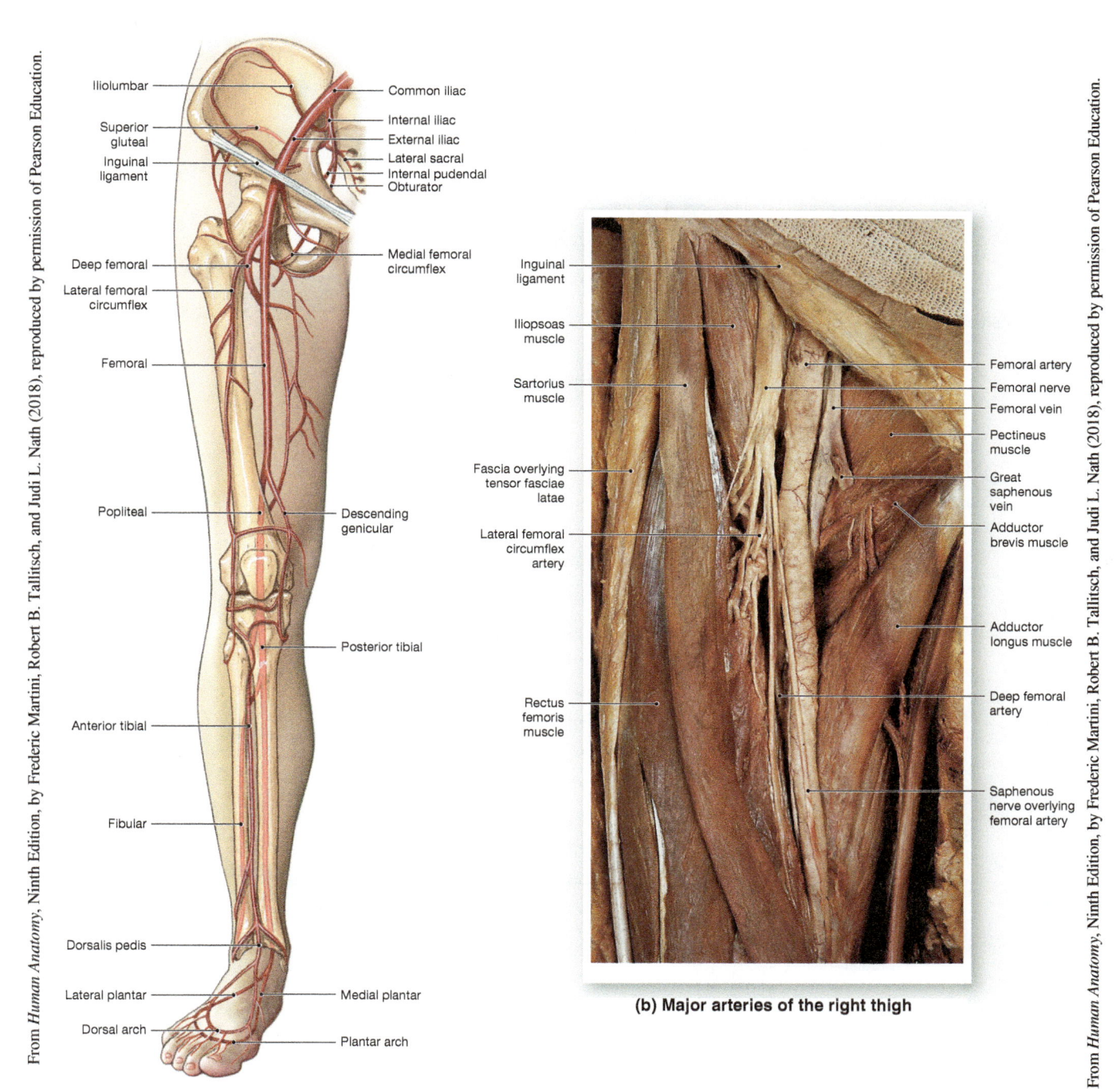

(a) Anterior view of the arteries supplying the right lower limb

(b) Major arteries of the right thigh

Figure 4.11   Major Arteries of the Lower Limb, Part I

CHAPTER FOUR   *Selected Muscles of the Appendicular & Axial Skeleton*   95

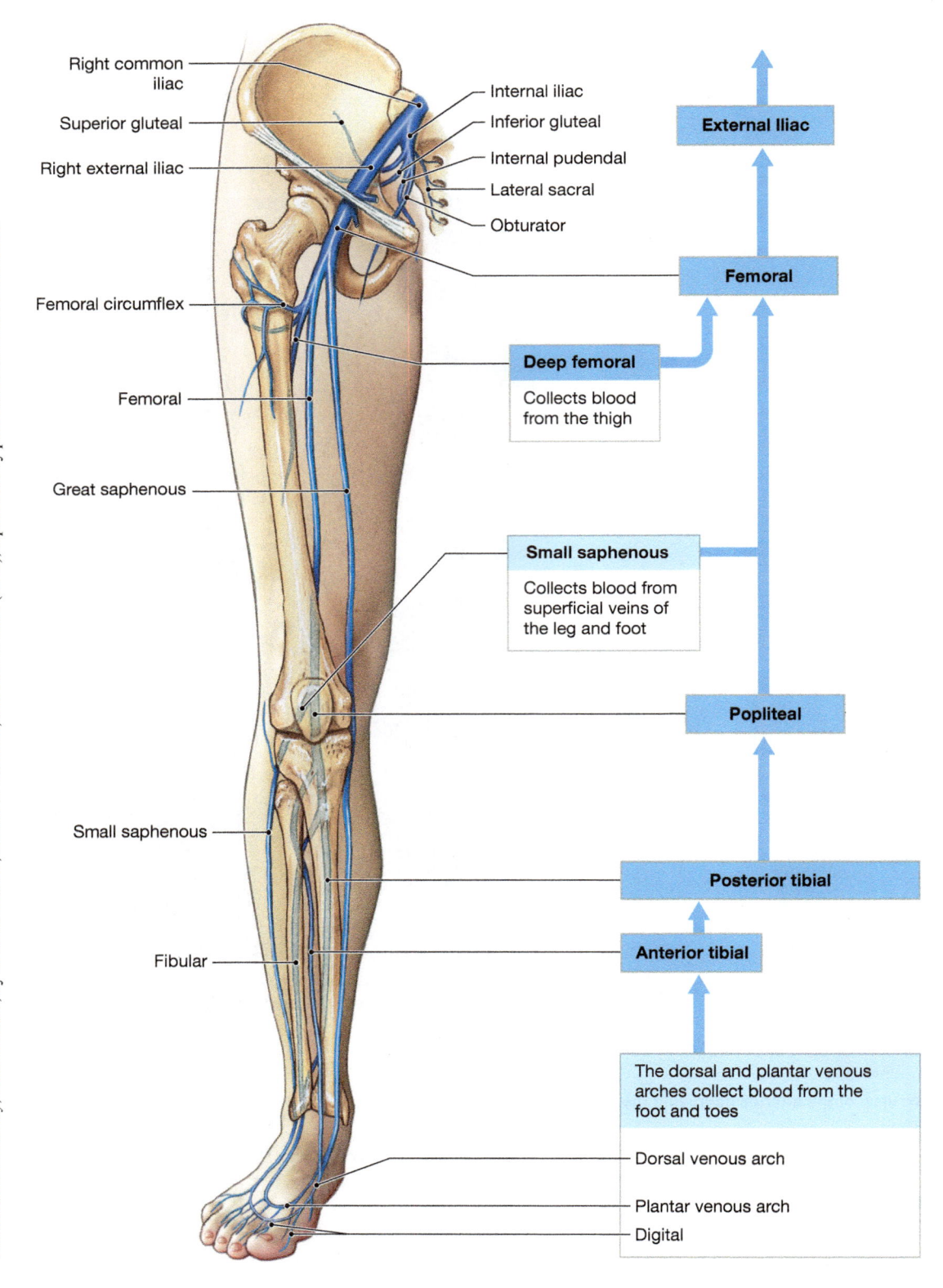

Figure 4.12 Anterior view showing the veins of the right lower limb

96   *Complete Introductory Human Anatomy Lab Guide*

VIII. INNERVATION OF MUSCLES OF THE LOWER EXTREMITY

The nerve supply to muscles of the lower extremity comes from branches of the **lumbar plexus** and **sacral plexus**. The **lumbar plexus** is formed from the ventral rami of lumbar spinal nerves 1-4 and the **sacral plexus** is formed from ventral rami of spinal nerves L4–L5 and S1–S4. These plexuses are sometimes referred to as the **lumbosacral plexus**.

You will examine the major nerves of these plexuses in the donor body. Identify the **obturator nerve, superior gluteal nerve, inferior gluteal nerve, femoral nerve** and the **sciatic nerve**. Also identify the two divisions of the **sciatic nerve**, the **tibial** and **common fibular nerves**.

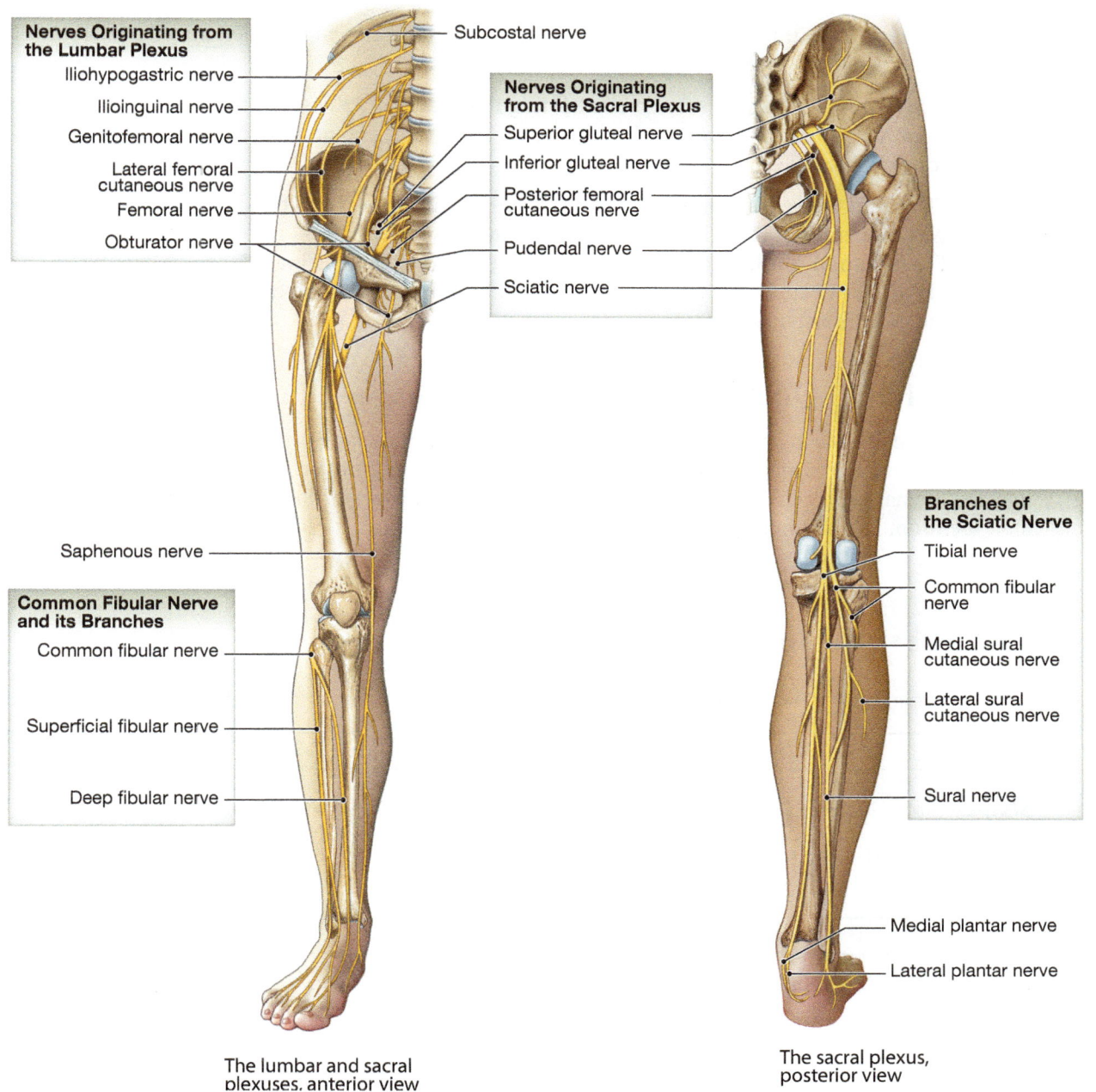

Figure 4.13 Peripheral Nerves Originating from the Lumbar and Sacral Plexuses

CHAPTER FOUR   *Selected Muscles of the Appendicular & Axial Skeleton*   97

NERVES BRANCHING FROM THE LUMBAR PLEXUS

1. The **femoral nerve** is found with the femoral artery and vein along the anteromedial surface of the thigh. The femoral nerve and its branches innervate the muscles of the anterior thigh.
2. The **obturator nerve** innervates muscles of the adductor group, including the adductor longus, adductor magnus and gracilis.

NERVES BRANCHING FROM THE SACRAL PLEXUS

1. The **superior gluteal nerve** innervates the gluteus medius and gluteus minimus as well as the tensor fasciae latae. It passes superior to the piriformis muscle.
2. The **inferior gluteal nerve** innervates the gluteus maximus. It is found inferior to the piriformis muscle.
3. The **sciatic nerve** is the largest nerve in the thigh. It is actually a combination of two nerves, the **tibial nerve** and the **common fibular nerve**. Its branches innervate many muscles of the posterior thigh and leg.
   - The **tibial nerve** is the more medial of these two divisions. The tibial nerve innervates the **gastrocnemius, soleus** and the **biceps femoris**.
   - The **common fibular nerve** (common peroneal nerve) is the lateral branch of the sciatic nerve. The deep fibular nerve, which branches from the common fibular nerve, innervates the **tibialis anterior**.

IX. METHODS OF NAMING MUSCLES

Muscles are named using a variety of criteria. It is important for students to recognize the descriptive nature of the names of muscles so that the names will be meaningful and easier to learn. Often muscles are named for their **size, shape, action, number of divisions,** their **fiber arrangement** or their **location**. List examples, where indicated, in the blanks below.

Size

List examples of muscles named for their size.

_____   _____
_____   _____
_____

Shape

List examples of muscles named for their shape.

_____   _____
_____   _____
_____

Action

List examples of muscles named for their action.

_____   _____
_____   _____
_____   _____

Number of Divisions

List examples of muscles named for the number of divisions.

_____
_____
_____

Location

List examples of muscles named for their location or one of their points of attachment.

_____   _____
_____   _____
_____   _____

X. COMPARTMENTS OF SKELETAL MUSCLES

Learning the names of the muscles is one of the greatest tasks of memorization in anatomy. If you are feeling overwhelmed by studying muscle charts, look for ways to make muscle action, origin, insertion, and nerve supply functionally relevant to you.

Most muscles are grouped into compartments or logical groups. These groups have important common features:

1. They are usually located on one side of a part of a limb.
2. Members of a compartment usually have the same nerve innervation.
3. Members of a compartment usually have similar functions, just act on different parts.

If you act out the actions of muscles, you will find that you remember their actions much better. Using a model of a human skeleton, you can use a rubber band placed on the origin and on the insertion of appendicular muscles to show muscle action.

You can easily learn nerve supplies to muscles when you realize how they are organized by compartments. Complete the worksheet below. Remember to learn the exceptions to these generalities!

Muscular Compartments Worksheet

Compartment	Innervation	General Functions
Anterior arm	_____	_____
Posterior arm	_____	_____
Anterior forearm	_____	_____
Posterior forearm	_____	_____
Gluteal	_____	_____
Posterior thigh	_____	_____
Medial thigh	_____	_____
Anterior thigh	_____	_____
Anterior leg	_____	_____
Posterior leg	_____	_____
Lateral leg	_____	_____

Study and Review Questions – Skeletal Muscles

CHAPTER FOUR

Answers to these questions are found in Chapter Four of this guide.

1. Match the muscle with its **origin**. Match the muscle in **column A** with the correct origin in **column B**. Write the letter of your answer in the blank by the appropriate term in column A.

   Column A

   _____ Pectoralis major

   _____ Supraspinatus

   _____ Rhomboid minor

   _____ Levator scapulae

   _____ Teres major

   Column B

   A. Spinous processes of C7-T1

   B. Inferior angle of scapula

   C. Lateral clavicle, spine, and acromion process of scapula

   D. Supraspinous fossa

   E. C1 –C4 or C5

   F. Sternum, clavicle and costal cartilage of ribs 2-6

2. Match the muscle with its **nerve supply**. Match the muscle in column A with the correct nerve supply in **column B**. Write the letter of your answer in the blank by the appropriate term in column A. Some nerves might not be used.

   Column A

   _____ Biceps brachii

   _____ Infraspinatus

   _____ Deltoid

   _____ Triceps brachii

   Column B

   A. Axillary nerve

   B. Median nerve

   C. Suprascapular nerve

   D. Radial nerve

   E. Musculocutaneous nerve

3. Match the muscle with its **origin**. Match the muscle in **column A** with the correct origin in column B. Write the letter of your answer in the blank by the appropriate term in column A.

   Column A

   _____ Gluteus medius

   _____ Tensor fascia latae

   _____ Piriformis

   _____ Superior gemellus

   Column B

   A. Anterior surface of the sacrum

   B. Spine of the ischium & ischial tuberosity

   C. Posterior surface of the ilium

   D. Iliac crest and anterior superior iliac spine

4. Match the muscle with its **action**. Match the muscle in **column A** with the correct action in **column B**. Write the letter of your answer in the blank by the appropriate term in column A.

   Column A　　　　　　　　　　**Column B**

   _____ Gluteus maximus　　A. Adducts, flexes, and rotates thigh medially

   _____ Sartorius　　　　　　B. Extends leg

   _____ Rectus femoris　　　C. Extends and rotates thigh laterally

   _____ Adductor longus　　D. Flexes leg, flexes thigh and rotates it medially

   　　　　　　　　　　　　　　E. Extends leg; flexes thigh

5. Match the muscle with its insertion. Match the muscle in **column A** with the correct insertion in **column B**. Write the letter of your answer in the blank by the appropriate term in column A.

   Column A　　　　　　　　　　**Column B**

   _____ Biceps femoris　　　A. Calcaneus by way of the calcaneal tendon

   _____ Gastrocnemius　　　B. 1st metatarsal

   _____ Semitendinosus　　C. Head of the fibula; lateral condyle of tibia

   _____ Peroneus longus　　D. Medial surface of the body of the tibia

   _____ Soleus

6. Match the muscle with its nerve supply. Match the muscle in column A with the correct nerve supply in column B.

   Column A　　　　　　　　　　　**Column B**

   _____ Rectus femoris　　　　　　A. Superior gluteal nerve

   _____ Biceps femoris short head　B. Common fibular nerve

   _____ Gastrocnemius　　　　　　C. Obturator nerve

   _____ Adductor longus　　　　　D. Femoral nerve

   _____ Gluteus medius　　　　　　E. Tibial nerve

   _____ Tibialis anterior　　　　　F. Deep fibular nerve

FIVE
The Central Nervous System: The Brain & Spinal Cord

LABORATORY MATERIALS

Brain and spinal cord models
Human donor brains and spinal cords
Donor body with spinal cord dissection
Sagittal head model
Photomicrographs

I. HISTOLOGY OF NEURAL TISSUE

The central nervous system includes the brain and spinal cord. **Peripheral nerves** are located outside the CNS. These micrographs focus primarily on tissues of the central nervous system.

1. **Spinal cord**—cross-section through the cervical region:
   a. Compare the anterior and dorsal (posterior) horns.
   b. Note the **gray matter** that makes up the anterior and posterior horns. Gray matter is composed of neuronal cell bodies.
   c. **White matter** surrounds gray matter in the spinal cord. White matter is composed of myelinated neuronal axons.
   d. Distinguish between the **anterior median fissure** and **posterior median sulcus**.
   e. Locate the central canal of the spinal cord.

2. **Cross section of spinal cord:**

   Identify the **anterior** (ventral) and **posterior** (dorsal) horns. Locate the anterior median fissure and posterior median sulcus. Compare the anterior and posterior horns at the thoracic region to those on the slide of the cervical region.

3. **Anterior horn motor neuron** (Lower motor neuron):
   a. Note chromatophilic substance and the nucleus within the neuron.
   b. Locate the nerve cell processes.
   c. Note the small nuclei of neuroglial cells (non-conductive nerve cells) surrounding the anterior horn motor neuron (lower motor neuron).

4. **Neuron showing axon hillock:**
   a. **Chromatophilic substance** (Nissl substance) is contained within the cell body (soma) and is responsible for the gray color of "gray matter."
   b. Chromatophilic substance (Nissl substance) is *absent* from the axon. Therefore, due to the type of staining, dendrites and the cell body take up stain and the axon does not.

c. The **axon hillock** shows up as a depression in the cell body.

d. The **perikaryon** is the cytoplasm around the nucleus of a nerve cell.

5. **Neuron stained to show Nissl substance:**

   a. Nissl substance is made up of rough endoplasmic reticulum and ribosomes and is located within the perikaryon (cytoplasm surrounding the nucleus) and in the dendrites of neurons.

   b. Nissl substance is absent from the axon.

6. **Dorsal root ganglion:**

   a. The **dorsal root ganglion** contains the cell bodies of sensory neurons.

   b. The dorsal root carries **sensory impulses** toward CNS processing centers.

   c. The ventral root has no ganglion and carries **motor impulses** away from the CNS.

   d. Note the cross-sections of cell bodies in the dorsal root ganglion.

   e. Neurons in ganglia are typically **pseudounipolar neurons**, which are almost always **sensory neurons**.

   f. The **dorsal** and **ventral roots** join to form a spinal nerve, which exits through the intervertebral foramen.

7. **Myelinated fibers** (axons) within white matter of the spinal cord:

   a. The myelin sheath is stained, but the axon itself does not stain.

   b. The axon is in the center of each ring of dark stain.

8. **Longitudinal section of a nerve:**

   a. The myelin sheath is stained purple and wraps around the nerve cell processes.

   b. The myelin sheath increases the speed of nerve transmission.

   c. Gaps along the section of nerve are called **Nodes of Ranvier** (ron-VE-ay).

9. **Motor unit:**

   a. The motor unit is made up of one motor neuron and all the muscle cells it innervates.

   b. The single axon has **telodendria** and **synaptic knobs**.

   c. The junction between the synaptic knobs and a muscle fiber is called the **neuromuscular junction**. Note the skeletal muscle cells that are innervated by the synaptic knobs.

10. **Pyramidal cells** are located in the primary motor area of the cerebral cortex.

    a. Pyramidal cells are neurons for voluntary motor impulses and are named for their pyramid-shaped cell bodies.

    b. The corticospinal pathways begin with pyramidal cells.

11. **Purkinje cells:**

    a. Purkinje cells are found in the cortex of the cerebellum.

    b. Branching dendrites extend from the cell. The single axon is not visible.

    c. The small nuclei seen around the Purkinje cell belong to small neurons of the cerebellum.

12. **Astrocytes:**
    a. **Astrocytes** are star-shaped **neuroglial cells**. They are found throughout **gray** and **white matter** of both brain and spinal cord.
    b. The numerous, thin, branching processes of the astrocytes associate with blood vessels in the CNS to form the blood brain barrier that protects neurons in the CNS.
13. **Tongue papillae:**
    a. Tongue papillae are structures located on the dorsal surface of the tongue that contain taste buds.
    b. Taste buds are imbedded in the lateral surface of all types of tongue papillae, except filiform papillae.
    c. Taste buds are "gustatory" (taste) receptors.
14. **Taste buds:** Note the taste buds within the epithelium of the tongue papillae.

II. HISTOLOGICAL COMPONENTS OF THE CENTRAL NERVOUS SYSTEM

Neurons

Neurons are cells that transmit messages (nerve impulses) to other neurons or to target organs.

Define the following terms related to neurons:

1. **Nerve cell body** _____
2. **Axon** _____
3. **Dendrite** _____
4. **Nucleus** _____
5. **Tract** _____
6. **Ganglion** _____
7. **Nerve** _____

Types of Neurons

1. **Anaxonic neuron** _____
2. **Bipolar neuron** _____
3. **Pseudounipolar neuron** _____
4. **Multipolar neuron** _____

III. THE CENTRAL NERVOUS SYSTEM & RELATED STRUCTURES

The central nervous system consists of the brain and spinal cord. We will begin with the protective coverings of the brain and spinal cord before covering the spinal cord itself. The brain will be covered in lab by the five subdivisions that reflect the embryonic development: Telencephalon, Diencephalon, Mesencephalon, Metencephalon and Myelencephalon. Refer to the textbook for a complete explanation of the relationships of these subdivisions.

MENINGES

The meninges are layers of connective tissue membranes that surround the brain and spinal cord and act to support and protect them. The meninges are discussed below, beginning with the outermost layer.

1. **Dura mater** ("tough mother") is the outermost of the meninges. This dense irregular connective tissue layer is a tough protective covering of the brain. In the cranium, the dura mater is made up of two layers, between which are formed the "dural venous sinuses." The dural venous sinuses function as veins that take deoxygenated blood away from the brain. One of the sinuses is the **superior sagittal sinus**, which courses between the layers of the cranial dura mater. The outer layer of the dura mater is tightly attached to the internal surface of the skull. Meningeal arteries lie between the dura and the bone of the skull. The dura mater surrounding the spinal cord is comprised of a single layer and therefore there are no dural venous sinuses associated with the spinal cord. Another difference is that the dura around the spinal cord is not attached to the inner surface of the vertebral canal. This creates an **epidural space** between the dura and the bone of the vertebral canal. Dura mater around the spinal cord covers spinal nerves into the intervertebral foramen where it merges into the periosteum of the bone. The epidural space contains epidural fat and network of veins, the **epidural venous plexus**. Epidural anesthetics can be administered into this space.

2. **Arachnoid mater** ("spidery mother") is the middle meninx (singular of meninges). It is attached to the inner surface of the dura mater around both the brain and spinal cord. It has a gauzy, cobweb-like consistency. Arachnoid mater is distinguishable at the gross level. Observe this layer covering the brain, deep to the dura mater. The **Subarachnoid space** is the space between the arachnoid mater and the pia mater in which cerebrospinal fluid (CSF; see below) circulates. In the cranial cavity cerebral veins cross the subarachnoid space and empty into the dural venous sinuses. The subarachnoid space is continuous around the brain and spinal cord.

3. **Pia mater** ("soft mother") is the innermost layer of the meninges. This thin, transparent layer is intimately associated with the neural tissue and is not distinguishable at the gross anatomical level. It is the connective tissue that holds the cerebral and spinal arteries and veins into place and adheres to the convolutions of the gyri and sulci of the cerebral hemispheres. Two specializations of the pia mater are found in association with the spinal cord.

    a. The filum terminale is a thin strand of pia that extends inferiorly from the conus medularis of the spinal cord to anchor the spinal cord to the sacrum and coccyx.

    b. Denticulate ligaments are extensions of pia mater that extend laterally from the spinal cord at regular intervals. These "teeth" of pia mater extend across the sub arachnoid space through the arachnoid mater and anchor the spinal cord to the dura mater.

4. **Falx cerebri** is a fold of the inner layer of the cranial dura that divides the cerebral hemispheres. It extends from the crista galli of the ethmoid bone anteriorly to the tentorium cerebelli and internal occipital crest. The superior sagittal venous sinus is found at the junction of the falx

cerebri and the dura attached to the skull. The inferior sagittal venous sinus is found along the inferior edge of the falx cerebri.

5. **Tentorium cerebelli** is a fold of dura similar in structure to the falx cerebri. It spans between the petrous ridges of the temporal bone, along the occipital bone to the midline where it attaches to the falx cerebri. It separates the occipital lobes of the cerebrum from the cerebellum.

6. **Tentorial insure** is the opening in the tentorium cerebelli for passage of the midbrain.

From *Human Anatomy*, Ninth Edition, by Frederic Martini, Robert B. Tallitsch, and Judi L. Nath (2018), reproduced by permission of Pearson Education.

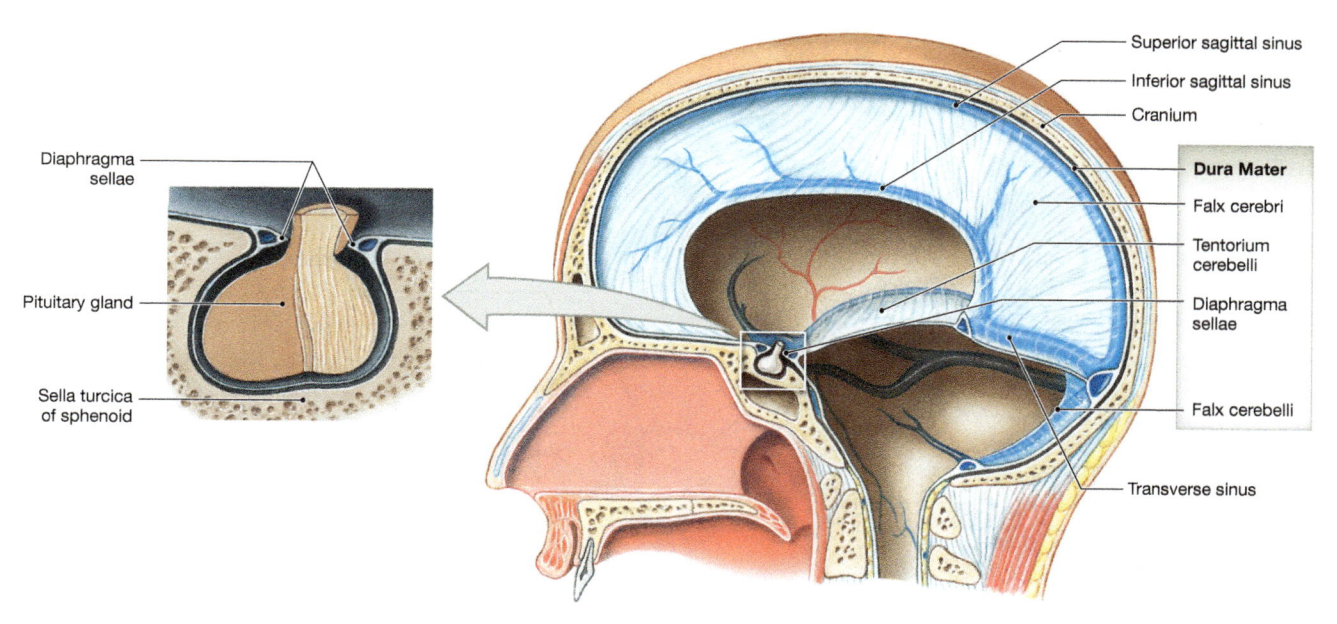

Figure 5.1 A corresponding view of the cranial cavity with the brain removed showing the orientation and extent of the falx cerebri and tentorium cerebelli.

IV. SPINAL CORD & RELATED STRUCTURES

THE SPINAL CORD

The **spinal cord** is continuous with the **medulla oblongata** of the brain. It is located within the vertebral canal and extends to the level of vertebrae L1 or L2. Locate these features on anatomical models or dissected spinal cords (Fig. 5.2).

1. External features of the spinal cord include:
   a. **Cervical** and **lumbosacral enlargements** are regions of the spinal cord with large cross-sectional areas, which correspond to the nerve plexuses and innervate the upper and lower limbs, respectively.
   b. The **conus medullaris** is the pointed inferior end of the spinal cord.
   c. The **anterior median fissure** is a longitudinal groove running vertically along the anterior midline of the spinal cord.
   d. The **posterior median sulcus** is a longitudinal groove running vertically along the posterior midline of the spinal cord.

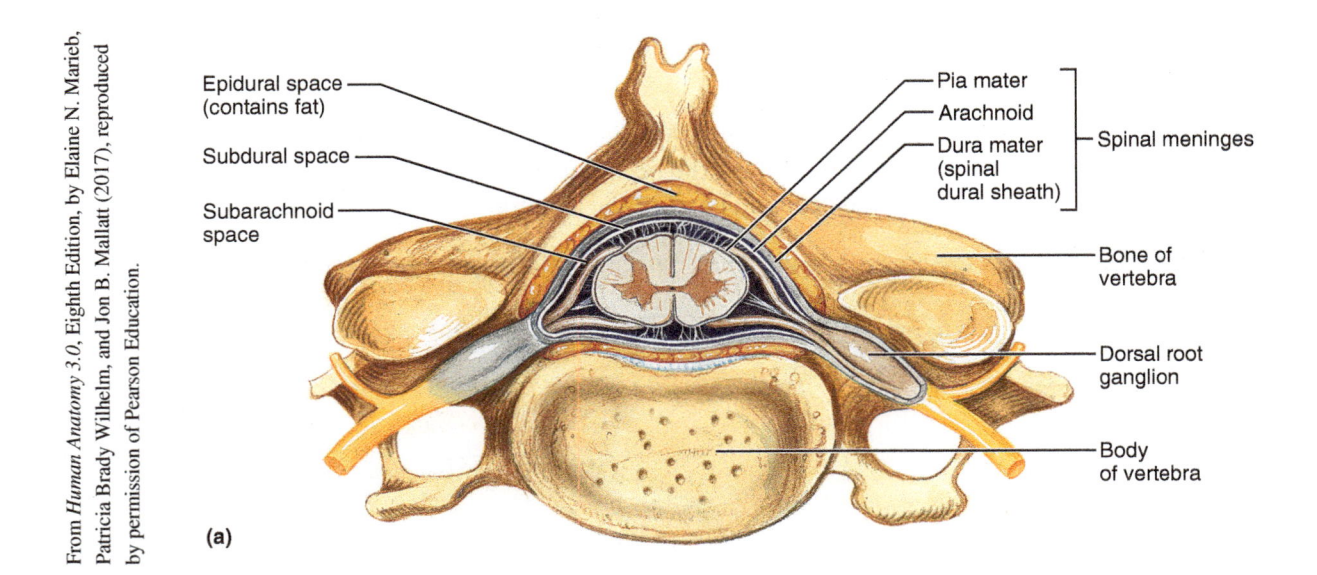

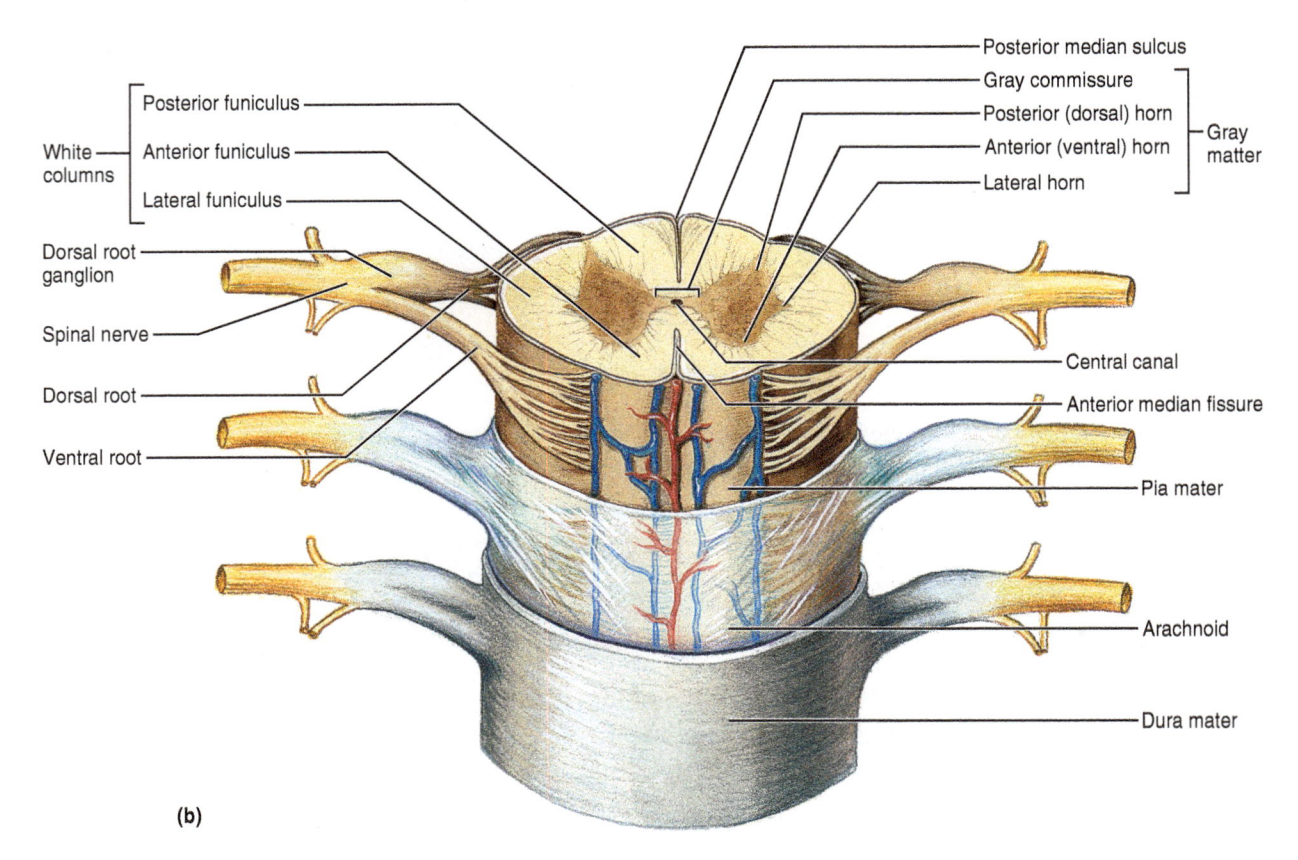

Figure 5.2 **Anatomy of the Spinal Cord.** (a) Cross section through the spinal cord in the cervical region illustrating its relationship to a surrounding cervical vertebra. (b) Three-dimensional ventral view of the spinal cord and its meningeal coverings. The dorsal direction is at the top in both these figures.

108 *Complete Introductory Human Anatomy Lab Guide*

2. In a cross-section of the spinal cord, **gray matter** forms the H-shaped central region, which is made up primarily of neuronal cell bodies. Note the central region of **gray matter** on a cross-sectional spinal cord model and on photomicrographs. (Fig. 5.2)

3. **White matter** of the spinal cord surrounds the central region of gray matter and consists of ascending and descending tracts. The tracts are comprised of functionally related bundles of **myelinated axons**.

4. **Spinal nerves** are nerves of the **peripheral nervous system** (PNS), which contain somatic sensory, somatic motor, visceral sensory and visceral motor (both sympathetic and parasympathetic) fibers. There are 31 pairs of spinal nerves, which are formed and distributed as follows:

    a. **Dorsal** and **ventral roots** of spinal nerves join to form short (approximately 1 cm.) **spinal nerves,** which exit the vertebral canal through the **intervertebral foramina.**
       - **Dorsal roots** are formed by somatic and visceral sensory neurons. Their cell bodies are located in the **dorsal root ganglia**.
       - **Ventral roots** are formed by somatic motor neurons. Their cell bodies are located in the gray matter of the anterior (ventral) horn of the spinal cord.

    b. The spinal nerve branches into a **dorsal** and a **ventral ramus** after exiting through the intervertebral foramen. Spinal nerves and their dorsal and ventral rami are mixed nerves, that is, they contain both **motor** and **sensory fibers**. The **dorsal rami** innervate muscles and skin of the back area. The **ventral rami** form the following structures:
       - The **cervical plexus** (ventral rami of spinal nerves C1-C4) innervates structures of the neck. The phrenic nerve is the most important nerve of the cervical plexus.
       - The **brachial plexus** (ventral rami of spinal nerves C5-T1) innervates structures of the upper limb.
       - **Intercostal nerves** (ventral rami of spinal nerves T1-T12) innervate structures of intercostal regions.
       - The **lumbosacral plexus** (ventral rami of spinal nerves L1-S5) innervates structures of the lower limb.

    c. The **cauda equina** (horse's tail) is made up of long dorsal and ventral roots of lumbar, sacral and coccygeal spinal nerves which pass through the vertebral canal to exit through the intervertebral foramen at the vertebral level corresponding to the spinal nerve level of origin.

V. BRAIN

The human brain has been considered the most complex functional structure in the known universe. It receives all sensory input from the body and coordinates and initiates active responses both at and below the level of consciousness. The brain has five major subdivisions. We will learn all of these, their major parts and their general functions.

TELENCEPHALON

Introduction

The telencephalon consists of the **cerebral hemispheres,** two convoluted masses of neural tissue separated in the sagittal plane by the **longitudinal fissure**. In the intact brain the cerebral hemispheres are separated by the falx cerebri, located in the longitudinal fissure. In the whole brain, gently spread the longitudinal fissure and look from above to see the superior surface of the corpus callosum (Fig. 5.3).

(a) A sagittal section through the brain

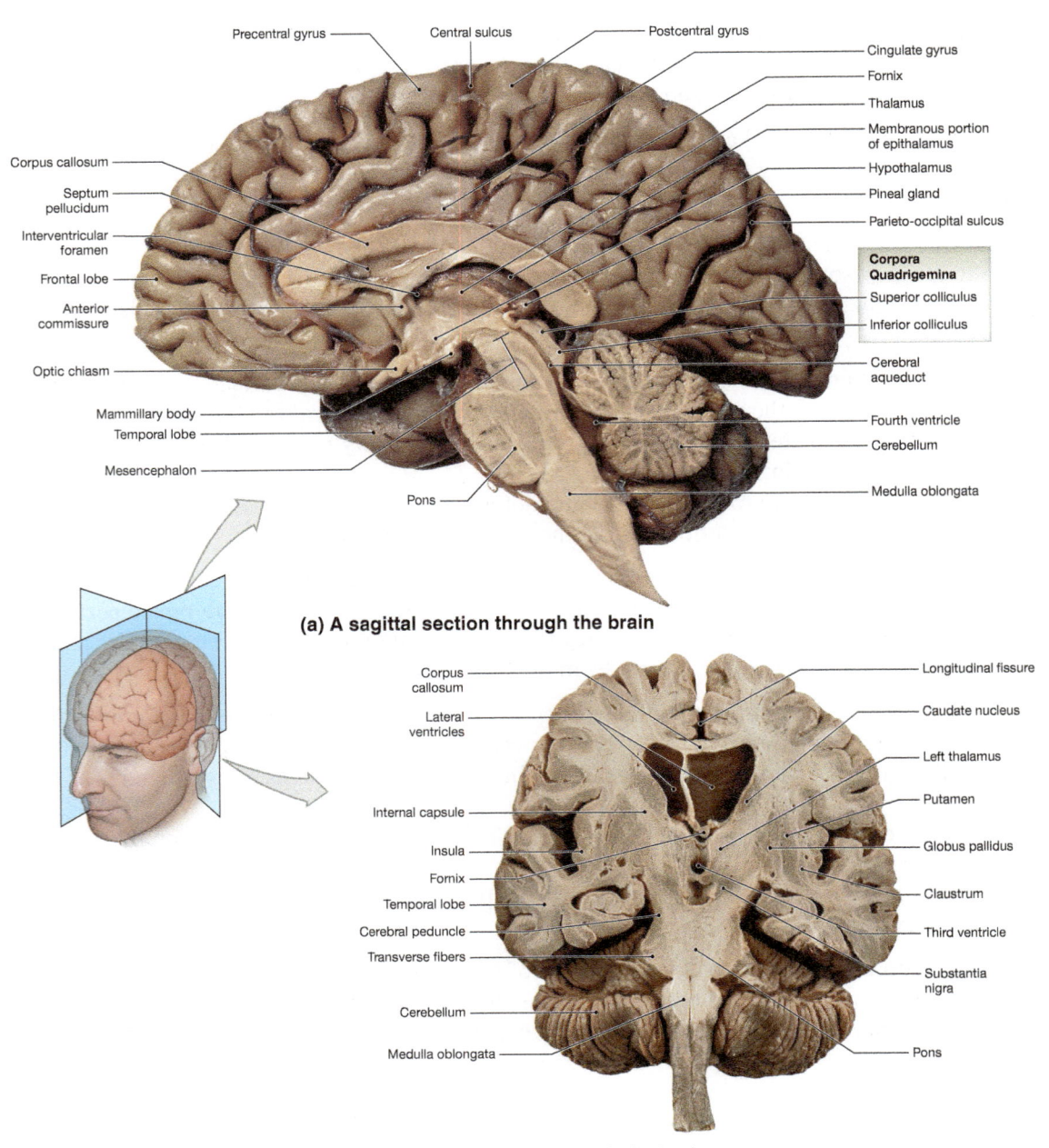

(b) A coronal section through the brain

From *Human Anatomy*, Ninth Edition, by Frederic Martini, Robert B. Tallitsch, and Judi L. Nath (2018), reproduced by permission of Pearson Education.

Figure 5.3 **Sectional Views of the Brain**

Gray matter of the cerebral hemispheres comprises the cerebral cortex. The cerebral cortex is made up primarily of neuronal cell bodies. Note the following features:

1. **Gyri** (singular=gyrus) are the "ridges" which rise between the sulci of the cerebral cortex. Two important gyri are discussed below:

    a. The **precentral gyrus** is located just anterior to the central sulcus. The precentral gyrus is the location of the primary motor cortex, which functions in conscious, voluntary movements

Complete Introductory Human Anatomy Lab Guide

of the skeletal muscles. **Pyramidal cells** (discussed in the histology section) are a type of neuron located in the precentral gyrus.

    b. The **postcentral gyrus** is located just posterior to the central sulcus. The postcentral gyrus is the location of the primary somatosensory cortex. The postcentral gyrus receives sensory information from touch, pressure, pain and temperature receptors.

2. **Sulci** (singular = sulcus) are conspicuous "grooves" etched in the cerebral cortex. Especially deep sulci are termed "fissures." Two significant sulci are the central sulcus and lateral sulcus.

    a. The **central sulcus** is a deep groove between the precentral and postcentral gyrus. The central sulcus separates the frontal and parietal lobes of the brain.

    b. The **lateral sulcus** is a deep groove separating the parietal and frontal lobes from the temporal lobe. The insula lobe of the brain is located deep to the lateral sulcus.

Lobes of the Cerebral Hemispheres

Each hemisphere is divided into five lobes based primarily on structural landmarks, such as gyri, and sulci that provide the boundaries. Some specific functions can be scribed to parts of lobes, but the boundaries between functional areas are less clearly defined. Areas of the cerebral cortex designated as "primary cortex" have direct connections to the thalamus, either sensory or motor. Association areas provide links between motor and sensory input. They help to put sensory stimuli into context and coordinate motor responses.

1. The **frontal lobe** is anterior to the central sulcus. The precentral gyrus in the frontal lobe controls such tasks as voluntary movement and learned motor skills. The frontal lobe is found in the anterior cranial fossa. The frontal lobe contains primary somatic motor cortex and somatic motor association areas.

2. The **parietal lobe** is located between the central sulcus and the occipital lobe. The parietal lobe contains the primary sensory cortex and somatic sensory association cortex.

3. The **occipital lobe** is posterior to the parietal lobe. The occipital lobe contains the primary visual cortex and the visual association area.

4. The **temporal lobe** is inferior to the lateral sulcus and is found in the middle cranial fossa. The temporal lobe contains the primary auditory cortex, the auditory association area, the olfactory cortex, and a portion of the region for speech interpretation.

5. The **insula** is located deep within the lateral sulcus, between the parietal and temporal lobes. Our understanding of its functions are incomplete, but include self-awareness, homeostasis and interoception.

White Matter of the Cerebral Hemisphere

White matter of the cerebral hemispheres is located in the deep regions of the cerebral hemispheres. The white matter of the cerebral hemispheres is made up primarily of neuronal axons grouped in functionally related **tracts** that pass to other areas of the central nervous system.

1. **Association tracts** connect structures within a single cerebral hemisphere.

2. **Commissural tracts** connect structures between the two cerebral hemispheres. The **corpus callosum** is an example of a commissural tract.

3. **Projection tracts** connect structures between one cerebral hemisphere and the spinal cord.

Lateral Ventricles

Lateral ventricles are spaces within each cerebral hemisphere that are filled with cerebrospinal fluid (CSF).

The two lateral ventricles are separated from each other in the midsagittal plane by a thin layer of tissue called the **septum pellucidum**.

All ventricles of the brain contain **choroid plexus**. Choroid plexus is composed of a collection of **permeable capillaries** overlain with a layer of **ependymal cells**. Choroid plexus is the tissue that produces CSF.

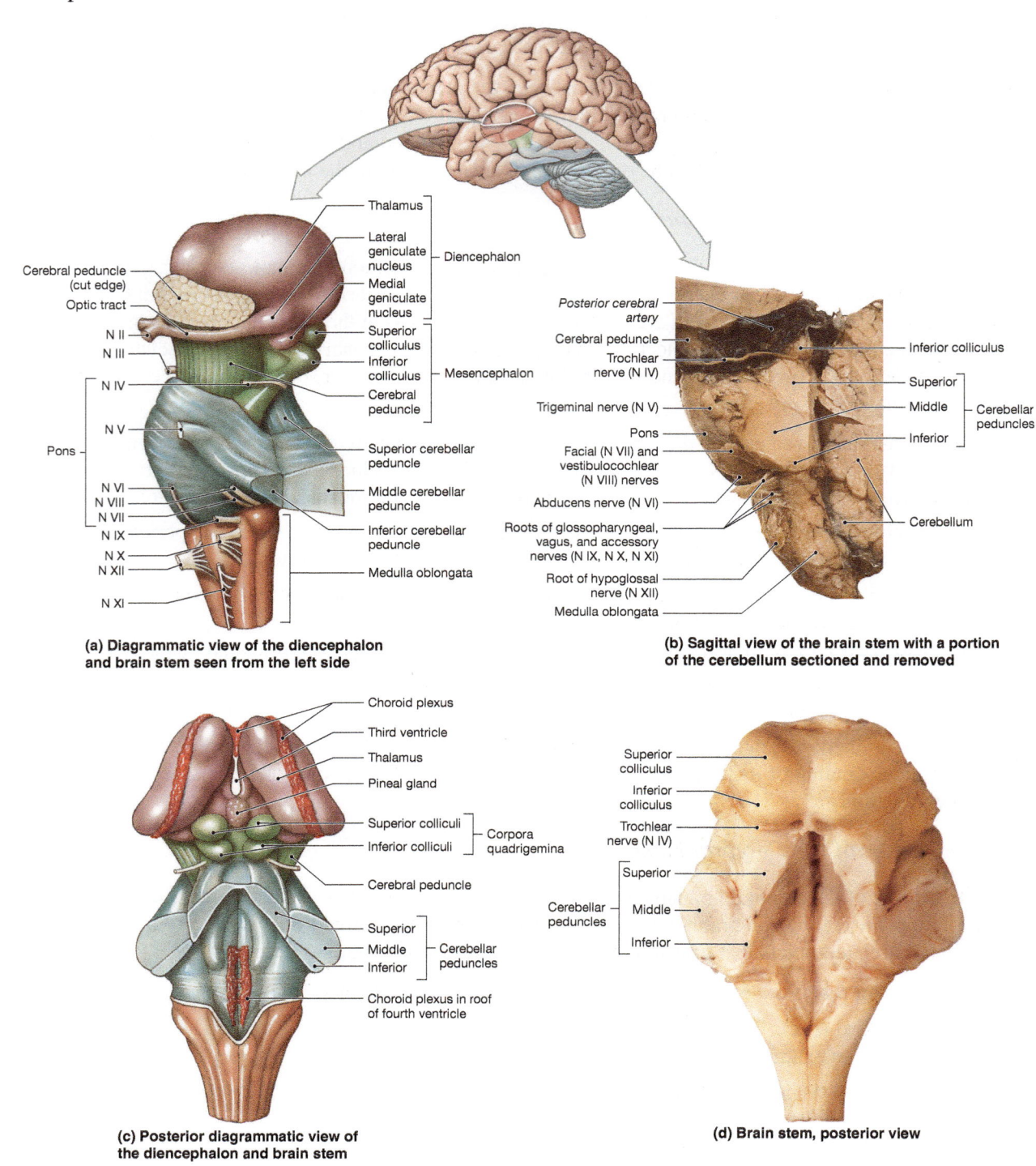

Figure 5.4   The Diencephalon and Brain Stem

112   *Complete Introductory Human Anatomy Lab Guide*

DIENCEPHALON

The **diencephalon** (the "between brain") consists mainly of two masses of nuclei, the **thalamus, epithalamus** and **hypothalamus**. (Fig. 5.4)

Thalamus

The **thalamus** is composed of two round structures, each comprised of over a dozen individual nuclei. The thalami are located just **rostral** (toward the nose) to the midbrain.

1. The thalami function primarily as "somatosensory relay stations." This means that the axons of somatosensory neurons synapse with the cell bodies of thalamic neurons and send somatosensory information to the cerebral cortex for processing.

2. The thalami also form part of the walls of the third ventricle (see third ventricle).

3. The **intermediate mass** (interthalamic adhesion) is a connection between the two thalami across the third ventricle. This structure is not present in all people.

Epithalamus
Pineal Gland

The **pineal gland** is involved in control of sleep-wake cycles (circadian rhythm). The pineal gland secretes the hormone **melatonin**. The pineal gland is the small, cone-shaped gland located posterior to the thalamus.

Hypothalamus

The **hypothalamus** is a bilaterally located group of nuclei lying inferior to the thalamus. It also forms part of the wall of the third ventricle.

The hypothalamus controls the release of a number of hormones and controls the output of the autonomic nervous system. Three structures related to the hypothalamus are discussed below.

1. The **optic chiasm** is formed by the decussation (crossing) of fibers of the optic nerve (cranial nerve II) and is located inferior to the hypothalamus. The optic chiasm forms the anterior boundary of the hypothalamus.

2. The hypothalamus is attached to the **pituitary gland** (hypophysis) by the neural connections of the **infundibulum**. The **infundibulum** of the hypothalamus is the neural connection with the pituitary gland. The infundibulum is located along inferior aspect of hypothalamus (see above). Recall that the pituitary gland sits in the sella turcica of the sphenoid bone.

3. The **mammillary bodies** are a pair of rounded nuclear masses located inferior to the hypothalamus. They relay signals between the limbic system and the thalamus.

Third Ventricle

The **third ventricle** is a thin slit at the midline, formed between the thalamus and hypothalamus on the right and left sides. The third ventricle is connected to the lateral ventricle on each side by an **interventricular foramen,** and with the fourth ventricle by the cerebral aqueduct. The third ventricle contains a choroid plexus for CSF production.

Mesencephalon

The **Mesencephalon (or midbrain)** is the portion of the brain between the diencephalon and metencephalon. It passes through the tentorial incisure. The midbrain contains the nuclei of the oculomotor and trochlear nerves (cranial nerves III and IV).

1. The **cerebral peduncles** are columns of neural tissue consisting primarily of descending **motor tracts**. The cerebral peduncles form the "neck" of the midbrain and are located between the pons and thalamus.

2. The **substantia nigra** is pigmented tissue located deep to the cerebral peduncles on the anterior side of the midbrain consisting of dopamine-producing cells.

3. The **corpora quadrigemina** (qwa-dri-JEM-in-ah) are two pairs of rounded structures containing the nuclei involved in visual and auditory pathways. They are located along the dorsal aspect of the midbrain.

    a. The **superior colliculi** are involved in eye movement when tracking a moving object.
    b. The **inferior colliculi** are involved with head movement in response to auditory stimuli.

4. The **cerebral aqueduct** is the passageway connecting the third and fourth ventricles; located just ventral to the **superior** and **inferior colliculi**. Cerebrospinal fluid flows from the third ventricle to the fourth ventricle via the cerebral aqueduct.

Metencephalon

Cerebellum

The **cerebellum** is part of the Metencephalon located inferior to the occipital lobe of the cerebrum. It is found in the posterior cranial fossa under cover of the tentorium cerebelli.

1. Functions of the cerebellum include aiding in balance, posture and coordination below the level of consciousness.

2. The cerebellum has two small hemispheres separated by a small dural fold, the **falx cerebelli**.

3. **Arbor vitae** is the white matter of the cerebellum. The arbor vitae branches extensively within the cerebellum.

4. Folia are ridges forming the grey matter of the cerebellum.

5. The cerebellum communicates with the **pons** and **medulla oblongata** through the cerebellar peduncles (see Pons below).

Pons

The **pons** is the anterior part of the Metencephalon, inferior to the midbrain. The pons contains nuclei of three cranial nerves, the **trigeminal** (V), **abducens** (VI) and **facial** (VII) nerves. The pons also includes projection fibers that make connections between various parts of the brain, especially with the cerebellum.

1. **Cerebellar peduncles** are three paired (superior, middle, inferior) bundles of tracts, which pass to and from the cerebellum. The middle cerebellar peduncle is the largest.

2. The dorsal surface of the pons forms part of the ventral wall of the fourth ventricle.

MYELENCEPHALON

Medulla Oblongata

The **medulla oblongata** comprises the myelencephalon, the most primitive part of the brain. It is inferior to the pons and contains the nuclei of the **vestibulocochlear (VIII), glossopharyngeal (IX), vagus (X), spinal accessory (XI) and hypoglossal (XII) nerves.**.

1. The **pyramids of the medulla** are ventrally located columns containing descending motor neurons. The left and right pyramids meet in the ventral midline of the medulla. Two prominences lateral to the pyramids are the **olives**. These are important landmarks for the identification of cranial nerves.

2. The medulla oblongata houses nuclei of the respiratory and cardiovascular control centers.

Fourth Ventricle

The **fourth ventricle** is a pyramidal space located between the pons and medulla, and the cerebellum. It is connected to the third ventricle by the **cerebral aqueduct** (see above). The fourth ventricle contains choroid plexus and three foramina which allow CSF to flow into the subarachnoid space. These foramina are the **median aperture** and two **lateral apertures**.

VI. CRANIAL NERVES

Cranial nerves are (with one exception) peripheral nerves that originate from the brain and extend to peripheral organs. Cranial nerves contain sensory, somatic motor or parasympathetic fibers, either singly or in some combination. Their nuclei are located within the brainstem and the fibers of cranial nerves III-XII appear to emerge from the brainstem along its ventral and lateral surfaces. (Fig. 5.5; Table 5.1)

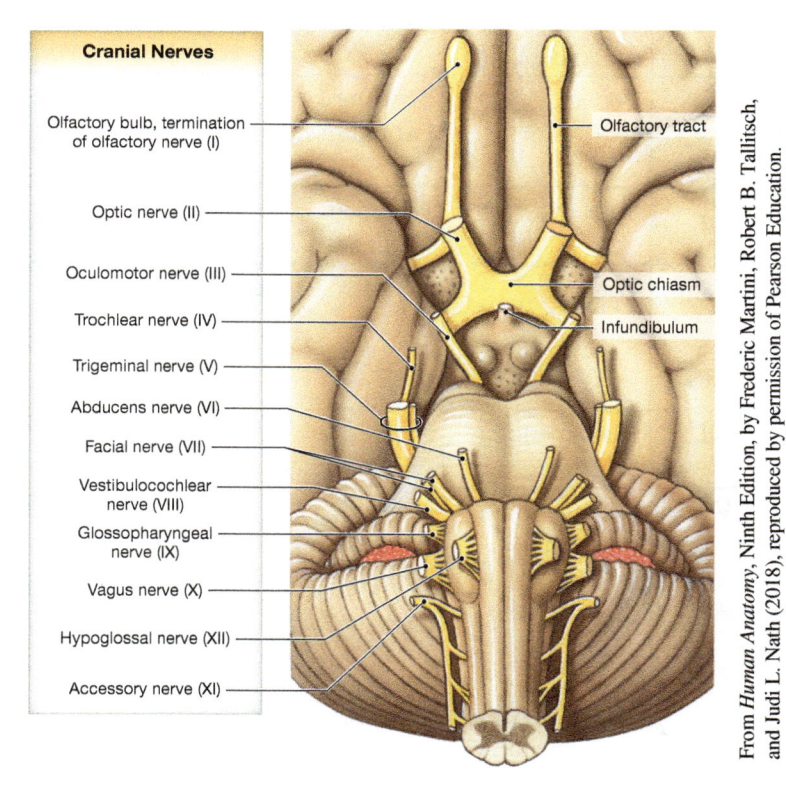

Figure 5.5 **Ventral view of the human brain, showing the cranial nerves.**

You are responsible for the following information about all cranial nerves:

1. The name and number of each cranial nerve (numbers of cranial nerves are always written in Roman numerals)
2. The function(s) of each cranial nerve
3. The point at which each cranial nerve emerges from the brain.
4. The opening in the skull through which the nerve passes.

The table above provides a concise method of studying **cranial nerves**. The mnemonic device, "O, o, o, to touch and feel very green vegetable, AH" will help you remember the *name* of each cranial nerve.

Table 5.1 – Cranial Nerves

Name	No.	Attachment to Brain	Skull opening	Functional Categories	Functions
Olfactory	I	Olfactory bulb	Cribriform plate	Special Sensory	Sense of smell
Optic	II	Lateral Geniculate body of Thalamus	Optic canal	Special Sensory	Vision
Oculomotor	III	Mesencephalon	Superior Orbital fissure	Somatic Motor, Visceral Motor	Eye movement, pupillary constriction
Trochlear	IV	Dorsal surface of mesencephalon	Superior Orbital fissure	Somatic Motor	Eye movement (superior oblique m.)
Trigeminal-Ophthalmic Div.	V_1	Pons	Superior Orbital fissure	Somatic Sensory	Sensory to face and eye
Trigeminal-Maxillary Div.	V_2	Pons	Foramen Rotundum	Somatic Sensory	Sensory to face, upper teeth and nasal cavity
Trigeminal-Mandibular Div.	V_3	Pons	Foramen Ovale	Somatic Sensory; Somatic Motor	Sensory to face, lower teeth and oral cavity. Motor to muscles of mastication
Abducens	VI	Pons-medulla junction	Superior Orbital fissure	Somatic Motor	Eye movement (lateral rectus m.)
Facial	VII	Pons-medulla junction	Internal Acoustic meatus	Special Sensory, Somatic Motor, Visceral Motor	Taste (ant. $\frac{2}{3}$ tongue), Motor to muscles of facial expression, Motor to salivary and lacrimal glands
Vestibulocochlear	VIII	Pons-medulla junction	Internal Acoustic meatus	Special Sensory	Hearing & equilibrium

Name	No.	Attachment to Brain	Skull opening	Functional Categories	Functions
Glossopharyn-geal	IX	Medulla dorsal to Olive	Jugular foramen	Special Sensory, Somatic Sensory, Visceral Sensory, Somatic Motor Visceral Motor	Taste (post. $\frac{1}{3}$ tongue), Sensory to middle ear cavity, Sensory to pharynx, carotid body, Motor to Stylopharyngeus muscle, Motor to parotid salivary gland
Vagus	X	Medulla dorsal to Olive	Jugular foramen	Somatic Sensory, Visceral Sensory, Somatic Motor, Visceral Motor,	Sensory to skin near ear, Sensory to pharynx, larynx, thoracoabdominal organs, Muscles of pharynx, larynx, Motor to thoraco-abdominal organs
Spinal Accessory	XI	Medulla dorsal to Olive	Jugular foramen	Somatic Motor	Motor to Trapezius and sternocleido-mastoid
Hypoglossal	XII	Medulla ventral to Olive	Hypoglossal canal	Somatic Motor	Motor to intrinsic muscles of tongue

VII. BLOOD SUPPLY OF THE BRAIN

1. Arterial blood reaches the brain from two sources, the **internal carotid** and the **vertebral arteries**.
   a. The **internal carotid artery** is a branch of the common carotid artery, which enters the cranium through the carotid canal. The internal carotid artery reaches the base of the brain to either side of the sella turcica.
   b. The **vertebral artery** is the first branch of the subclavian artery. The vertebral artery passes through the transverse foramina of cervical vertebrae to enter the cranium through the foramen magnum.

2. **Cerebral arterial circle** (Circle of Willis) is a circular anastomosis between the internal carotid and the vertebral arteries, which provides a continuous blood supply to the brain. The circle consists of specifically named branches and communicating arteries (Fig. 5.6):
   a. **Vertebral arteries** enter the cranial cavity through the foramen magnum.
   b. The **basilar artery** forms from the union of the vertebral arteries. The basilar artery passes over the ventral surface of the pons.
   c. **Posterior cerebral arteries** are the terminal branches of the basilar arteries. They supply the posterior region of the cerebrum.
   d. **Posterior communicating arteries** are branches of the posterior cerebral arteries. They join the internal carotid arteries.
   e. **Internal carotid arteries** enter the cranium through the carotid canal.
   f. **Middle cerebral arteries** are direct continuations of the internal carotid artery.

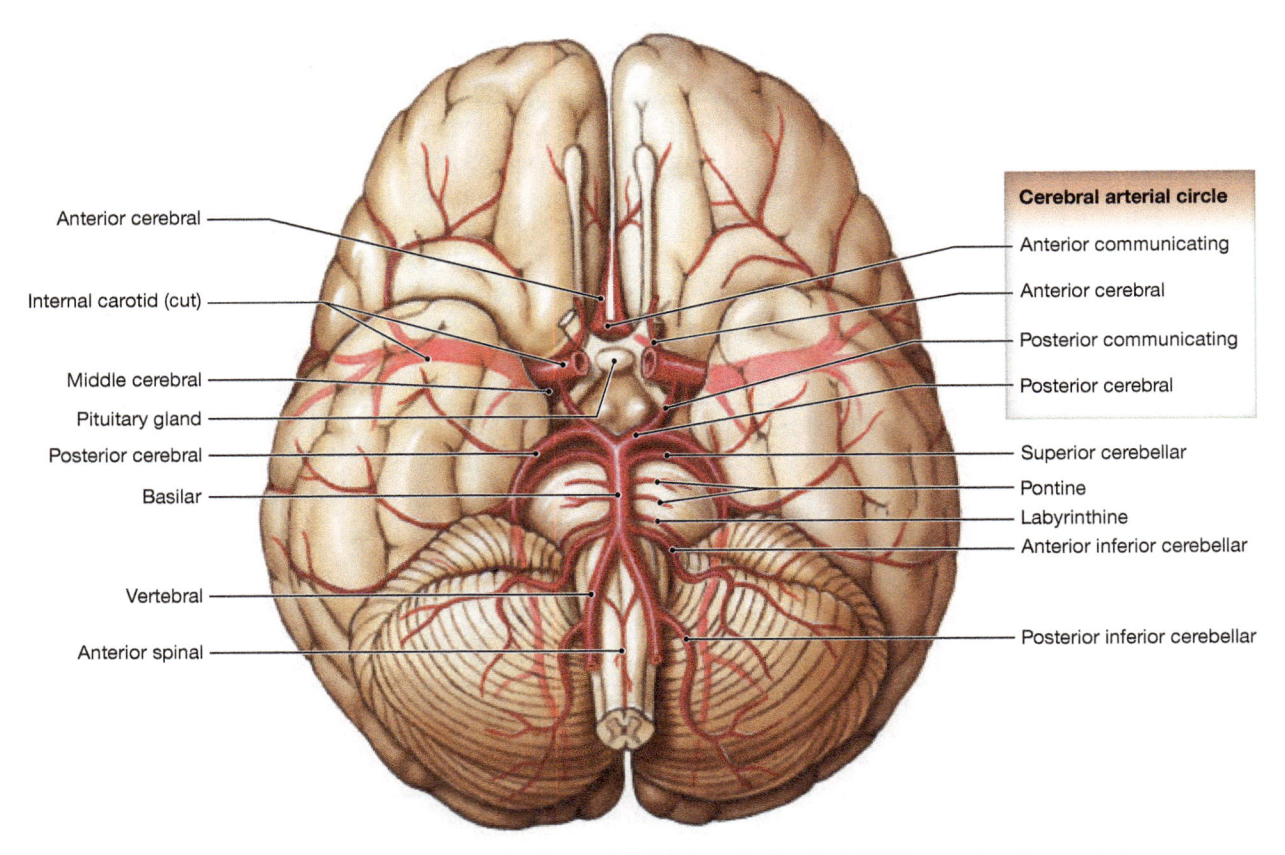

Figure 5.6 Major arteries serving the brain (ventral view).

From *Human Anatomy*, Ninth Edition, by Frederic Martini, Robert B. Tallitsch, and Judi L. Nath (2018), reproduced by permission of Pearson Education.

      g. **Anterior cerebral arteries** are also branches of the internal carotid artery.

      h. **Anterior communicating artery** connects the anterior cerebral arteries with each other.

3. Route of drainage of venous blood from the brain:

      a. The **cerebral veins** carry deoxygenated blood from the brain into the system of dural venous sinuses. They cross the subarachnoid space to reach the dural venous sinuses (Fig. 5.1).

      b. Dural venous sinuses form a network of channels formed between the two layers of dura mater. Only the cranial dura mater contains dural venous sinuses.

      c. These sinuses receive venous drainage from the cerebral veins and ultimately carry the deoxygenated blood out of the cranium through the jugular foramina and into the internal jugular veins.

d. Locate the grooves formed on the inner surface of the cranium by some of the dural venous sinuses.
e. Identify the following structures on models and within the cranial meninges:
- Superior sagittal sinus
- Transverse sinuses
- Jugular foramen
- Internal jugular vein

VIII. AUTONOMIC NERVOUS SYSTEM

FUNCTION

The autonomic nervous system provides motor innervation to smooth muscle, cardiac muscle, arrector pili muscles and all glands. As such it is the motor control over the cardiovascular, digestive, urogenital and endocrine systems. These are visceral organs and a synonym of "autonomic" is "visceral motor". Visceral organs also have sensory innervation, but this is visceral sensory, not autonomic. The autonomic nervous system has two subdivisions that are functionally and structurally distinct. These are the **parasympathetic** and **sympathetic** divisions.

For the autonomic nervous system, you need to know the origin, pathways, target organs, point of synapse and function.

ANATOMY AND DISTRIBUTION

Autonomic pathways consist of two nerve cells that communicate with a synapse. The first cell starts in the central nervous system, either the brain or spinal cord and extends to synapse in a ganglion outside the CNS. It is called the **preganglionic** nerve. The second cell extends from the ganglion to the organ that it innervates. This is called the **postganglionic** nerve.

1. **Parasympathetic** nerves serve the functions of "rest and digest." They help maintain homeostasis in the body, the ability of the body to maintain stable internal conditions.

    a. Origins—Brainstem nuclei of Cranial nerves III, VII, IX, X, and lateral column of sacral spinal cord segments 2-4.

    b. Pathways—Preganglionic fiber, Cranial nerves III, VII, IX to parasympathetic ganglia in head; Cranial nerve X to ganglia on effector organs; Pelvic splanchnic nerves to ganglia on effector organs

    c. Synapse—on effector organs

    d. Targets—Salivary glands, lacrimal glands, mucous glands in head; Smooth muscle, cardiac muscle and glands in thoracic and abdominal organs; Smooth muscle of lower abdominal and pelvic organs; External genitalia.

2. **Sympathetic** nerves prepare the body for an increase in activity, sometimes called "fight or flight" responses (Fig 5.7).

    a. Origin—Lateral column of gray matter in spinal cord segments T1-L2.

    b. Pathways

        i. Preganglionic fiber, spinal cord to sympathetic trunk; Postganglionic fiber, rejoins spinal nerve and distributes to territory of that spinal nerve. Postganglionic fibers to thoracic organs go directly from sympathetic trunk.

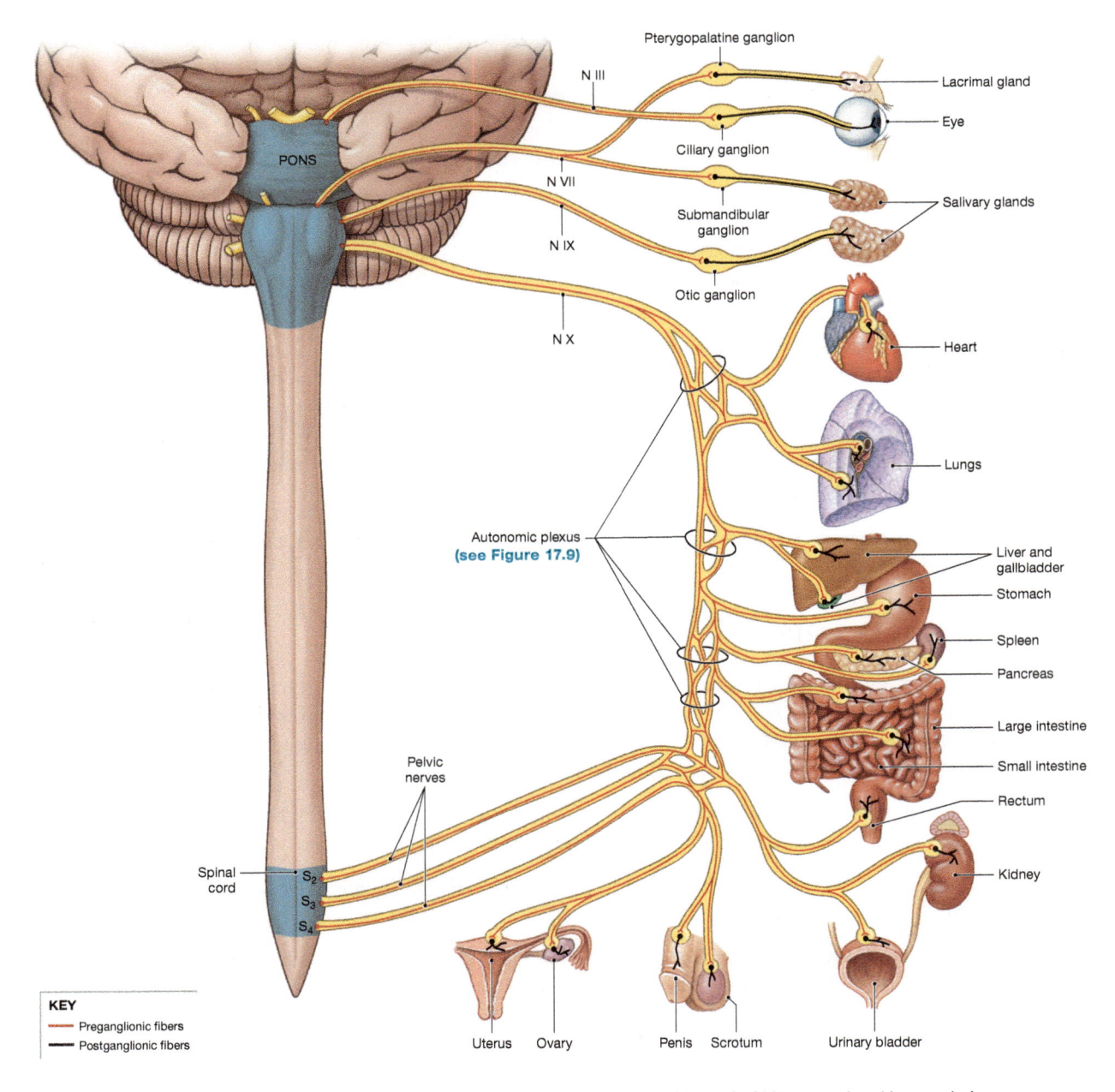

Figure 5.7 **Parasympathetic (Craniosacral) Division of the Autonomic Nervous System.** Red lines indicate preganglionic nerve fibers. Black lines indicate post-ganglionic fibers. Terminal ganglia of the vagus nerve and pelvic splanchnic nerves fibers are not shown; most of these ganglia are located in or on the target organ. (Note: S = sacral nerve.)

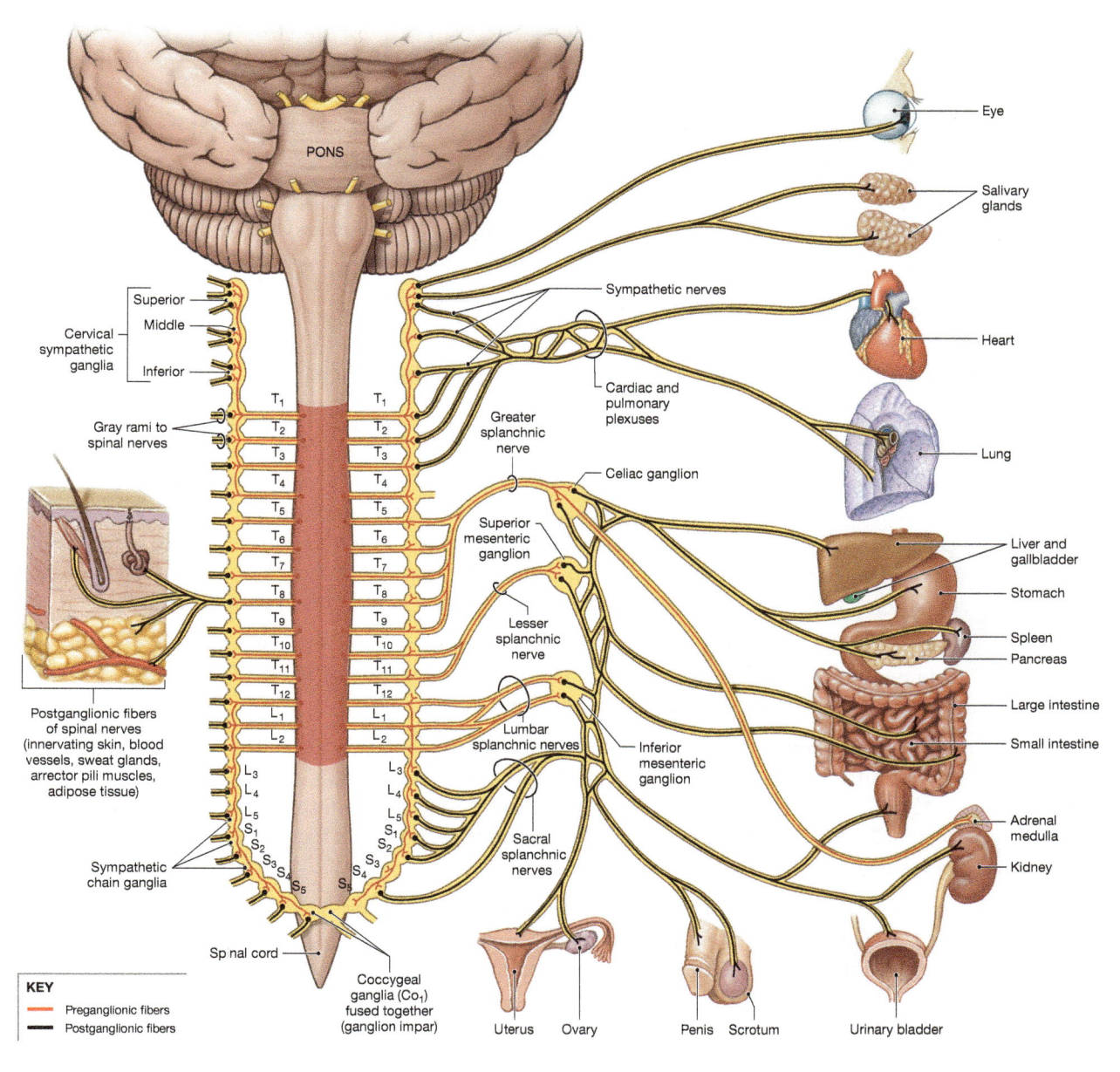

From *Human Anatomy*, Ninth Edition, by Frederic Martini, Robert B. Tallitsch, and Judi L. Nath (2018), reproduced by permission of Pearson Education.

Figure 5.8 **Sympathetic (Thoracolumbar) Division of the Autonomic Nervous System.** Red lines indicate preganglionic fibers; black lines indicate postganglionic fibers.

CHAPTER FIVE   *The Central Nervous System: The Brain & Spinal Cord*   121

ii. Preganglionic fiber, spinal cord to sympathetic trunk, then via splanchnic nerves to aortic autonomic ganglia in abdomen. Postganglionic fiber, follows arteries to effector organ in abdomen

c. Synapse—Sympathetic trunk for distribution to peripheral and thoracic organs; Aortic ganglia for distribution to abdominal and pelvic organs.

d. Targets: Peripheral blood vessels, sweat and sebaceous glands, arrector pili muscles; Thoracic organs (heart, lungs, great vessels); Smooth muscle and glands in abdominal organs.

IX. NERVOUS SYSTEM PATHWAYS

ASCENDING & DESCENDING TRANSMISSION OF INFORMATION

Somatosensory (Ascending) Pathways

1. Pathways begin in the periphery with stimulus to a **somatosensory receptor**. Receptors transmit somatosensory stimuli (e.g., fine discriminative touch, pressure, vibration, pain, temperature, proprioception) to first-order somatosensory neurons. These first-order neurons travel to the CNS within a peripheral nerve and enter the spinal cord along the **dorsal root**. Somatosensory neurons are pseudounipolar neurons and their cell bodies are located in the **dorsal root ganglia.**

2. Somatosensory pathways which continue to the **postcentral gyrus** of the parietal lobe synapse in the thalamus before continuing to ascend; hence the designation of the thalamus as a "somatosensory relay station." Review material on the thalamus.

3. The **first-order neuron** synapses (communicates) with a second-order neuron somewhere within the CNS. The information carried in somatosensory pathways ascends along a "chain" of 2-3 neurons to end in higher brain control centers, including the cerebellum and the postcentral gyrus (primary somatosensory cortex). In the postcentral gyrus, conscious recognition of a particular sensation takes place.

4. Most somatosensory pathways cross to the **contralateral** (opposite) side of the body somewhere within the CNS and continue to ascend to higher brain levels on that side. This crossing over is called **decussation**; it can be clinically important, but has no functional significance.

Somatomotor (Descending) Pathways

1. Somatomotor pathways begin in several higher brain nuclei, most notably the precentral gyrus (primary motor cortex) of the frontal lobe. They are arranged in two-neuron chains called upper and lower motor neurons.

2. The first neuron of a descending motor pathway is called an upper motor neuron. Cell bodies of many upper motor neurons are located in the cerebral cortex of the precentral gyrus. They send their myelinated axons through the brain and spinal cord as tracts within the white matter.

3. Upper motor neurons synapse on lower motor neurons within either cranial nerve nuclei of the brainstem or within nuclei of the gray matter of the anterior (ventral) horn of the spinal cord. Lower motor neurons are the motor neurons of peripheral nerves.

4. Axons of lower motor neurons exit the spinal cord through the ventral root. They travel to skeletal muscles within peripheral nerves and innervate skeletal muscle fibers at the **neuromuscular junction**.

5. Some somatomotor pathways cross (decussate) to the **contralateral** (opposite) side of the body somewhere within the CNS and continue to descend to brainstem or spinal cord levels on that side.

Study and Review Questions – The Nervous System

CHAPTER FIVE

Answers to these questions are found in Chapter Five of this Lab Guide.

1. From the definitions that you wrote down in Chapter Five concerning neurons, define the following:

    a. Nucleus _____

    b. Tract _____

    c. Bipolar neuron _____

    d. Multipolar neuron _____

2. List the three layers of meninges from external to internal _____, _____, and _____.

Answer the following questions regarding the ventricular system of the brain:

3. What are ventricles and where are they located? _____

4. What tissue produces the cerebrospinal fluid? _____

5. What are the functions of CSF? _____

6. Trace a drop of cerebrospinal fluid from its superior-most site of production to its site of drainage into subarachnoid space.
   _____
   _____
   _____
   _____
   _____

7. Name the lobes of the brain and one cortical processing area associated with each.

    a. The _____ lobe contains cortical processing for: _____ .

    b. The _____ lobe contains cortical processing for: _____ .

    c. The _____ lobe contains cortical processing for: _____ .

    d. The _____ lobe contains cortical processing for: _____ .

8. What hormone is secreted by the **pineal gland** and what is the hormone's function?
   _____

EXERCISES IN HUMAN ANATOMY

9. What are three functions of the **cerebellum**? _____,
   _____, and _____.

10. What are the 2 parts of the **corpora quadrigemina** and their respective functions?

    a. _____

    b. _____

11. What is the function of the **pyramids of the medulla**? _____

12. List the two arteries that are the arterial supply to the brain. _____ &
    _____.

13. What are two specializations of pia mater? _____ &
    _____

14. Describe the location of white matter and gray matter in the spinal cord.
    _____

15. Why are dural sinuses located in the cranial dura mater, but not in the spinal dura mater? _____
    _____

16. Which cranial nerves have a purely sensory function?
    _____, _____, _____.

17. Which brain structure is a "somatosensory relay station?"
    _____.

18. What type of nuclei are housed in the medulla oblongata?
    _____ and _____.

19. The corpus callosum is an example of what type of tract? _____.

126   *Complete Introductory Human Anatomy Lab Guide*

SIX

Organs & Muscles of the Head

LABORATORY MATERIALS

Sagittal head model
Models of ear, eye and tooth

I. MUSCLES OF THE HEAD REGION

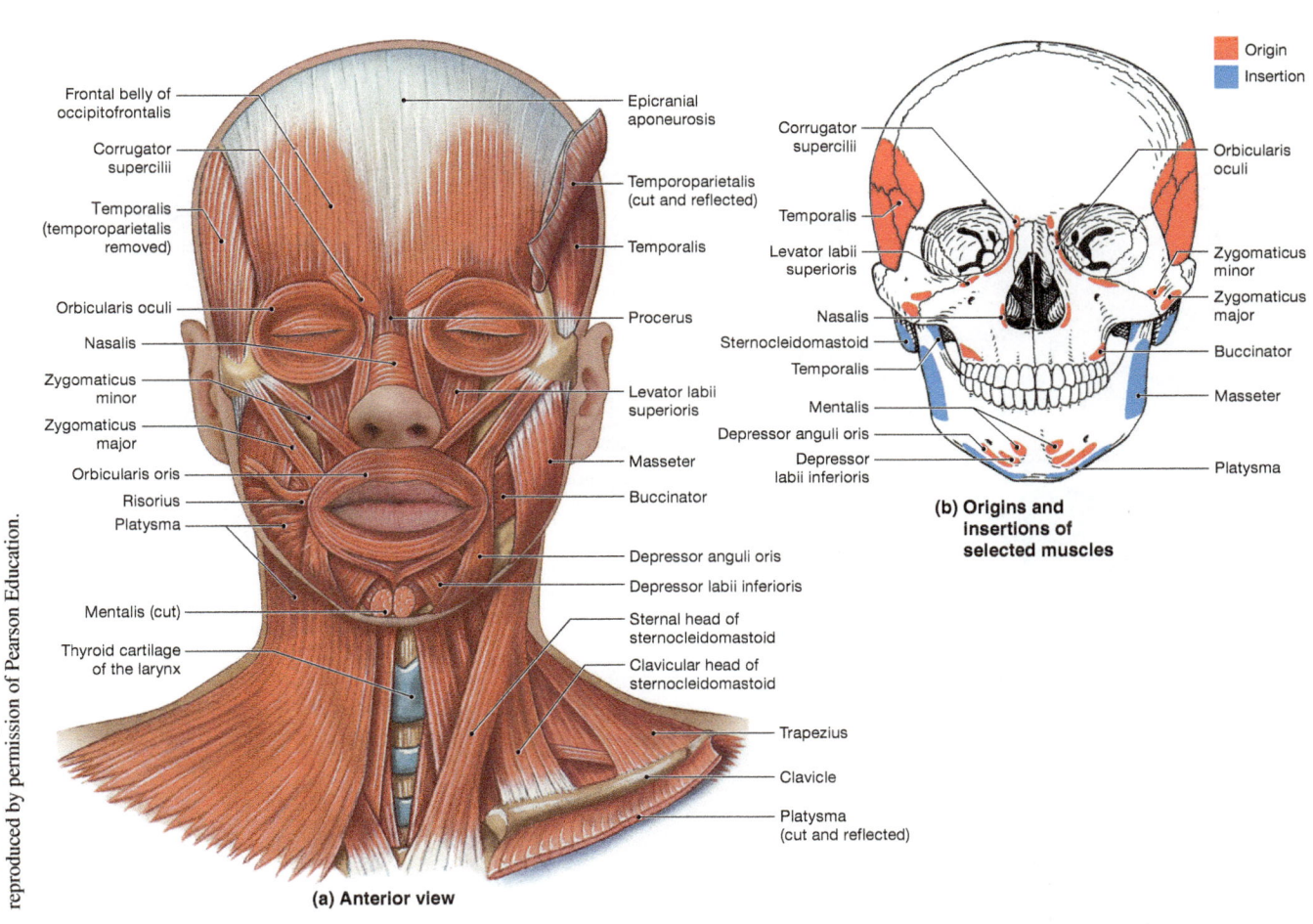

Figure 6.1 Muscles of the Head and Neck

MUSCLES OF FACIAL EXPRESSION

Many of these superficial muscles originate and insert within the subcutaneous tissue of the face. Their actions include the wide range of facial expressions that humans are able to produce. Muscles of facial expression are innervated by the **facial nerve** (cranial nerve VII). (Fig. 6.3)

127

1. The **epicranius** (also known as occipitofrontalis) is located under the scalp from forehead to occipital region. It includes a central aponeurosis. The epicranius acts to raise eyebrows and wrinkle the brow. The epicranius is formed from two muscles, the frontalis and occipitalis.

    a. The **frontalis** is the portion of this muscle at the forehead.
    b. The **occipitalis** is the portion of the epicranius at the occipital region.

2. The **orbicularis oculi** is a sphincter muscle of the eye, which acts to close the eyelids.

3. The **orbicularis oris** is a sphincter muscle of the oral region, which acts to close the lips.

4. The **buccinator** (BUK-sin-a-tor) acts to compress the cheek.

5. The **platysma** acts to draw the angle of mouth and the lower lip inferiorly. This muscle creates ridges of skin along lateral aspects of the neck.

6. The **zygomaticus major** acts to draw the angle of the mouth superiorly as in smiling.

7. The **depressor labii inferioris** acts to draw the lower lip inferiorly as in frowning or pouting.

(a) The temporalis and masseter are prominent muscles on the lateral surface of the skull. The temporalis passes medial to the zygomatic arch to insert on the coronoid process of the mandible. The masseter inserts on the angle and lateral surface of the mandible.

(b) The location and orientation of the pterygoid muscles can be seen after removing the overlying muscles, along with a portion of the mandible.

(c) Selected insertions on the medial surface of the mandible. See also Figures 6.3 and 6.14.

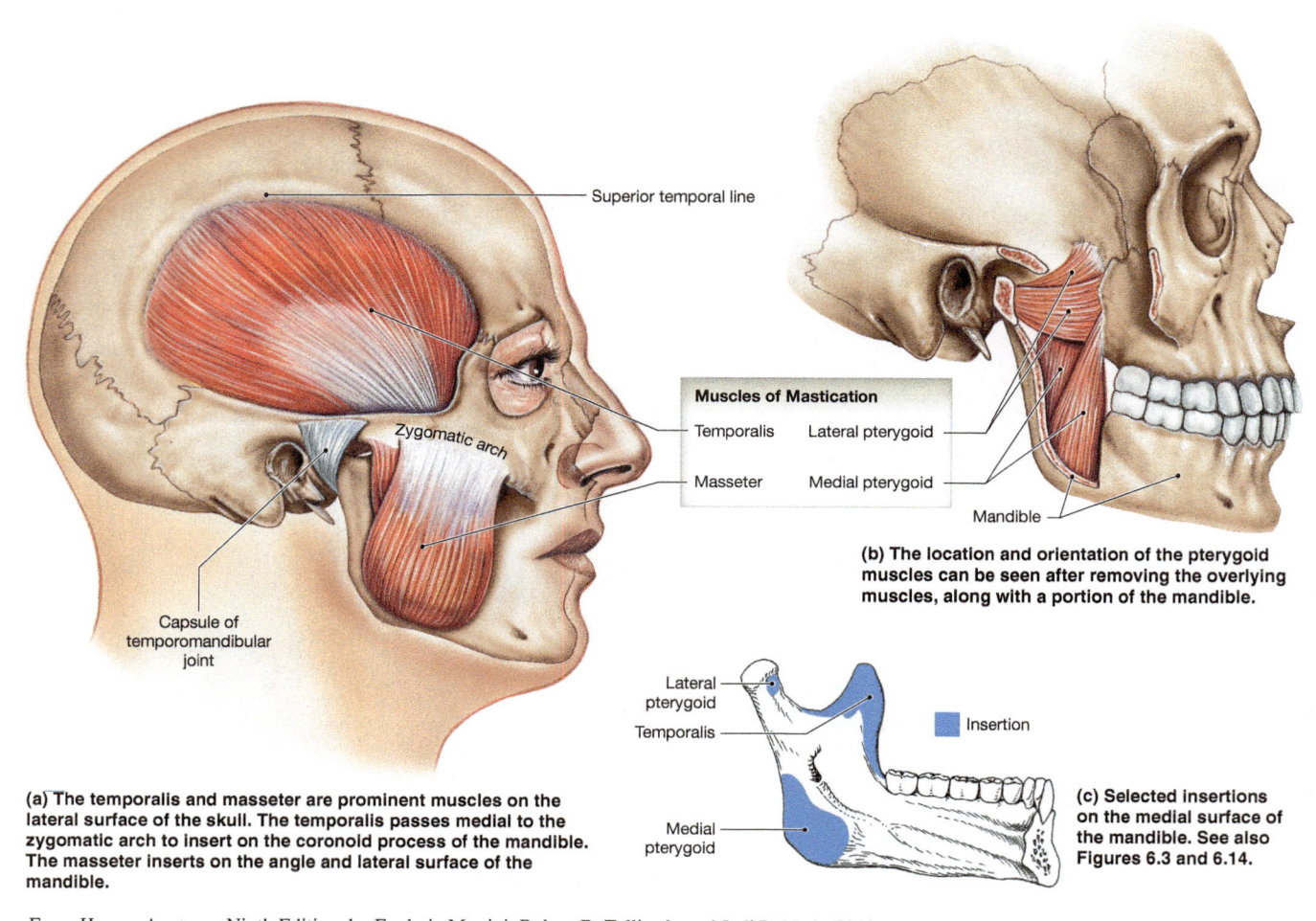

From *Human Anatomy*, Ninth Edition, by Frederic Martini, Robert B. Tallitsch, and Judi L. Nath (2018), reproduced by permission of Pearson Education.

Figure 6.2 **Muscles of Mastication.** The muscles of mastication move the mandible during chewing.

MUSCLES OF MASTICATION

Muscles of mastication act to move the mandible relative to the maxillae to produce the movements required for chewing. The mandibular division of the **trigeminal nerve** (cranial nerve V_3) innervates the four muscles of mastication. The muscles of mastication are the masseter, temporalis and medial and lateral pterygoids.

1. The **masseter** arises from the zygomatic arch and inserts on the lateral side of the mandible. It acts to close the jaws by raising or elevating the mandible towards the maxillae.
2. The **temporalis** elevates and retracts the jaw. It inserts on the coranoid process and acts to close the jaws and to pull the mandibular condyle back into the mandibular fossa of the temporal bone following wide jaw opening.
3. The **medial pterygoid** arises from the medial surface of the lateral pterygoid plate and inserts on the medial side of the mandible near the angle. It protracts and elevates the mandible, and deviates the mandible to one side when contracting unilaterally.
4. The **lateral pterygoid** arises from the lateral surface of the lateral pterygoid plate and inserts on the neck of the mandible and on the articular disc of the mandible. It protracts the mandible and deviates the mandible to one side when acting unilaterally (Fig. 6.2).

MUSCLES OF THE PHARYNX AND PALATE

The pharynx and palate are made of many small muscles and function in swallowing. These muscles are innervated primarily by the **vagus** nerve (cranial nerve X).

II. ORGANS OF THE HEAD

NASAL REGION

The **nasal region** includes cartilaginous and bony structures of the nose and structures within the nasal cavity.

1. Structures of the nose

    a. **External nares** (nostrils) are the openings to the outside.
    b. The **vestibule of the nose** is located just internal to the external nares and is lined with skin (non-keratinized stratified squamous epithelium) and hairs.

2. Structures of the nasal cavity

    a. **Superior, middle** and **inferior nasal conchae** are scrolls of bone projecting from the lateral nasal wall into the corresponding nasal cavity. They are covered with **nasal mucosa** (pseudostratified ciliated columnar epithelium).
    b. **Superior, middle** and **inferior meatuses** are the regions of the lateral nasal wall located beneath the corresponding nasal conchae. The **nasolacrimal duct** and the **paranasal sinuses** open into the nasal cavity within these meatuses. Recall that a meatus is a space or opening.
    c. The **olfactory region** is the area above the superior nasal concha. This area is covered with **olfactory epithelium**.
    d. The nasal septum is composed of the perpendicular plate of the ethmoid bone, vomer and nasal septal cartilage. These bones divide the nasal cavity into left and right halves and are also covered with nasal mucosa.

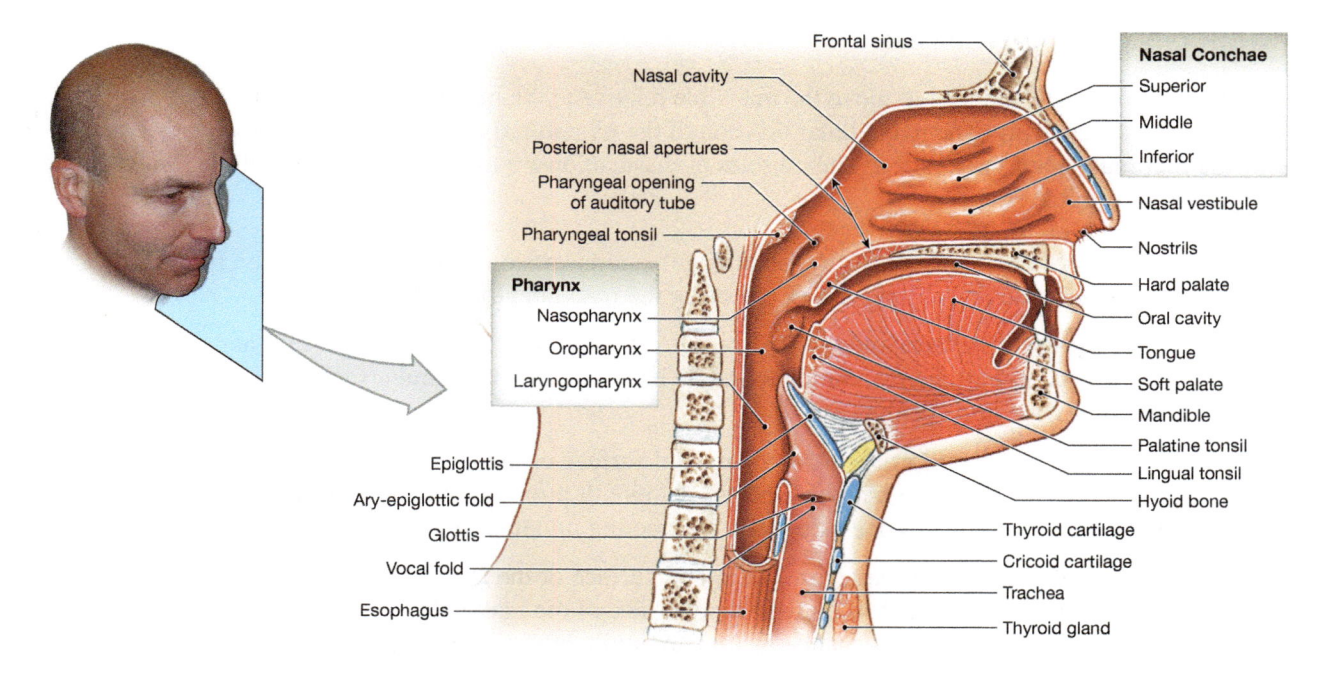

Figure 6.3 **The Anatomy of the Upper Respiratory Tract.** Sagittal section of the head and neck.

THE ORAL REGION

(Fig. 6.3)

1. The **oral orifice** and **lips** define the boundary of the oral cavity.

2. The **vestibule** is the space between the teeth and the inside of the lips and cheeks.

3. **Teeth** are located within the alveolar region of the mandible and maxilla. **Gingivae** (the gums) surround the base and root of each tooth.

4. The **oral cavity** is lined with oral mucosa, which includes non-keratinized stratified squamous epithelium.

5. The **fauces** frame the opening into the **oropharynx**. The borders of the fauces are the uvula, the palatoglossal and palatopharyngeal arches and the base of the tongue.

6. The **tongue** is covered on its dorsal surface with papillae. Taste buds (gustatory receptors) are located within many of the papillae.

7. **Lingual tonsils** are located at the base of the tongue.

8. The **hard palate** is the "roof" of the mouth. The hard palate is formed from the palatine process of the maxilla anteriorly, and the horizontal plate of the palatine bone posteriorly. The hard palate is covered with oral mucosa.

9. The **soft palate** is a muscular, posterior extension of the hard palate covered with oral mucosa. Note the **uvula** hanging from the posterior midline of the soft palate.

10. The **palatine tonsil** is a lymphatic organ located between the palatoglossal and palatopharyngeal arches. These arches are the anterior and posterior limbs of the fauces.

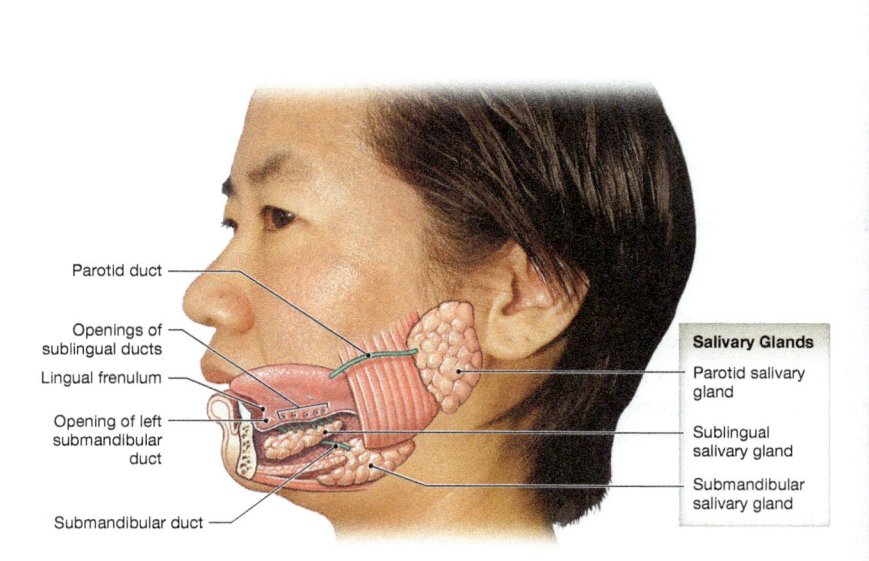

(a) Lateral view showing the relative positions of the salivary glands and ducts on the left side of the head. Much of the left half of the body and the left ramus of the mandible have been removed. For the positions of the ducts inside the oral cavity, see Figure 26.3.

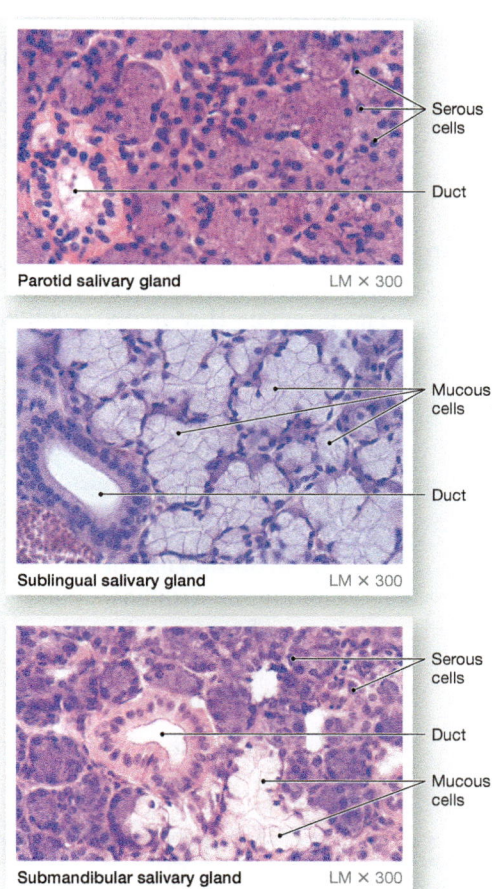

(b) Histological detail of the parotid, submandibular, and sublingual salivary glands. The parotid salivary gland produces saliva rich in enzymes. The gland is dominated by serous secretory cells. The sublingual salivary gland produces saliva rich in mucins. This gland is dominated by mucous secretory cells. The submandibular salivary gland produces saliva containing enzymes and mucins, and it contains both serous and mucous secretory cells.

From *Human Anatomy*, Ninth Edition, by Frederic Martini, Robert B. Tallitsch, and Judi L. Nath (2018), reproduced by permission of Pearson Education.

Figure 6.4 **The Salivary Glands**

CHAPTER SIX   *Organs & Muscles of the Head*   131

SALIVARY GLANDS

Salivary glands produce saliva that contains salivary enzymes. These enzymes initiate chemical digestion of food within the oral cavity. They are exocrine glands that secrete their products through ducts. Identify the following glands and associated structures.

1. The **parotid gland** is located anterior to the ear and superficial to the masseter muscle. The **parotid duct** crosses the masseter muscle and pierces the tissues of the cheek adjacent to the second maxillary molar.

2. The **submandibular gland** is located inferior to the mandible. The submandibular duct enters the floor of the oral cavity to either side of the **lingual frenulum** (a sheet of tissue connecting the tongue to the floor of the oral cavity).

3. The **sublingual gland** is located inferior to the tongue along the inner surface of the body of the mandible. Its multiple ducts open into the floor of the oral cavity along either side of the inferior surface of the tongue.

THE PHARYNX

The **pharynx** (**far**-ingks) is a tube of skeletal muscle that encloses the posterior aspect of the "throat." The three divisions of the pharynx are anatomically distinct and are defined below.
(Fig. 6.3)

1. The **nasopharynx** surrounds the posterior aspect of the nasal cavity, superior to the soft palate. Included within the nasopharynx are the openings to the **auditory tubes** and the **pharyngeal tonsils**.

2. The **oropharynx** surrounds the posterior aspect of oral cavity inferior to the soft palate, and is continuous with nasopharynx above. It receives ingested bolus of food from the oral cavity and inspired air from the nasopharynx. **Palatine tonsils** are located at its junction with the oral cavity and lingual tonsils are located at the base of the tongue. The inferior boundary of the oropharynx is the epiglottis.

3. The **laryngopharynx** surrounds openings into airway (larynx) and esophagus.

III. SELECTED SPECIAL SENSE ORGANS OF THE HEAD

AUDITORY & VESTIBULAR APPARATUS

The special senses of **audition** (hearing) and **equilibrium** are transmitted to the brain by receptors located within the inner ear. The **external**, **middle** and **inner ear** all contribute to the sense of hearing.

1. **External ear:** note the auricle and external auditory meatus.

2. The **middle ear** is an air-filled cavity bounded laterally by the tympanic membrane and houses the three auditory ossicles, the malleus, incus and stapes.

   a. The **tympanic membrane** (eardrum) is a delicate membrane separating the external from the middle ear.
   b. The **malleus** is attached to the tympanic membrane and articulates with the **incus**.

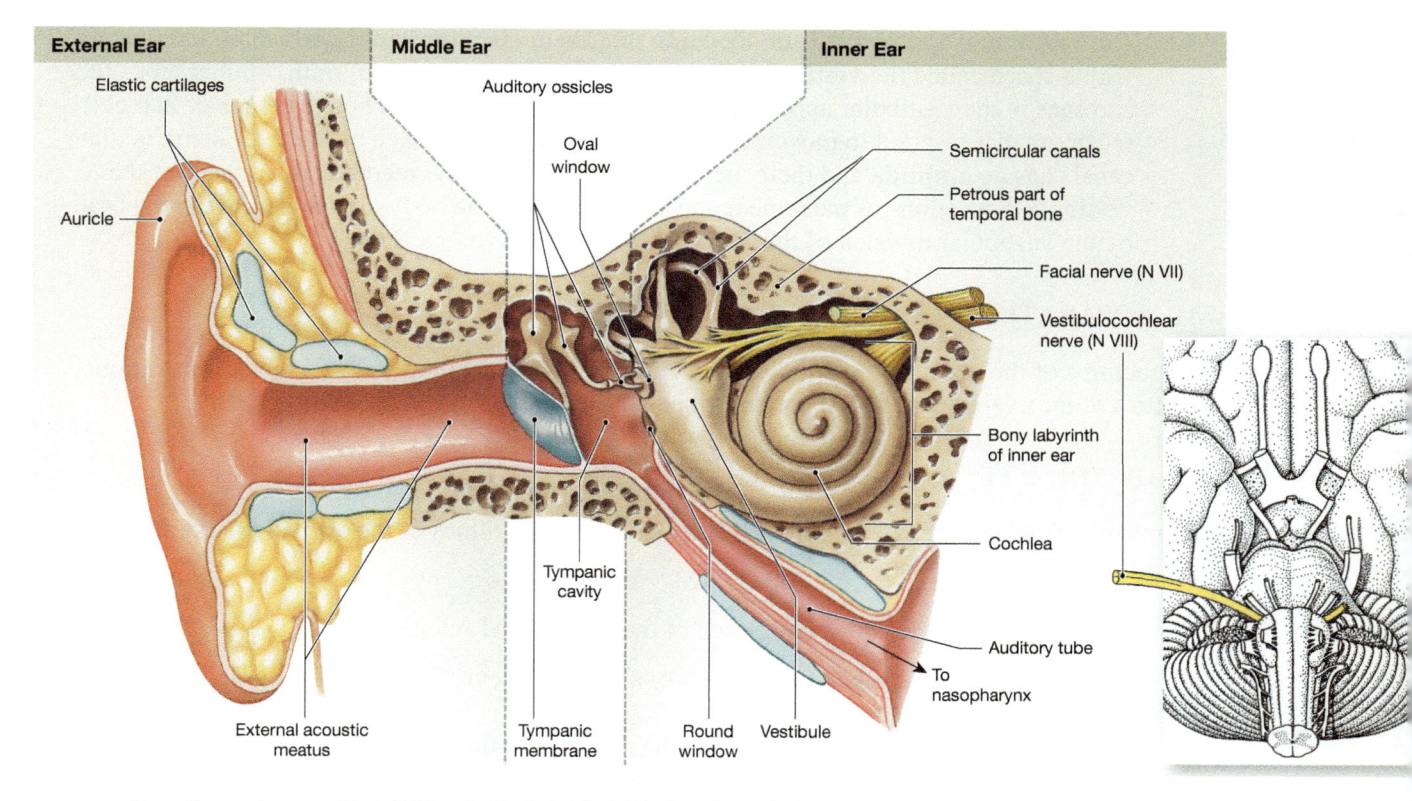

Figure 6.5 **Anatomy of the Ear.** A general orientation to the external, middle, and inner ear.

- c. The **stapes** articulates with the incus and the footplate of the stapes inserts into the **fenestra ovalis**, which is the opening into the inner ear.
- d. The **auditory tube** (Eustachian tube) is a passage that connects the tympanic cavity with the nasopharynx. This passageway allows air pressure in the middle ear cavity to be equal to atmospheric air pressure.

3. The inner ear consists of fluid-filled spaces in the petrous part of the temporal bone. The cavities are divided into the **cochlea** for hearing and the **vestibular apparatus** for equilibrium (Fig. 6.5).

    a. The cavities in the bone are filled with **perilymph**, a fluid similar to cerebrospinal fluid. These spaces are called the **bony labyrinth**.

    b. Within the perilymph-filled bony labyrinth are a series of interconnected membranous tubes and sacs filled with **endolymph,** which has a different chemical composition than perilymph. These spaces are collectively referred to as the **membranous labyrinth** and they house the **hair cell receptors** that transduce the stimuli that we perceive as sound and motions of the body.

    c. The **cochlea** is a spiral, snail-shaped structure that houses the hair cell receptors responsible for hearing. Collectively they are called the **Organ of Corti** and are found in the part of the membranous labyrinth called the cochlear duct. Movements of the fluids in the cochlea caused by sounds stimulate the Organ of Corti and these neuronal impulses are relayed to the brain by the cochlear division of the **Vestibulocochlear nerve** (cranial nerve VIII).

CHAPTER SIX   *Organs & Muscles of the Head*

d. The **vestibular apparatus** is divided into three **semicircular canals,** which all interconnect with a space called the **vestibule**. These are spaces of the bony labyrinth. Membranous tubes and sacs in the vestibular apparatus (also filled with endolymph) house groups of hair cell receptors that respond to movements of the head and body. Each of the three semicircular canals has an **ampulla** and there are two **maculae** within the membranous spaces of the vestibule. Sensations of movement and acceleration of the body are transmitted to the brain by the vestibular division of the Vestibulocochlear nerve.

VISUAL APPARATUS

The structures of the eye are studied most easily using anatomical models or textbook illustrations. Structures of the eyeball and vision are described below (Fig. 6.6).

TUNICS OF THE EYE

The three layers of the eyeball are referred to as "tunics." The tunics of the eyeball are the **fibrous, vascular** and **nervous tunics**.

1. The **fibrous tunic** of the eye is composed of the **cornea** and **sclera**.

   a. The **cornea** is the transparent anterior covering of the eye. The cornea is curved and helps to focus light entering the eye.
   b. The **sclera** ("white of the eye") covers the majority of the eyeball, with the exception of the region covered by the cornea. The sclera is composed primarily of collagen fibers. The extrinsic muscles of the eye (extraocular muscles) attach to the sclera.

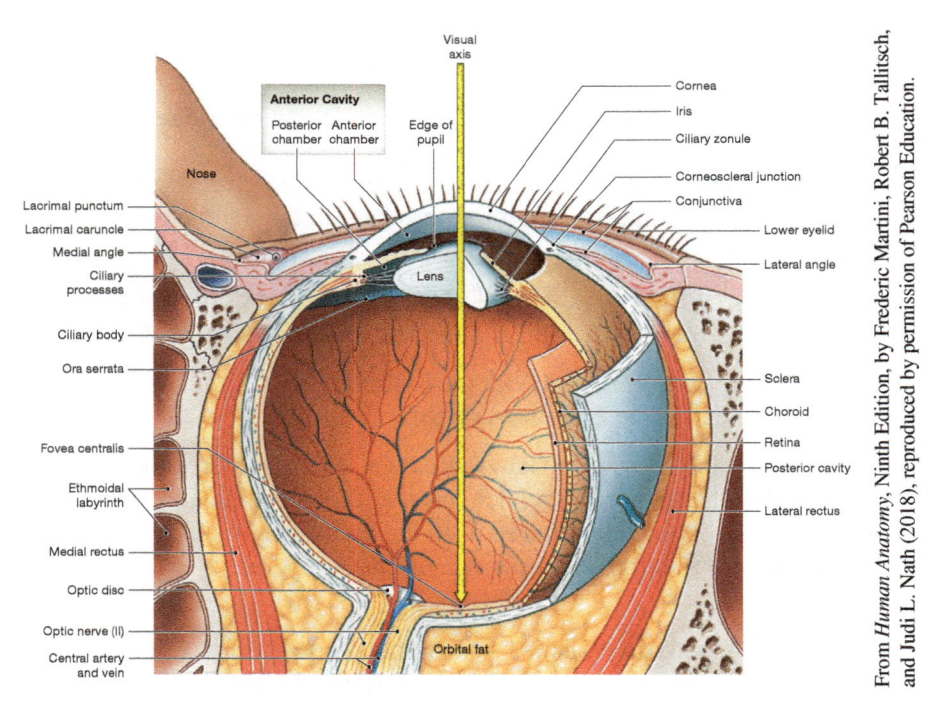

Figure 6.6 **Internal Structure of the Eye** (Sagittal Section). Diagrammatic view. The vitreous humor is illustrated only in the bottom half of the eyeball.

Complete Introductory Human Anatomy Lab Guide

2. The **vascular tunic** is composed of the **iris, choroid,** and **ciliary bodies**.
    a. The **iris** is the colored area of the eye surrounding the pupil. The diameter of the pupil is changed by the action of muscles in the iris.
    b. The **choroid** is a highly vascularized layer of the eye and provides nourishment to the retina.
    c. The **ciliary bodies** begin at the junction of the sclera and cornea. The ciliary bodies are connected to suspensory ligaments, which attach to the lens.

3. The **nervous tunic** consists of the **retina**, which is made up of receptors called **rods** and **cones.** The **optic nerve** (cranial nerve II) receives impulses from these receptors and passes this visual information along the optic tracts to the primary visual cortex within the occipital lobe of the brain.

OTHER STRUCTURES IN THE EYEBALL

1. **Aqueous humor** is a thin fluid located in the anterior cavity of the eye, between the cornea and the lens. The anterior cavity is formed from the anterior and posterior chambers of the eye. The **anterior chamber** of the eye is the space between the cornea and the iris. The **posterior chamber** is the space between the iris and the lens of the eye.

2. **Vitreous humor** is the gelatinous material in the **posterior** cavity. The posterior cavity extends from behind the lens of the eye to the retina.

3. The **pupil** is the opening in the **iris.** Light passes through the pupil to reach the retina.

4. The **lens** focuses images on the retina. It is a clear, almost spherical structure that is attached by suspensory ligaments to the ciliary body. Ciliary muscles change the shape of the lens based on whether one is focusing on objects at a distance or viewing nearby objects.

ACCESSORY STRUCTURES OF THE EYES

1. **Extraocular muscles** (extrinsic muscles of the eye) are small skeletal muscles attached to the bony orbit and directly to the eyeball. The extrinsic muscles of the eye produce eye movements. These muscles are innervated by the **oculomotor, trochlear,** and **abducens nerves** (cranial nerves III, IV and VI, respectively). A good mnemonic device for remembering the nervous innervation of the extraocular muscles is: $3(LR_6-SO_4)$. This means that the muscles receive their nerve from cranial nerve III (Oculomotor) except for the Lateral Rectus (CN VI) and the Superior Oblique (CN IV).

    The names of the six extraocular muscles are the **superior rectus, medial rectus, lateral rectus, inferior rectus, superior oblique,** and **inferior oblique.**

2. **Eyebrows** and **eyelashes** serve to prevent debris from entering the eyes.

3. **Eyelids** also prevent dust and debris from entering the eyes. Eyelids also keep the eyes lubricated with tears.

(a) Muscles on the lateral surface of the right eye

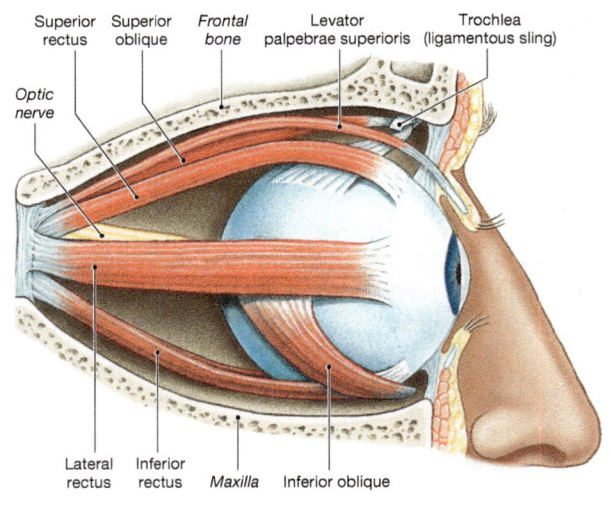

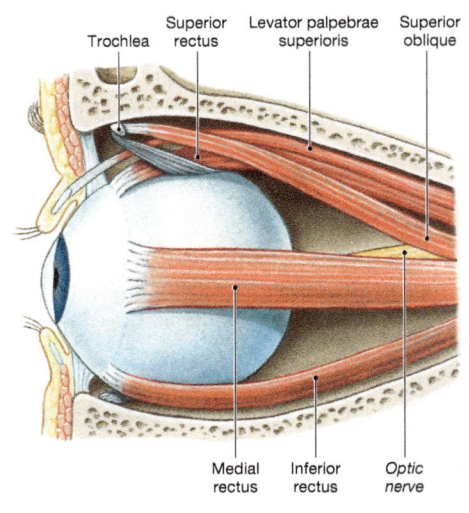

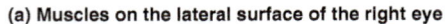

(b) Muscles on the medial surface of the right eye

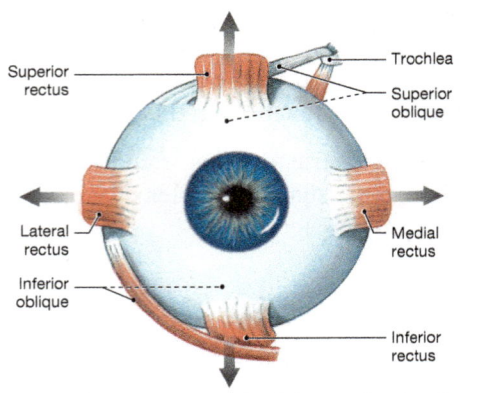

(c) Anterior view of the right eye showing the orientation of the extra-ocular muscles and the directions of eye movement produced by contractions of the individual muscles

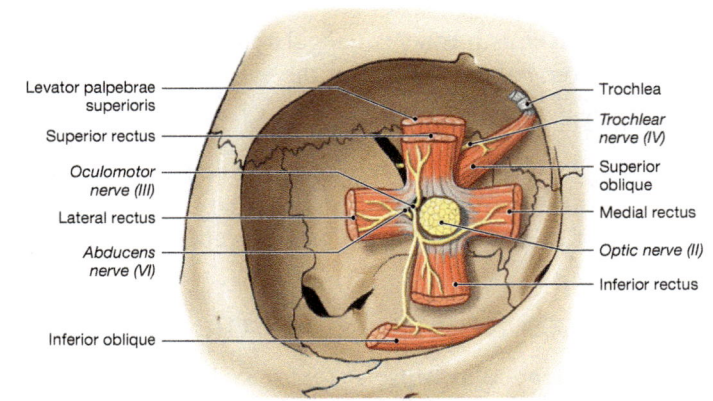

(d) Anterior view of the right orbit showing the origins of the extra-ocular muscles.

From *Human Anatomy*, Ninth Edition, by Frederic Martini, Robert B. Tallitsch, and Judi L. Nath (2018), reproduced by permission of Pearson Education.

Figure 6.7 **Extra-ocular Muscles.**

MUSCLE TABLE 6.1: EXTRA-OCULAR MUSCLES

Muscle	Origin	Insertion	Action	Innervation
Inferior rectus	Sphenoid around optic canal	Inferior, medial surface of eyeball	Eye looks down	Oculomotor nerve (CN III)
Medial rectus	As above	Medial surface of eyeball	Eye looks medially	As above
Superior rectus	As above	Superior surface of eyeball	Eye looks up	As above
Lateral rectus	As above	Lateral surface of eyeball	Eye looks laterally	Abducens nerve (CN VI)
Inferior oblique	Maxilla at anterior portion of orbit	Inferior, lateral surface of eyebal	Eye rolls, looks up and laterally	Oculomotor nerve (CN III)
Superior oblique	Sphenoid around optic canal	Superior, lateral surface of eyeball	Eye rolls, looks down and laterally	Trochlear nerve (CN IV)

4. The **conjunctiva** is the epithelial layer covering the inner surface of the eyelids and the outer covering of the eyeball. (Fig. 6.6)

5. The **lacrimal apparatus** includes the lacrimal glands, lacrimal ducts, lacrimal sac and the nasolacrimal duct. The lacrimal apparatus produces tears and allows them to drain from the eye to the nose.

IV. TEETH

1. The **crown** of the tooth extends above the **gingivae** (gums) and consists of the following regions.

    a. An outer layer of **enamel**.
    b. An inner core of **dentin**, a material similar to bone except that it does not contain osteocytes.
    c. The enamel and dentin surround the pulp cavity. The **pulp cavity** is the hollow region in the center of the crown that contains the neurovascular structures of the tooth.

2. The **neck of the tooth** is the constricted portion of the tooth which is covered by the **gingivae** and marks the boundary between the root and crown.

3. **Roots** of teeth are processes extending within the alveolar bone and help to anchor the tooth to the bone. The root consists of the following structures and material.

    a. The outer layer is composed of **cementum.** It is a highly innervated layer and softer than enamel.
    b. The inner layer of **dentin** is continuous with the dentin of the crown and neck of the tooth.
    c. A **root canal** is a hollow passage within the root and is continuous with the pulp cavity. The root canal conducts blood vessels and nerves (neurovascular structures) of the tooth from the alveolar bone to the pulp cavity.
    d. The **periodontal ligament** consists of collagenous fibers that connect the tooth root firmly to the alveolar bone.

CHAPTER SIX   *Organs & Muscles of the Head*

Study and Review Questions – Organs of the Head

CHAPTER SIX

Answers to these questions are found in Chapter Six of this guide.

1. What two muscles form the **epicranius**? _____ & _____

2. List the four muscles of mastication, their functions and their innervation.

   a. _____

   b. _____

   c. _____

   d. _____

3. List the three **salivary glands**, their types of secretion, and their location.

   a. _____

   b. _____

   c. _____

4. List the three cranial nerves involved in tasting.

   a. _____

   b. _____

   c. _____

5. What is the function of the **cochlea**? _____

6. What is the function of the **semicircular canals**? _____

7. What two structures comprise the fibrous tunic of the eye? _____ & _____

EXERCISES IN HUMAN ANATOMY

8. What three structures make up the vascular tunic of the eye?

   a. _____

   b. _____

   c. _____

9. Where is **vitreous humor** located? _____

10. Which tonsils are located in the oropharynx?
    _____ and _____.

11. The _____ contains the receptors for hearing.

12. Which eye structures are within or part of the anterior segment? _____
    _____.

13. The _____ is a tube connecting the tympanic cavity with the nasopharynx.

SEVEN

The Thoracic Cavity & Structures in the Neck

LABORATORY MATERIALS

1. Supine donor body and torso models
2. Preserved human hearts, lungs and dissected larynx
3. Models of hearts and trachea
4. Photomicrographs

I. HISTOLOGY OF THE THORACIC CAVITY

1. **Cross-section of trachea:**

    a. The mucous membrane of the trachea is composed of
        - **pseudostratified ciliated columnar epithelial tissue**
        - **lamina propria,** a type of connective tissue.
    b. Note the C-shaped cartilage ring of **hyaline cartilage** located around the anterior two-thirds of the trachea and external to the pseudostratified ciliated columnar epithelium.
    c. Observe the region of **smooth muscle** on this slide. The **trachealis muscle** is located between the two ends of the C-shaped hyaline cartilage rings in the trachea and primary bronchi.

2. **Section of primary bronchus:**

    a. Pseudostratified ciliated columnar epithelium lines the luminal surface of both the primary bronchi and the trachea.
    b. Hyaline cartilage forms part of bronchial tissue. Lacunae contain mature chondrocytes.

3. **Pseudostratified ciliated columnar epithelial tissue**

    a. **Goblet cells** are "wine glass" shaped single-celled glands found within pseudostratified ciliated columnar epithelium. The goblet cells secrete **mucin,** which, when mixed with water becomes mucus.
    b. Note the **cilia** at the apical surface of the columnar cells. Cilia are hair-like structures that beat to prevent pollutants from entering the respiratory tract.
    c. Not all the columnar cells reach the free surface, which contributes to the "stratified" appearance of pseudostratified ciliated columnar epithelium.

4. **Pseudostratified ciliated columnar epithelial tissue** (higher magnification)

    Identify:
    - Goblet cells
    - Cilia
    - Columnar cells
    - Lamina propria

5. **Pseudostratified ciliated columnar epithelium & lamina propria:**
   a. Pseudostratified ciliated columnar epithelium lines the trachea and primary bronchi.
   b. **Goblet cells** are located among the columnar cells and are characteristic of the epithelial layer in the trachea.
   c. Note lamina propria, which is a type of areolar connective tissue.

6. **Cross-section of secondary bronchus within the lung:**
   a. Note that **hyaline cartilage plates** have replaced the C-shaped rings. The cartilage plates are located around the circumference of the bronchus.
   b. Smooth muscle is also located in secondary bronchi.
   c. The structures of this secondary bronchus are also characteristic of segmental bronchi.

7. **Cross-section of bronchiole**:
   a. Hyaline cartilage is *absent* in bronchioles and from all more distal structures of the respiratory tract.
   b. This type of bronchiole is lined with **ciliated simple columnar epithelial tissue**.
   c. Cilia are present to prevent mucus from collecting in the respiratory bronchioles and alveoli.
   d. Goblet cells are **absent** from the bronchiole and all more distal regions of the respiratory tract.
   e. Smooth muscle surrounds the bronchiole.

8. **Section of bronchiole and branches of the pulmonary artery:**
   a. **Ciliated simple columnar epithelium** is the tissue lining these bronchioles.
   b. Locate the branch of the pulmonary artery within this micrograph.

9. **Terminal bronchiole:**
   a. Terminal bronchioles are the last part of the "conducting" portion of the respiratory tract.
   b. Locate examples of where respiratory bronchioles interrupt the smooth muscle of the terminal bronchiole.
   c. In regions where respiratory bronchioles interrupt the smooth muscle, gas exchange occurs between the epithelium of the respiratory tract and the surrounding capillaries.

10. **Respiratory bronchiole with branch of the pulmonary artery:**
    a. Gas exchange first occurs at the level of the respiratory bronchiole. **Gas exchange** occurs in the regions of the respiratory bronchiole in which smooth muscle is absent.
    b. Locate a branch of the pulmonary artery within this micrograph.
    c. Cells called **club cells** (Pneumocyte type II cell) secrete surfactant, which is a substance that reduces surface tension and prevents the walls of bronchioles from collapsing.
    d. **Respiratory bronchioles** are continuous with the distal end of the terminal bronchioles.

11. **Respiratory bronchiole with alveolar ducts and alveoli:**
    a. **Smooth muscle** surrounds much of the respiratory bronchiole, but certain areas have walls thin enough for gas exchange to occur. Respiratory bronchioles are the first structures in which gas exchange occurs.
    b. **Alveolar ducts** are continuous with the **respiratory bronchioles** and **alveolar sacs** branch from the walls of the alveolar ducts.
    c. **Alveoli** appear as out-pockets from the wall of the respiratory bronchiole and alveolar ducts.
    d. The lining of respiratory bronchioles is **simple cuboidal epithelium,** while alveoli and alveolar sacs are lined with **simple squamous epithelium.**

12. **Alveoli:**
    a. Alveoli are composed of **simple squamous epithelium.**
    b. Adjacent capillaries are also formed from simple squamous epithelium.
    c. The walls of alveoli and capillaries are the only tissues separating the blood in the capillaries from the air in the alveoli.
    d. Gas exchange occurs across the epithelial tissue of the alveoli and adjacent capillaries.

13. **Cross-sections of an artery, vein and nerve:**
    a. Note the thick-walled artery (muscular walls).
    b. Observe that the thin-walled vein has collapsed.
    c. Arteries and veins are composed of three tissue layers:
        - **tunica interna** (tunica intima)
        - **tunica media**
        - **tunica externa** (tunica adventitia).
        Arteries have a thick tunica media that is composed of smooth muscle.
    d. Compare the relative thickness of the tunica interna, tunica media and tunica externa (adventitia) of the artery and vein.
    e. Locate nerves within this micrograph, if possible. The nerve is solid, unlike veins or arteries.

14. **Cross-sections of an artery, vein and nerve:**
    a. Again, compare the flattened vein to the thick-walled muscular artery.
    b. Note the cross-section of three nerves and the adipose tissue surrounding these structures.

15. **Vasa vasorum within a large artery**
    a. Large blood vessels require their own blood supply.
    b. **Vasa vasorum** are the "vessels of vessels" and supply the outer region of the tunica media with oxygen.

16. **Elastic artery with vasa vasorum**
    a. The **tunica intima** is easily distinguished in a highly magnified artery. The tunica intima is formed from simple squamous epithelium.
    b. The **tunica media** is composed of smooth muscle and is very thick in an elastic artery.
    c. The **tunica externa** (tunica adventitia) contains the vasa vasorum. The vasa vasorum supply the outer region of the tunica media. The adventitia is continuous with surrounding connective tissues.

17. **Cross-section of a large vein:**
    a. Note the thick tunica externa of the vein. The **tunica externa** is the outer layer of veins and arteries. Veins have a very thick tunica externa (tunica adventia). The tunica externa is comprised of connective tissue.
    b. The small "holes" in the wall of the vein are the **vasa vasorum,** vessels of vessels. Vasa vasorum are found both in large veins and large arteries.
    c. Oxygen reaches large arteries and veins through the **vasa vasorum.** These large vessels must have their own blood supply because the walls of veins and arteries are too thick for gas exchange to occur across them.

18. **Cross-section of vein showing a valve:**
    a. Valves are located within veins, but not in arteries.
    b. The function of valves is to prevent the backflow of blood, and are usually seen only in the veins in the limbs.
    c. Valves can become incompetent and allow blood to pool. Pooling of blood in the veins of the thighs and legs is visible as varicose veins.

19. **Cortex and medulla of thymus:**
    a. A = Cortex of thymus. The cortex is the outer layer of the thymus
    b. B = Medulla of thymus. The medulla is in the center of the thymus.
    c. Arrow = Hassall's corpuscle. (Degenerating medullary epithelium)

20. **Medulla of thymus:**
    a. The thymus is an important organ in lymphocyte maturation.
    b. Note the large Hassall's (thymic) corpuscles. Hassall's corpuscles are limited to the medulla of the thymus.
    c. Hassall's corpuscles can be found in the infant thymus, but increase in number with age. These corpuscles are composed of degenerated medullary epithelial cells.
    d. The small, dark cells are lymphocytes. Among the lymphocytes are those that are attacked by the HIV virus.

II. ORGANS AND TISSUES IN THE NECK

LARYNX

The **larynx** consists of a cartilaginous framework with the vocal apparatus inside. It is located distal to the pharynx and is continuous with the proximal end of the trachea. The most important cartilages of the larynx are the **thyroid, cricoid, arytenoid,** and the **epiglottic cartilage**.

1. The **epiglottis** is a cartilaginous flap that closes over the trachea when food is swallowed, preventing food from entering the lungs.

2. **Thyroid cartilage** is the shield-shaped cartilage known as the "Adam's apple" and is located just inferior to the hyoid bone.

3. **Cricoid cartilage** is inferior to the thyroid cartilage. It is the only cartilage to make a complete ring.

4. A pair of **arytenoid cartilages** articulate with the cricoid cartilages. The vocal ligaments span between the arytenoid and thyroid cartilages. Movements of the cartilages and the ligaments open and close the rima glottidis

The **rima glottidis** is located within the larynx. It is the *space* between the right and left vocal folds through which air passes during breathing. **Note:** The **glottis** refers to the space **and** the vocal ligaments.

1. **Vestibular folds** do not act in sound production, but prevent substances from entering the glottis.

2. **Vocal folds** are located inferior to the ventricular folds. Sound is produced when the vocal folds vibrate, and the frequency (or pitch) of the sound depends on the diameter, length and tension of the vocal folds. Just inferior to the vocal folds, the epithelial tissue changes from stratified squamous to pseudostratified ciliated columnar epithelium.

Trachea

The **trachea** begins inferior to the larynx and lies anteriorly in the neck. It is made up of **C-shaped cartilage rings, fibroelastic membrane,** and the **trachealis muscle.** The **trachealis** is smooth muscle located between the ends of the c-shaped cartilage at the posterior surface of the trachea. The luminal surface of the trachea is lined with pseudostratified ciliated columnar epithelium. The trachea ends in the thorax when it bifurcates (divides) to make the primary bronchi.

Thyroid Gland

The **thyroid gland** is an endocrine gland located around the proximal end of the trachea, inferior to the thyroid cartilage. It is composed of two lateral lobes connected at the midline by an isthmus. Follicles of the thyroid gland secrete thyroid hormones.

Esophagus

The **esophagus** is a flattened muscular tube that connects distally with the stomach. The esophagus lies posterior to the trachea. The epithelium of the esophagus is stratified squamous for its entire length.

Blood Vessels in the Neck

1. The **right** and **left common carotid arteries** are lateral to the trachea within the carotid sheath. The **external carotid** and **internal carotid arteries** branch from the common carotid arteries. The internal carotid artery supplies the brain and has no branches in the neck. The external carotid artery has several branches in the neck and serves important structures in the neck, face and head. The branches of the external carotid are:

    a. **Superior thyroid artery** – to the thyroid gland and larynx
    b. **Lingual artery** – to the tongue
    c. **Facial artery** – to the skin and muscles of the anterior face
    d. **Occipital artery** – to the posterior scalp
    e. **Posterior auricular artery** – to region near the external ear
    f. **Superficial temporal artery** – majority of scalp
    g. **Maxillary artery** – to maxilla, mandible, muscles of mastication and nasal cavity.

2. The **right** and **left internal jugular veins** are tributaries of the subclavian veins. The internal jugular veins are parallel to the common carotid arteries.

3. The **vertebral artery** is the first branch arising from the **subclavian artery**. It passes through the transverse foramina of cervical vertebrae and then enters the foramen magnum bringing blood to the brain.

Nerves

1. The **phrenic nerve** arises from cervical nerves 3, 4 and 5. It supplies the respiratory diaphragm and lies on the anterior surface of the anterior scalene muscle.

2. The **vagus nerve** (cranial nerve X) lies within the carotid sheath along with the carotid artery. The vagus nerve is the most widely distributed of the cranial nerves and plays a significant role in parasympathetic innervation to thoracic and abdominal organs.

3. The **sympathetic trunk** lies to either side of the vertebral column. It brings sympathetic innervation from the thorax to the neck and head.

4. The **brachial plexus** originates from spinal nerve branches C5–T1. The brachial plexus passes between the **anterior** and **middle scalene muscles** in the neck.

MUSCLES OF THE NECK

1. The **platysma** is a flat, thin muscle of facial expression. It lies superficially in the lateral aspect of the neck and is attached to the mandible clavicle and sternum.

2. The **sternocleidomastoid** originates at the manubrium of the sternum and the clavicle and inserts at the mastoid process of the temporal bone.

3. The **scalene muscles** originate at the transverse processes of cervical vertebrae 2–7 and insert on the superior surfaces of ribs 1 and 2. The **brachial plexus** passes between the anterior and middle scalene muscles.

4. The **suprahyoid muscle group** is located *superior* to the hyoid bone and move the larynx superiorly during swallowing. The suprahyoid muscles include the **digastric, stylohyoid, mylohyoid** and **geniohyoid** muscles. In general, these muscles move the hyoid bone and aid in swallowing.

5. The **infrahyoid muscle group** is located *inferior* to the hyoid bone and depresses the hyoid bone and larynx during swallowing. The infrahyoid muscles include the **sternohyoid, sternothyroid, omohyoid,** and **thyrohyoid** muscles. The infrahyoid muscles depress the larynx and depress and retract the hyoid bone.

III. THE THORACIC CAVITY

BOUNDARIES OF THE THORACIC CAVITY

1. The **superior boundary** is the cervical fascia above the first rib.

2. The **inferior boundary** is the diaphragm. The **diaphragm** originates at the xiphoid process, ribs 7–12 and the anterior surface of lumbar vertebrae.

3. The **anterior boundary** is the sternum and costal cartilages.

4. **Thoracic vertebrae** form the posterior boundary of the thoracic cavity.

5. **Ribs** and **intercostal muscles** form the lateral boundary of the thoracic cavity.

PLEURAE

The **pleurae** are a double-layered membrane formed from epithelium and connective tissue. Layers of the pleural membrane are named according to the structures to which they attach. The **pleural cavity** is the potential space formed between the visceral and parietal pleura. A potential space means that there is actually no space in life, but the two membranes are not physically attached and a space could exist between them (Fig. 7.1).

1. **Parietal pleura** is the portion of the pleura that lines the chest cavity.

2. **Visceral pleura** is the portion of the pleura that covers the surface of lungs.

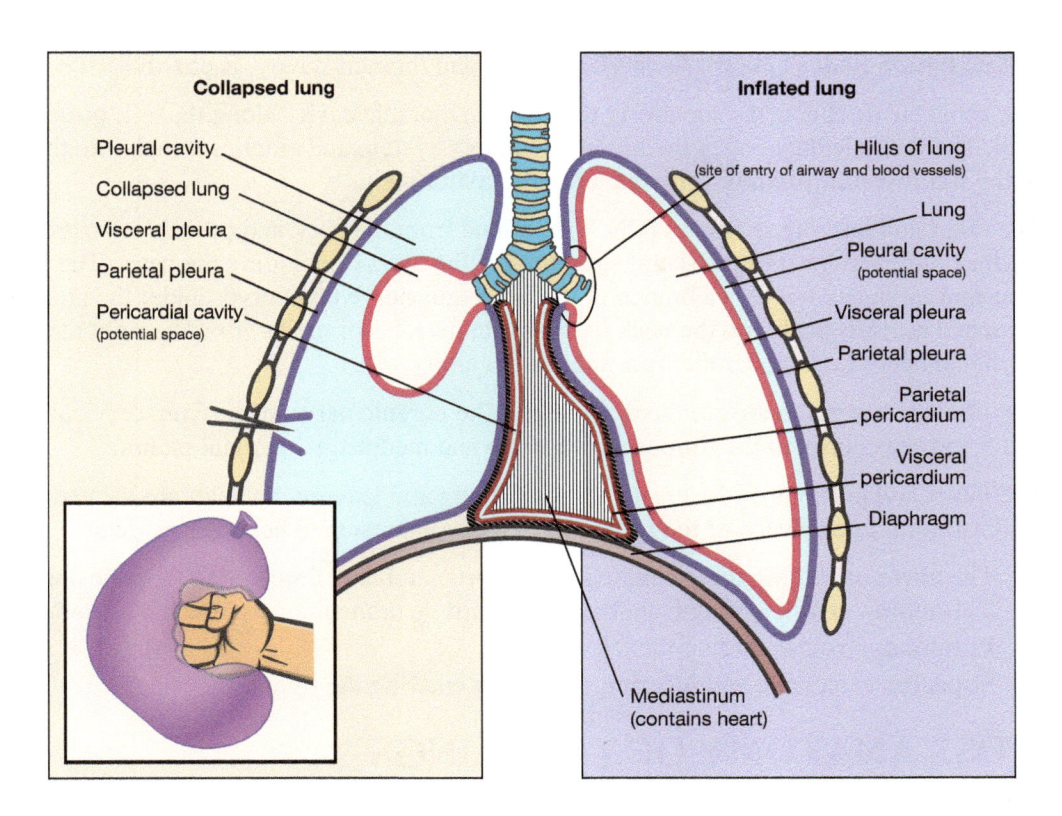

Figure 7.1 **Schematic of lining of pleural and pericardial cavities in a coronal section.** Under normal conditions no space exists between the visceral and parietal membranes (the pericardial cavity and lung on right). The collapsed lung (left) could result from a penetrating wound that would allow air to enter the pleural cavity. **Inset:** A fist pushing into an under-inflated balloon illustrates the concept of pleurae and pericardia. The surface of the balloon in contact with the fist represents the visceral membrane while the remainder of the balloon represents the parietal membrane. Although the surfaces have different designations, like the balloon, they are continuous with each other.

THE MEDIASTINUM

The **mediastinum** is the area between the right and left lung, which is bounded laterally by the lungs, anteriorly by the sternum, posteriorly by the thoracic vertebrae and inferiorly by the diaphragm. Structures found within the mediastinum include the heart and great vessels, trachea, esophagus, thoracic duct and important nerves.

1. The **thymus** is an endocrine gland overlying the anterior surface of the heart. The thymus of elderly people is usually reduced in size, and in prosected donor bodies any remaining thymus tissue has been removed to facilitate study of the heart and great vessels.

2. The **trachea** continues from the neck into the mediastinum and divides into the right and left primary bronchi.

3. The **esophagus** is posterior to the trachea (and heart) and is continuous at its inferior end with the stomach. The stomach and esophagus join at the esophageal (or cardiac) sphincter, just inferior to the diaphragm.

CHAPTER SEVEN   *The Thoracic Cavity & Structures in the Neck*

4. Locate **lymph nodes** in both the cervical region and thoracic cavity, if possible.

5. The **thoracic duct** courses superiorly through the thoracic cavity along the left, posterior chest wall. The thoracic duct enters the blood circulatory system and empties lymph into the junction of the **left internal jugular vein** and **left subclavian vein.**

6. The **right** and **left vagus nerves** (CN X) continue from the neck and pass through the mediastinum and innervate visceral structures of the thorax, including the heart. The left recurrent laryngeal nerve is a branch of the left vagus nerve that curves under the arch of the aorta and ascends back into the neck to innervate muscles of the larynx. The right recurrent laryngeal nerve turns under the right subclavian artery.

7. The **phrenic nerves** innervate the diaphragm. The phrenic nerve arises from cervical nerves 3, 4 and 5 and pass between the fibrous pericardium and mediastinal parietal pleura.

8. The **heart** and portions of the great vessels entering and leaving the heart are located within the mediastinum. Locate each of the following vessels on preserved hearts or models.

    - The **aorta**, including the ascending aorta, aortic arch and descending thoracic aorta
    - **Pulmonary trunk** arising from the right ventricle branching to pulmonary arteries
    - **Pulmonary veins** entering the left atrium
    - **Superior vena cava** and **inferior vena cava** entering the right atrium

IV. GROSS ANATOMY OF THE LUNGS

The **lungs** are paired organs consisting primarily of alveoli and branching bronchial tubes. The right and left lungs are structurally similar. The right lung has three lobes and the left lung has only two.

SURFACES AND REGIONS OF THE LUNG

- The **apex** of the lung is the superiorly pointing, cone-shaped part of the lung.
- The **hilus** is a passageway in the medial surface of each lung through which blood vessels and bronchi enter and exit the lung.
- The **root** of the lung consists of the pulmonary arteries, pulmonary veins, primary bronchi, nerves and lymph vessels. Each lung is anchored in the pleural cavity by these structures.
- The **costal surface** is the part of the lung that touches the inner side of the ribs and intercostal muscles.
- The **mediastinal surface** of each lung faces the heart. The mediastinal surface contains the hilus of the lungs.
- The **diaphragmatic surface** (base) of the lung is the concave, inferior surface of the lung that touches the superior border of the diaphragm.

STRUCTURE OF THE LEFT LUNG

The left lung has two lobes, the **superior lobe** and the **inferior lobe**.

a. The **oblique fissure** separates the inferior from the superior lobe.
b. The **cardiac impression** and **groove for the aorta** are two distinct impressions on the medial surface of the left lung.

STRUCTURE OF THE RIGHT LUNG

The right lung has three lobes, the **superior lobe, middle lobe** and **inferior lobe**.

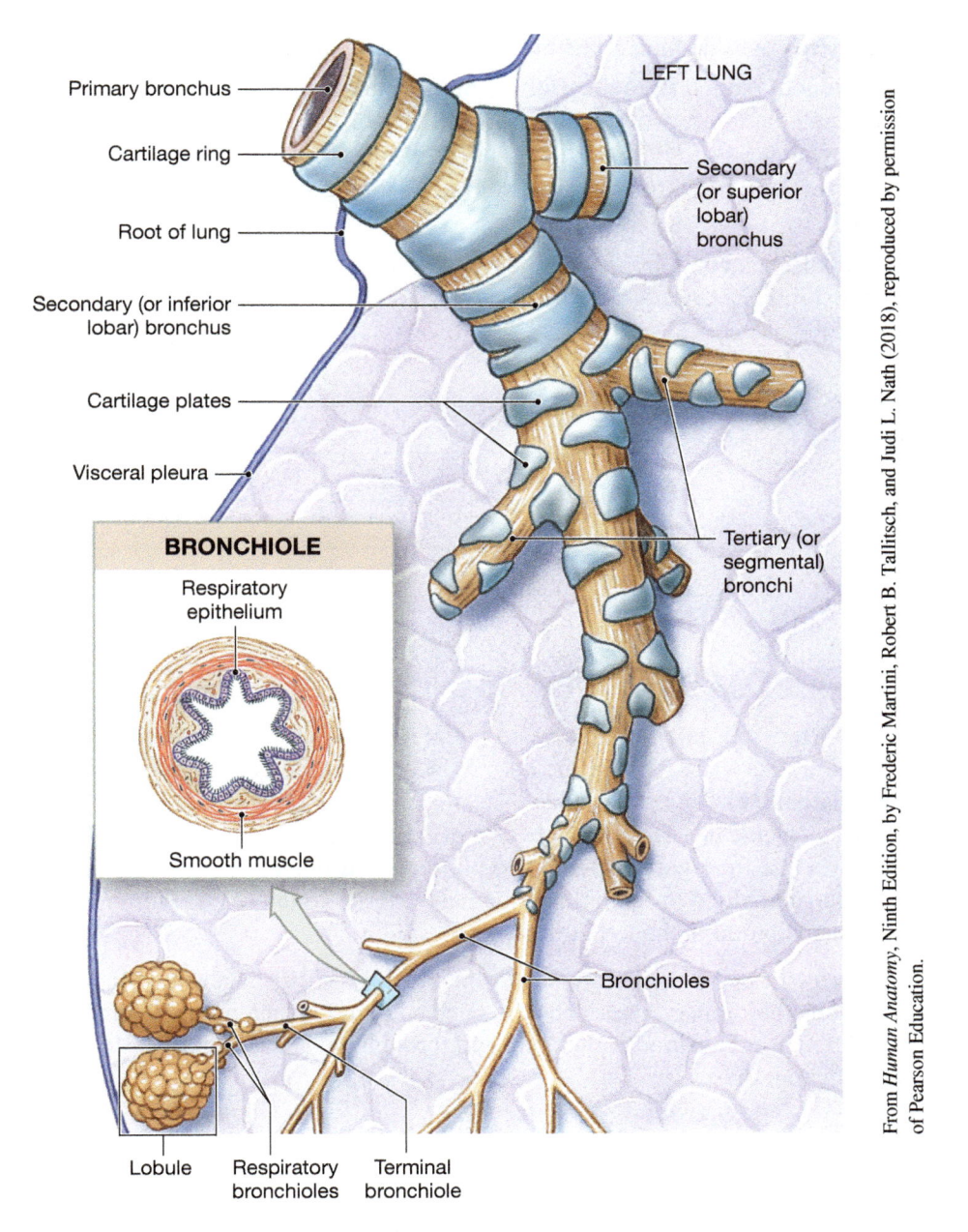

Figure 7.2 **Bronchi and Bronchioles.** For clarity, the degree of branching has been reduced; an airway branches approximately 23 times before reaching the level of a lobule.

  a. The **horizontal fissure** separates the superior and middle lobes.
  b. The **oblique fissure** separates the inferior lobe from the middle and superior lobes.

Bronchi & Bronchioles

Bronchi are a series of successively branching and progressively smaller passageways within each lung. Bronchi are part of the conduction portion of the lung and transport inhaled air to the *respiratory portion* of the lungs. Each specific type of bronchus has unique structural characteristics and functions.

CHAPTER SEVEN   *The Thoracic Cavity & Structures in the Neck*   149

- **Primary bronchi** enter the lung at the hilus. One primary bronchus enters each lung.
- **Secondary bronchi** branch from the primary bronchi to each lobe of the lung. The left lung has two lobes and therefore two secondary bronchi. The right lung has three lobes and three secondary bronchi.
- **Segmental** or **tertiary bronchi** are smaller tubes branching to each bronchopulmonary segment of lung tissue.

The largest bronchioles are continuous with the tertiary bronchi. **Note the characteristic tissue in each type of bronchiole.** Define each of the following and indicate tissue types present.

- Bronchioles: _____
- Terminal bronchioles: _____
- Respiratory bronchioles: _____
- Alveolar ducts: _____
- Alveolar sacs: _____
- Alveoli: _____

V. GROSS ANATOMY OF THE HEART

The **heart** is a fist-sized, muscular organ located in the mediastinum, which pumps blood through blood vessels to all organs and tissues of the body. The cardiovascular system is divided into **pulmonary** and **systemic** circuits.

- The **pulmonary circuit** involves the *right* side of the heart. Deoxygenated blood enters the right atrium and flows into the right ventricle. The pulmonary trunk leaves the right ventricle and carries deoxygenated blood through the pulmonary arteries to the lungs. Pulmonary veins return freshly oxygenated blood to the left atrium.
- The **systemic circuit** involves the left side of the heart. Freshly oxygenated blood enters the left atrium through the pulmonary veins. The oxygenated blood is then pumped through the bicuspid valve to the left ventricle. Blood is then pumped through the aortic semilunar valve, through the aorta and throughout the body.

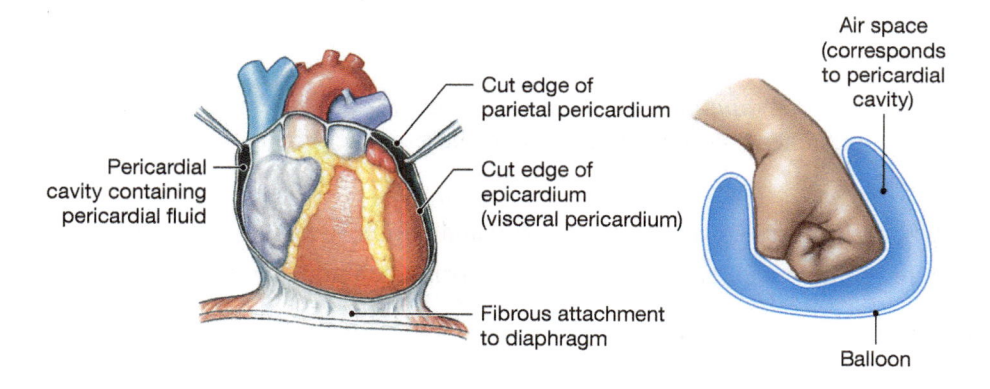

From *Human Anatomy*, Ninth Edition, by Frederic Martini, Robert B. Tallitsch, and Judi L. Nath (2018), reproduced by permission of Pearson Education.

Figure 7.3 **Relationships between the heart and the pericardial cavity.** The pericardial cavity surrounds the heart like the balloon surrounds the fist (right).

Pericardium

The heart is enclosed in a tough fibrous connective tissue sac. (see Fig. 7.3). The most external layer of the sac is called the **fibrous pericardium**. Beneath the fibrous pericardium is the serous pericardium. Similar to the pleural sacs, the **serous pericardium** is a double-layered sac comprised of the **parietal pericardium** and **visceral pericardium**. The visceral pericardium is also called the **epicardium** of the heart. The **pericardial cavity** is located between the visceral and parietal layers of the serous pericardium and contains a thin layer of serous fluid. The parietal pleura adjacent to the mediastinum is fused to the fibrous pericardium, and the phrenic nerves run between the layers.

Great Vessels

1. The **aorta** arises from the left ventricle. The aorta is a continuous vessel, but has separately named parts in each region of the body. The regions of the aorta within the thoracic cavity include the **ascending aorta, aortic arch** and **thoracic aorta**.

   The **coronary arteries** are the only branches from the ascending aorta.

   The **aortic arch** is the curved portion of the aorta. Branches extending from the aortic arch include the following arteries.

   a. The **brachiocephalic artery** is the first branch of the aortic arch. It divides again into the right subclavian and right common carotid artery.
   b. The **left common carotid artery** is the middle artery arising from the aortic arch. It splits further into the left external and left internal carotid artery in the neck.
   c. The **left subclavian artery** is the third branch arising from the aortic arch. It supplies blood to the upper limb and structures of the neck.

2. The **pulmonary trunk** arises from the right ventricle and divides into the right pulmonary and left pulmonary arteries.

3. The **pulmonary arteries** connect with the hilus of the lungs on their mediastinal surface.

4. The **superior vena cava** and **inferior vena cava** return blood to the right atrium. The **superior vena cava** is returning deoxygenated blood from the head, neck and upper extremities. The **inferior vena cava** is bringing deoxygenated blood from the abdomen, pelvis and the lower extremities.

5. The **azygos** and hemiazygos veins lie on either side of the thoracic vertebral bodies and return blood from the chest wall and drain into the superior vena cava.

A Schematic of Blood Flow Through the Heart and Body

The following flowchart provides a brief synopsis of blood flow through the heart. Trace blood from the superior and inferior vena cava into the right atrium of the heart and throughout the body.

Superior and inferior vena cava → right atrium → through the tricuspid valve → right ventricle → pulmonary semilunar valve → pulmonary trunk → pulmonary arteries → lungs → pulmonary veins → left atrium → through the bicuspid valve → left ventricle → aortic semilunar valve → ascending aorta → aortic arch → descending aorta → body.

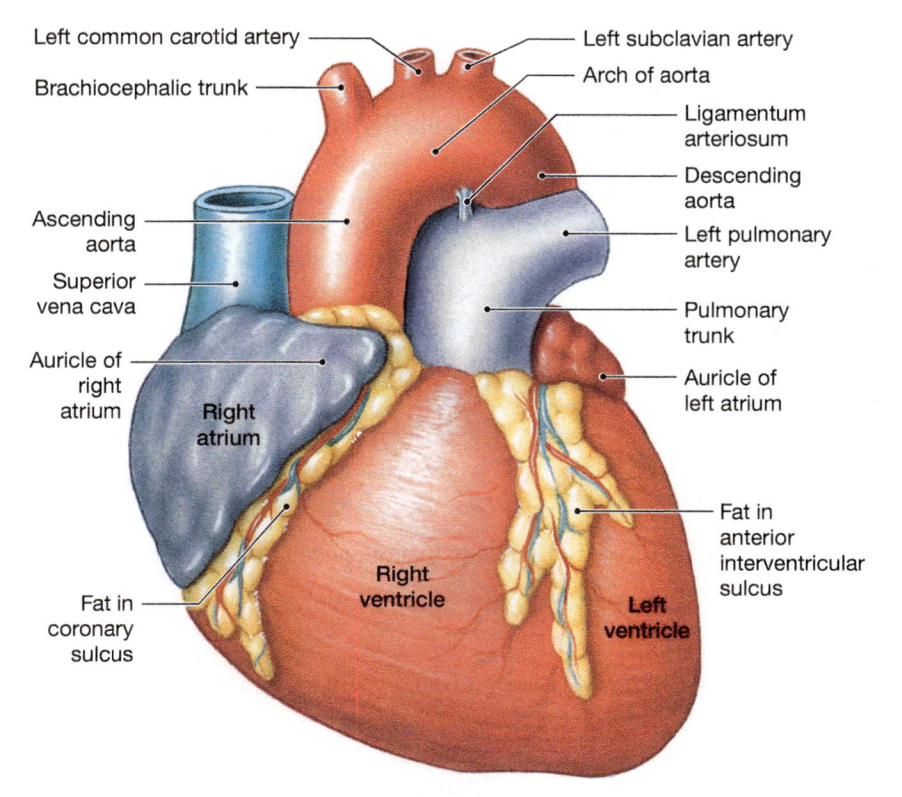

Figure 7.4   **Gross Anatomy of the Heart.** Anterior view.

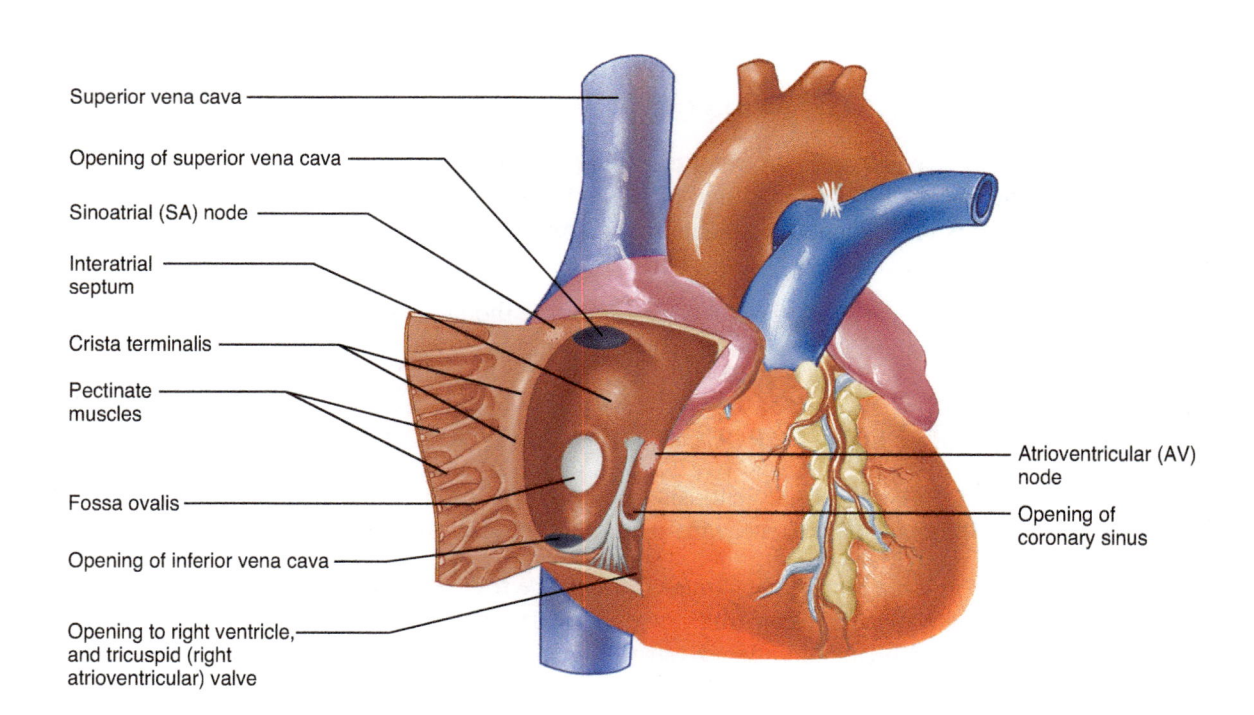

Figure 7.5a   **Gross Anatomy of the Heart.** Anterior view emphasizing the right atrium, which has been opened; the anterior wall of the atrium has been reflected to the side.

152   *Complete Introductory Human Anatomy Lab Guide*

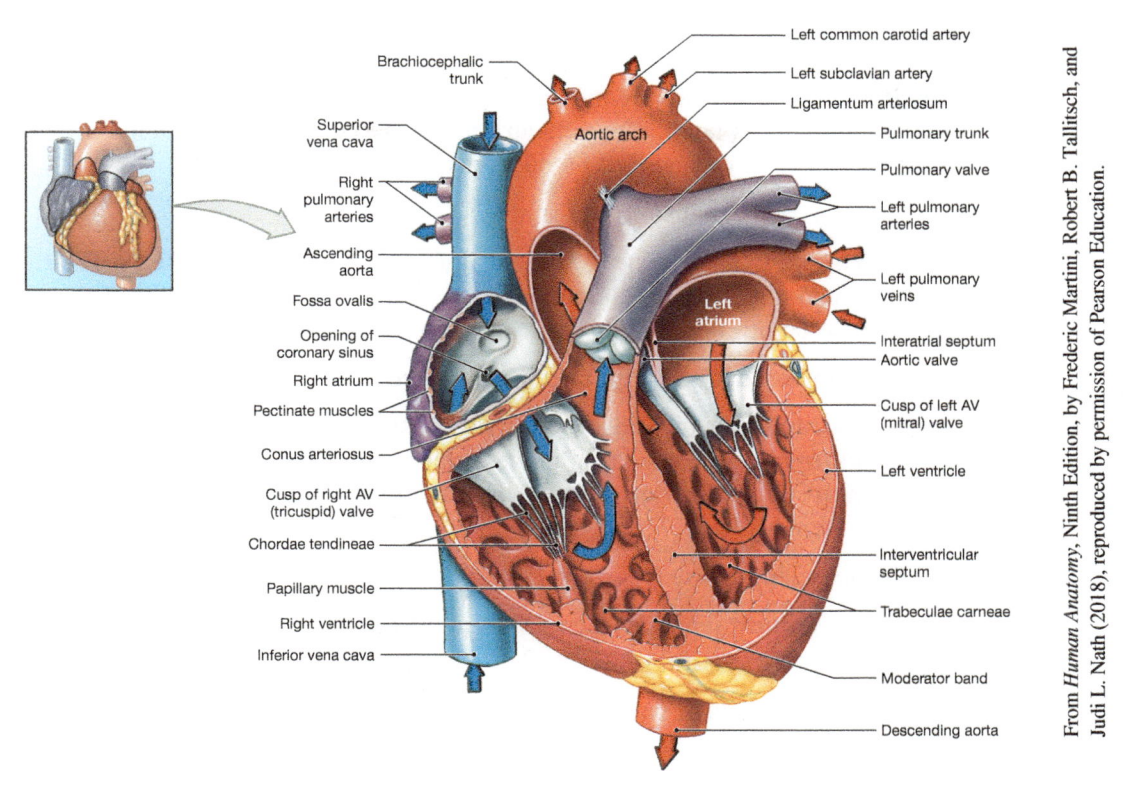

Figure 7.5b **Gross Anatomy of the Heart.** Frontal section of the relaxed heart showing the major landmarks and the path of blood flow (arrows) through the atria and ventricles.

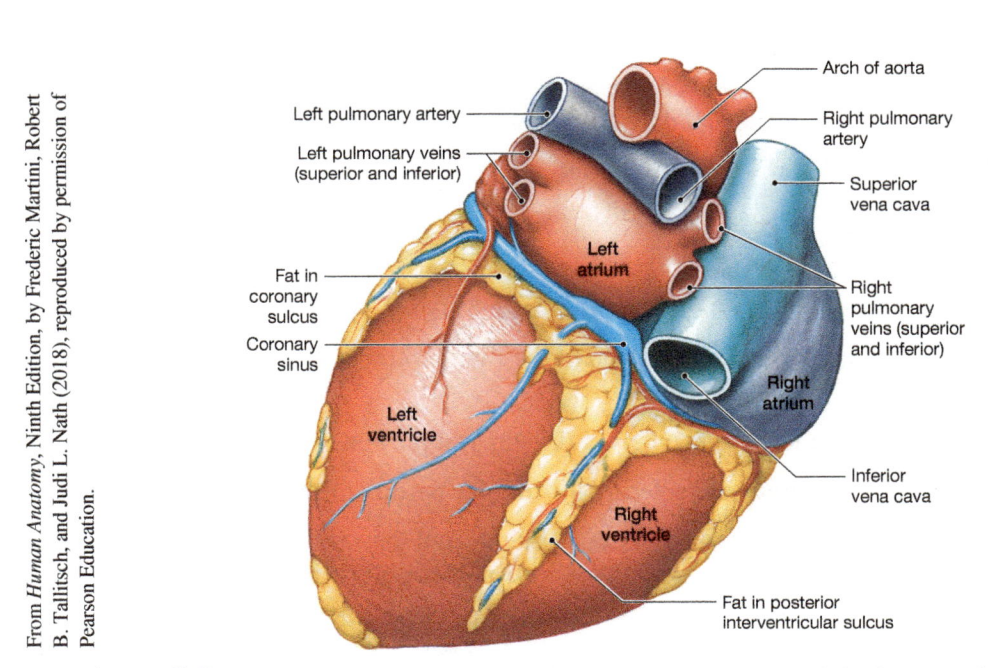

Figure 7.5c **Gross Anatomy of the Heart.** Posterior view of the heart and great vessels.

CHAPTER SEVEN   *The Thoracic Cavity & Structures in the Neck*   153

STRUCTURES OF THE HEART

1. The **right atrium** and **left atrium** are the two superior chambers of the heart. They are the "receiving chambers" of the heart. The right atrium receives deoxygenated blood from the body and the left atrium receives oxygenated blood from the lungs.

2. **Auricles** are "ear-shaped" expansions of the atria.

3. The **right ventricle** and **left ventricle** are the two inferior chambers of the heart. The right ventricle pumps blood through the pulmonary trunk into the pulmonary arteries and to the lungs and the left ventricle pumps blood through the aorta to the body.

4. The heart wall is composed of three intimately associated layers.
   - The **endocardium** is the innermost layer, made of simple squamous epithelial tissue.
   - The **myocardium** is the middle layer and is formed from cardiac muscle tissue.
   - The **epicardium** (visceral pericardium) is the outer layer of the heart, made of simple squamous epithelial tissue.

5. Septa divide the heart lengthwise (Fig. 7.5).
   - The **interatrial septum** separates the right atrium from the left atrium.
   - The **interventricular septum** separates the right ventricle from the left ventricle.

6. The heart possesses two types of valves. **Atrioventricular valves** are located between the atria and ventricles. **Semilunar valves** are located at the base of the aorta and the base of the pulmonary trunk.

REMNANTS OF FETAL CIRCULATION

Two notable features of the adult heart are remnants of functional structures of the fetal heart. The fossa ovalis (Figure 7.5a) is the remnant of the foramen ovale, located in the wall of the right atrium. The **ligamentum arteriosum** (Figures 7.5a and b) is the remnant of the ductus arteriosus. The ductus arteriosus was a connection between the pulmonary trunk and the arch of the aorta. The lungs of the fetus do not function in respiration and cannot accommodate all of the blood pumped out of the right ventricle. Both the foramen ovale and ductus arteriosus were shunts taking blood away from pulmonary circulation prior to birth.

CHAMBERS OF THE HEART

The Right Atrium

1. The **right auricle** is an "ear-shaped" expansion of the right atrium on the external surface of the heart.

2. The **superior vena cava** is a large vein entering the superior portion of the right atrium.

3. The **inferior vena cava** is a large vein entering the inferior portion of the right atrium.

4. The **coronary sinus** is the blood vessel that drains blood from the cardiac veins and back into the right atrium. It travels horizontally along the **posterior surface** of the heart between the atria and ventricles and enters the right atrium.

5. The **fossa ovalis** (oval fossa) is an oval depression in the wall of the right atrium. It is the remnant of a structure of fetal circulation, the **foramen ovale**. The foramen ovale was an opening between the right and left atria in the fetus.

6. **Pectinate muscles** are muscular ridges located on the inner surface of the right auricle and right atrium. Pectinate muscles are not present in the left atrium.

The Right Ventricle

1. The **tricuspid valve** has three cusps. It is the valve between the right atrium and right ventricle.

2. **Chordae tendineae** are tendinous cords that attach the inferior surface of the tricuspid valve to the papillary muscles of the ventricle.

3. **Papillary muscles** are cone-shaped extensions of the ventricular myocardium which attach the chordae tendineae, and thus the valve, to the internal surface of the heart wall (Fig. 7.5).

   When the ventricle contracts, the tricuspid valve closes because blood is forced against the valve. The papillary muscles contract simultaneously with the ventricles and the chordae tendineae tighten, preventing prolapse of the valve. This prevents blood from regurgitating into the right atrium.

4. **Trabeculae carneae** are muscular ridges within the ventricle. Purkinje fibers (part of the conducting system of the heart) pass through them.

5. The **pulmonary semilunar** valve has three cusps projecting inferiorly into the right ventricle. This valve does not have chordae tendineae or papillary muscles attached to it.

   The pulmonary semilunar valve opens as the right ventricle contracts and closes when the ventricle relaxes. The pulmonary semilunar valve guards the opening to the pulmonary trunk and prevents the back flow of blood into the right ventricle.

The Left Atrium

The **left atrium** receives oxygenated blood from four **pulmonary veins**.

1. The **pulmonary veins** enter the left atrium on the posterior surface of the heart, inferior to the pulmonary arteries (Figs. 7.4 & 7.5).

2. Locate the **left auricle** on the external surface of the left atrium. The left auricle and atrium lack pectinate muscles.

The Left Ventricle

The **left ventricle** has the same internal volume as the right ventricle, however it has a much thicker muscular wall.

1. The **bicuspid valve** (mitral valve) has two cusps and is located between the left atrium and left ventricle. The remainder of the anatomy and function of this valve is similar to the tricuspid valve.

2. Identify the **chordae tendineae** in the left ventricle. They are tendinous cords attached to the inferior surface of the bicuspid valve. The chordae tendineae in the left ventricle are usually larger than those in the right ventricle.

3. Locate the **papillary muscles** in the left ventricle. They are cone-shaped extensions of the ventricular myocardium which attach the chordae tendineae to the internal surface of the heart wall.

4. **Trabeculae carneae** are muscular ridges within the ventricle. The trabeculae carneae in the left ventricle are larger and more distinct compared to those in the right ventricle.

(a) Coronary vessels supplying the anterior surface of the heart.

(b) Coronary vessels supplying the posterior surface of the heart.

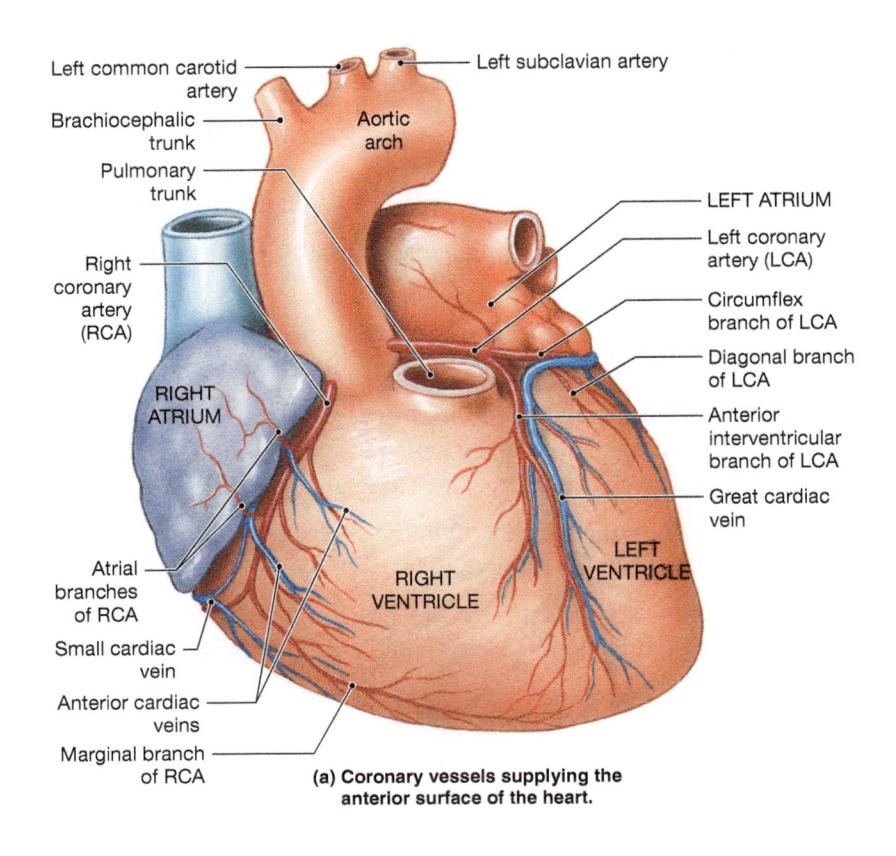

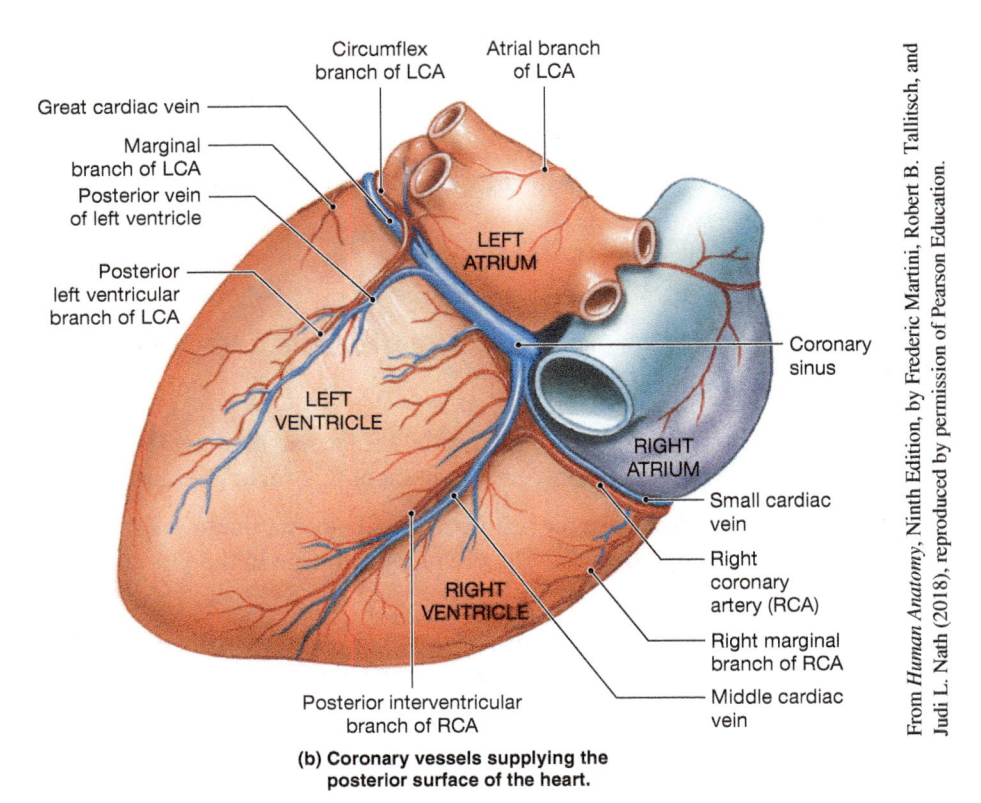

Figure 7.6   Coronary Circulation

From *Human Anatomy*, Ninth Edition, by Frederic Martini, Robert B. Tallitsch, and Judi L. Nath (2018), reproduced by permission of Pearson Education.

Complete Introductory Human Anatomy Lab Guide

When the left ventricle contracts, the bicuspid valve closes because blood is forced against the valve. The papillary muscles contract simultaneously with the ventricles and the chordae tendineae tighten, preventing prolapse of the valve. This prevents blood from regurgitating into the left atrium.

5. The **aortic semilunar valve** has three cusps and is located within the base of the aorta. The aortic semilunar valve does not have chordae tendineae or papillary muscles attached to it. It is similar in anatomy and function to the pulmonary semilunar valve.

The **aortic semilunar valve** has three cusps projecting inferiorly into the left ventricle. The aortic semilunar valve opens as the left ventricle contracts and closes when the ventricle relaxes. The aortic semilunar valve guards the opening to the aorta and prevents the back flow of blood into the left ventricle.

Coronary Circulation

1. The **right** and **left coronary artery** branch from the ascending aorta and distribute blood to the myocardium (Fig. 7.6).

2. Coronary arteries run in the groove between the atria and ventricles.

3. The right coronary artery supplies blood to the right atria and ventricles and turns around the posterior surface of the heart to run in the posterior interventricular sulcus.

4. The left coronary artery bifurcates 1-2 cm after is leaves the aorta. The anterior interventricular branch runs along the interventricular sulcus on the anterior (or sternocostal surface) of the heart. The other branch, the circumflex branch, turns around the left side of the heart giving branches to the left atrium and ventricle. This distribution of coronary arteries can be variable between individuals.

5. **Cardiac veins** drain the myocardium and into the coronary sinus.

6. The **coronary sinus** is a venous structure that drains blood into the right atrium.

THE CONDUCTION SYSTEM OF THE HEART

Specialized myocardial cells control heart muscle stimulation intrinsically. The electrical impulses originate in the right atrium and are passed into the walls of the myocardium.

1. The **sinoatrial node** (SA node) is the "pacemaker" of the heart. The sinoatrial node generates impulses, which are passed through the atrial walls to the atrioventricular node.

2. The **atrioventricular node** (AV node) is located at the inferior portion of the interatrial septum. It receives the electrical impulses of the sinoatrial node and passes the wave of depolarization into the atrioventricular bundle.

3. The **atrioventricular bundle** passes the impulse to the bundle branches.

4. **Bundle branches** are located in the interventricular septum and pass the impulse to the Purkinje fibers throughout the ventricular myocardium.

5. **Subendocardial conducting network** (Purkinje fibers) take the impulse simultaneously to the papillary muscles and the ventricular myocardium. Purkinje fibers run in the trabeculae carneae of the ventricles.

Components of the Conducting System

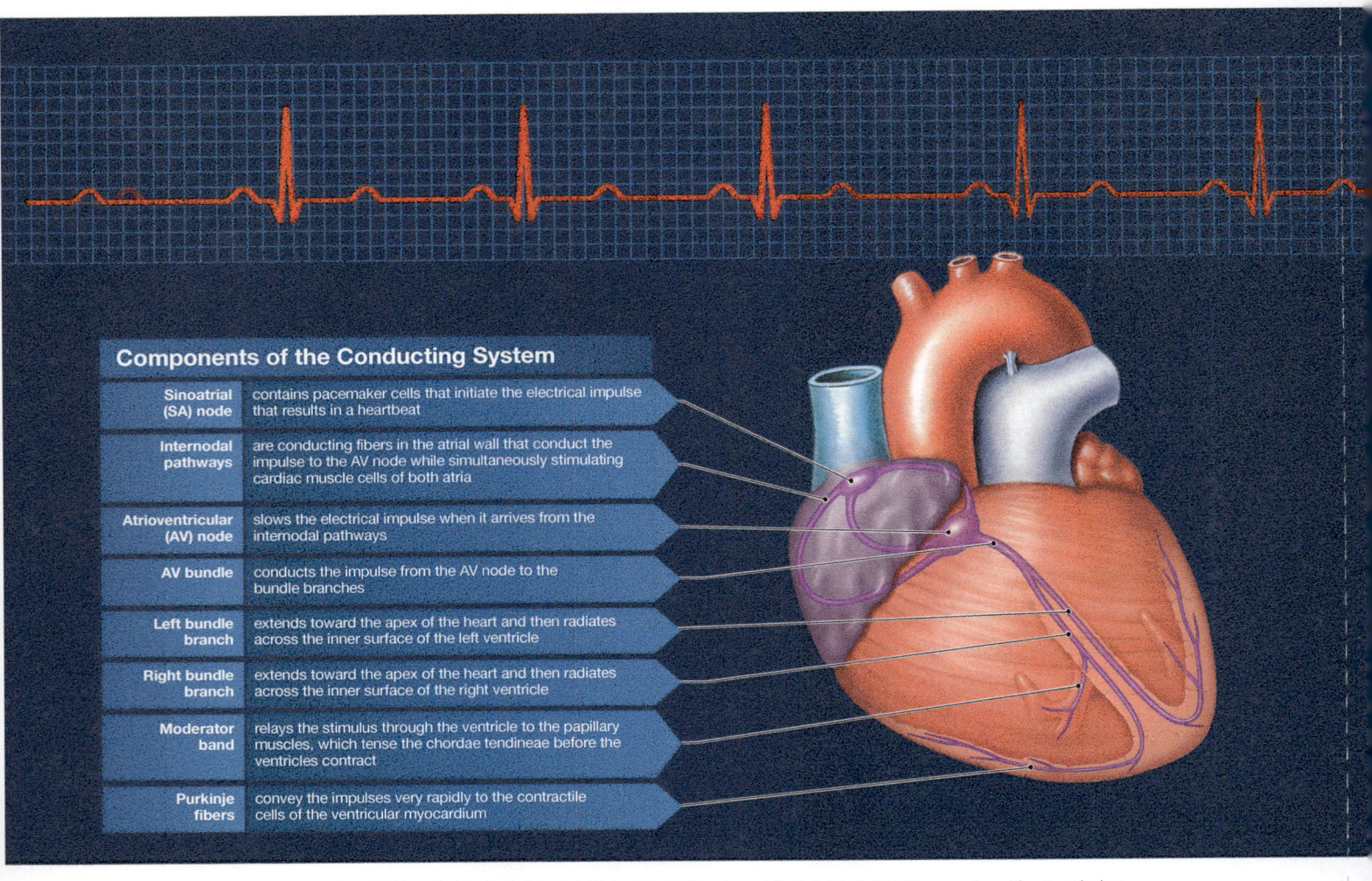

Sinoatrial (SA) node	contains pacemaker cells that initiate the electrical impulse that results in a heartbeat
Internodal pathways	are conducting fibers in the atrial wall that conduct the impulse to the AV node while simultaneously stimulating cardiac muscle cells of both atria
Atrioventricular (AV) node	slows the electrical impulse when it arrives from the internodal pathways
AV bundle	conducts the impulse from the AV node to the bundle branches
Left bundle branch	extends toward the apex of the heart and then radiates across the inner surface of the left ventricle
Right bundle branch	extends toward the apex of the heart and then radiates across the inner surface of the right ventricle
Moderator band	relays the stimulus through the ventricle to the papillary muscles, which tense the chordae tendineae before the ventricles contract
Purkinje fibers	convey the impulses very rapidly to the contractile cells of the ventricular myocardium

From *Human Anatomy*, Ninth Edition, by Frederic Martini, Robert B. Tallitsch, and Judi L. Nath (2018), reproduced by permission of Pearson Education.

Figure 7.7   Components of the Conducting System.

Study and Review Questions – The Thoracic Cavity

CHAPTER SEVEN

Answers to these questions are found in Chapter Seven of this guide.

1. Define **rima glottidis**. _____

2. List three of the major blood vessels located in the neck.

   a. _____

   b. _____

   c. _____

3. From where does the **phrenic nerve** arise? _____

4. The _____ is a thin, flat muscle of facial expression located in the neck.

5. Which of these structures is **not** located in the mediastinum.

   a. Heart

   b. Phrenic nerve

   c. Lung

   d. Thoracic duct

6. Define hilus of the lung. _____

7. List the three branches of the aortic arch.

   a. _____

   b. _____

   c. _____

8. List five structures associated with the **right atrium**.

   a. _____

   b. _____

   c. _____

   d. _____

   e. _____

EXERCISES IN HUMAN ANATOMY

9. List three structures associated with the **left ventricle**.

   a. _____

   b. _____

   c. _____

10. List three structures of **coronary circulation**.

    a. _____

    b. _____

    c. _____

11. Which cranial nerve supplies parasympathetic innervation to the heart? _____

12. Where does the **thoracic duct** empty lymph into blood circulation? _____

13. What are two remnants of fetal circulation located on the adult heart?
    _____ & _____ .

14. Define trabeculae carneae. _____
    _____ .

15. Trace the path of cardiac conduction. _____
    _____
    _____
    _____ .

UPPER RESPIRATORY AND BRONCHIAL TREE WORKSHEET.

Use this worksheet to learn the cavities and the subdivisions and boundaries of the pharynx and bronchial tree. Know the following:

1. Names of all the parts that are labeled

2. The identifying characteristic of each part

3. The type of epithelium found in each area.

160 Complete Introductory Human Anatomy Lab Guide

A. _____

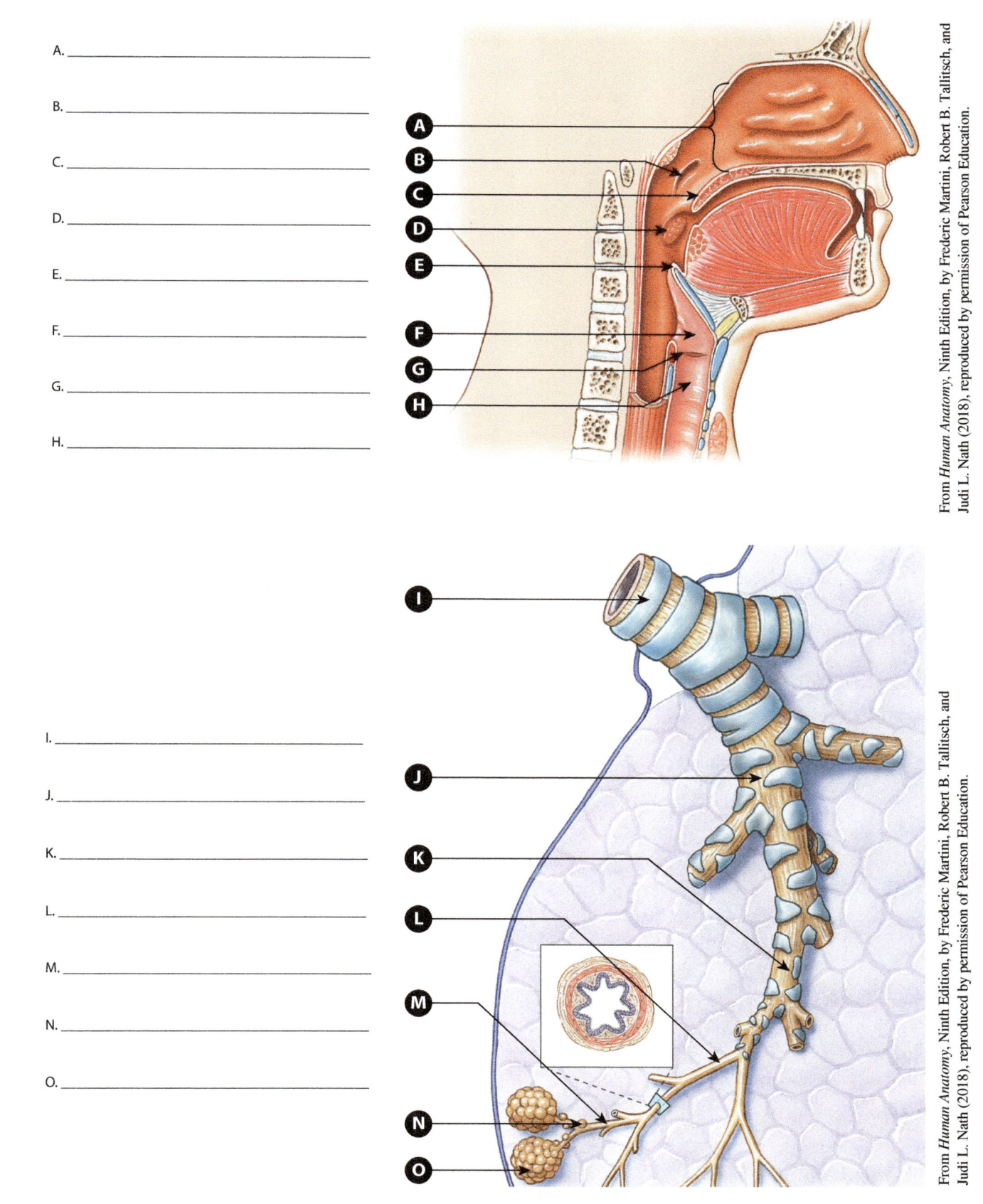

B. _____

C. _____

D. _____

E. _____

F. _____

G. _____

H. _____

I. _____

J. _____

K. _____

L. _____

M. _____

N. _____

O. _____

CHAPTER SEVEN   *The Thoracic Cavity & Structures in the Neck*   161

EIGHT

The Abdominopelvic Cavity: The Digestive & Urinary Systems

LAB MATERIAL
1. Cadaver: Supine
2. Dissected human kidneys and models
3. Torso model
4. Models of digestive organs
5. Photomicrographs

I. HISTOLOGY OF ABDOMINOPELVIC ORGANS

1. **Cross-section of the small intestines:**

   The small intestine has five distinct layers when viewed in cross-section. The layers from external to internal are: **visceral peritoneum, longitudinal muscularis, circular muscularis, submucosa** and **mucosa.** The epithelium of the **mucosal layer** is made of simple columnar epithelial tissue.

   a. **Visceral peritoneum** is a serous membrane that surrounds the intestines.
   b. The **longitudinal muscularis** is the outer layer of smooth muscle that helps propel food through the gut.
   c. The **circular muscularis** is the inner layer of smooth muscle that helps propel food through the gut. The spindle-shaped cells are distinguishable in this layer.
   d. The **submucosa** connects the mucosa to the muscular layers.
   e. Mucosa forms the lining of the small intestines and is composed of simple columnar epithelial tissue. Goblet cells are located among the columnar cells.

2. **Villi of the small intestine:**

   a. Recall familiar structures such as villi, goblet cells and simple columnar epithelial tissue.
   b. Locate the **lacteal** within each villus. Lacteals absorb triglycerides from digested food.

3. **Lobules of the liver**

   a. Locate the **central vein** within each lobule and the **connective tissue** separating the lobules from each other.
   b. The liver has a multitude of functions. Some basic liver functions include **bile manufacture** and **cholesterol synthesis**. The liver also **detoxifies** harmful substances and **processes nutrients**.

4. **Liver lobule** (higher magnification)

   a. **Hepatocytes** are cells that make up the liver.
   b. **Sinusoids** are spaces between liver cells.
   c. The **central vein** appears as an opening in the center of the slide.
   d. A **portal triad** is a branch of the hepatic artery, a portal venule, and a bile duct.

5. **Renal corpuscles within the kidney:**
   a. The renal corpuscle is composed of the **glomerular capsule** (Bowman's capsule) and the **glomerulus**.
   b. Kidney tubules are made of **simple cuboidal epithelial tissue**.

6. **Renal corpuscle:**
   a. Recall that the glomerular capsule is the external layer and the glomerulus is the tuft of capillaries inside the capsule.
   b. The **glomerulus** is a tuft of capillaries through which blood passes.
   c. Wastes are removed from the blood through the glomerulus and kidney tubules.

II. BOUNDARIES OF THE ABDOMINOPELVIC CAVITY

Anterior and lateral boundaries of the abdominopelvic cavity are the **abdominal muscles** and the **bony pelvis**. In males the **spermatic cord** penetrates the abdominal muscles inferiorly as it passes through the inguinal canal.

The posterior boundary includes the **vertebral column, bony pelvis, iliopsoas** and **quadratus lumborum muscles** and **fascia**.

The superior boundary of the abdominopelvic cavity is the **diaphragm** and the inferior boundary is the **pelvic diaphragm**, which is formed from the **levator ani** and **coccygeus muscles**.

III. MUSCLES OF THE ABDOMINOPELVIC CAVITY

ANTERIOR ABDOMINAL WALL MUSCLES

1. The **rectus abdominis** originates at the pubis and inserts at the xiphoid process of the sternum. The rectus abdominis muscles are enclosed within two aponeuroses called the rectus sheaths; one superficial and one deep. These aponeuroses are the tendons of the muscles of the lateral abdominal wall and meet in the midline at the **linea alba**.

2. The **external abdominal oblique** originates at the borders of ribs 5–12 and inserts at the linea alba. The **external abdominal oblique** is the most superficial of the anterolateral abdominal muscles.

3. The **internal abdominal oblique** originates at the thoracodorsal fascia and iliac crest. It inserts at the inferior surface of ribs 9–12, the linea alba and the pubis. The **internal abdominal oblique** lies just deep to the external abdominal oblique.

4. The **transversus abdominis** originates on the cartilage of lower ribs, thoracodorsal fascia and iliac crest. It inserts at the linea alba and pubis. The transversus abdominis is the innermost of the abdominal muscles and lies deep to the internal abdominal oblique.

Observe how the fibers of each of these abdominal muscles run in a different direction (Fig. 8.1).

POSTERIOR ABDOMINAL WALL MUSCLES

1. The **quadratus lumborum** originates on the iliac crest and runs superiorly to attach to rib 12 and the transverse processes of lumbar vertebrae.

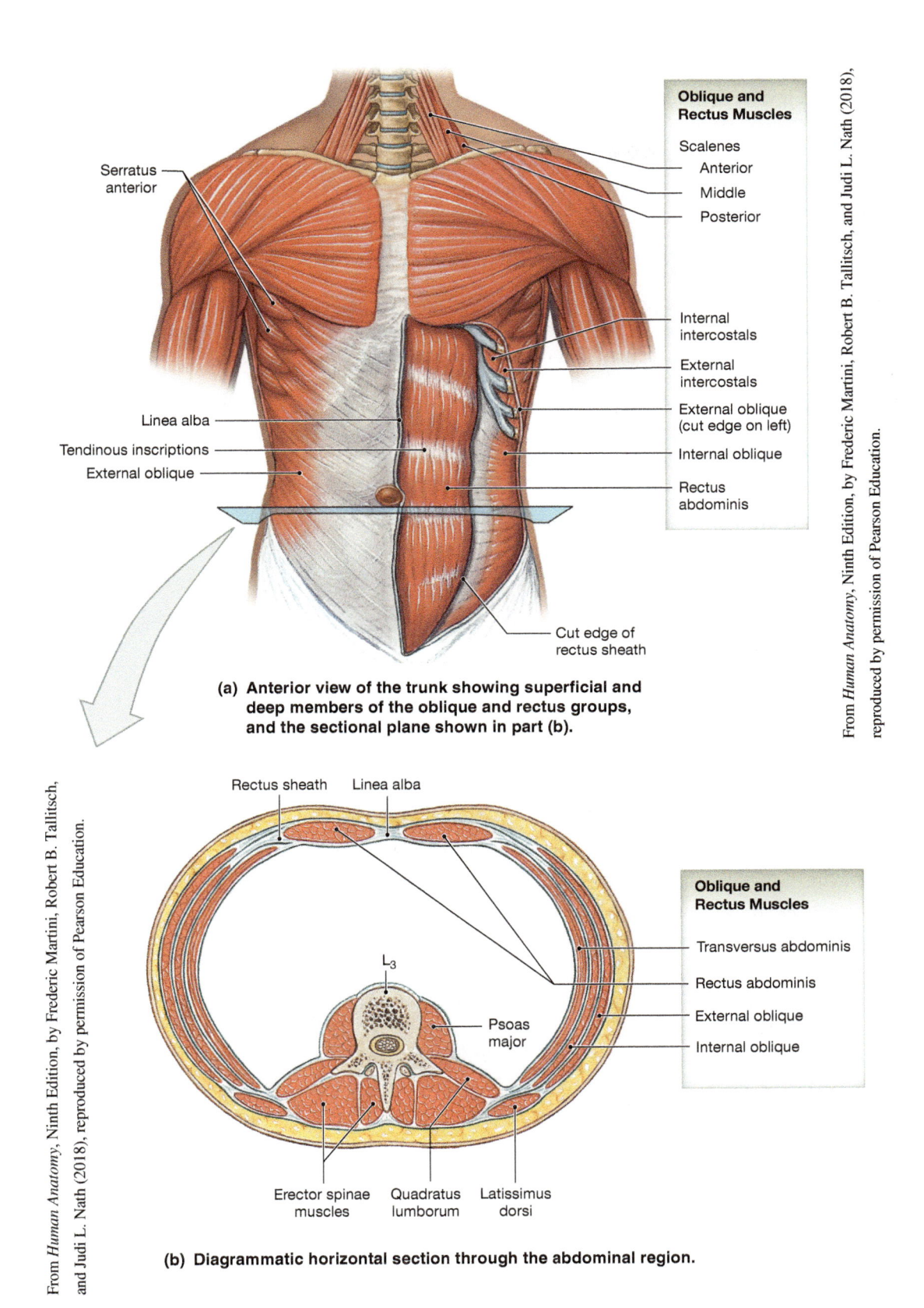

(a) Anterior view of the trunk showing superficial and deep members of the oblique and rectus groups, and the sectional plane shown in part (b).

(b) Diagrammatic horizontal section through the abdominal region.

Figure 8.1 **The Oblique and Rectus Muscles.** Oblique muscles compress underlying structures between the vertebral column and the ventral midline; rectus muscles are flexors of the vertebral column.

CHAPTER EIGHT *The Abdominopelvic Cavity: The Digestive & Urinary Systems* 165

2. The **psoas major** originates on the anterior surfaces of the transverse processes of vertebrae T12–L5 and inserts at the lesser trochanter of the femur.

3. The **iliacus** originates at the iliac fossa and fuses with the psoas major proximal to their insertion on the lesser trochanter of the femur. The **iliacus** and **psoas major** muscles are often called the **iliopsoas** muscle because of their common insertion.

MUSCLES OF THE PELVIC FLOOR AND PERINEUM

The muscles of the pelvic floor provide support for the internal pelvic organs (digestive, urinary and reproductive), and the structures of the perineum and external genitalia attach to them inferiorly. These muscles are responsible for anal and urinary continence.

1. The levatores ani muscles (singular = levator ani) form a funnel-shaped layer of muscle, which tapers to surround the anal canal and the external anal sphincter. These muscles form part of the pelvic diaphragm and support the pelvic organs. The levatores ani muscles are formed from two distinct muscles, the **pubococcygeus** and the **iliococcygeus**.

   The origins of the levator ani are the inner wall of the pelvis from the pubis to the spine of the ischium. The insertions of the levator ani are the inner wall of the coccyx and the medial part of the opposite levator ani (See figure 8.2).

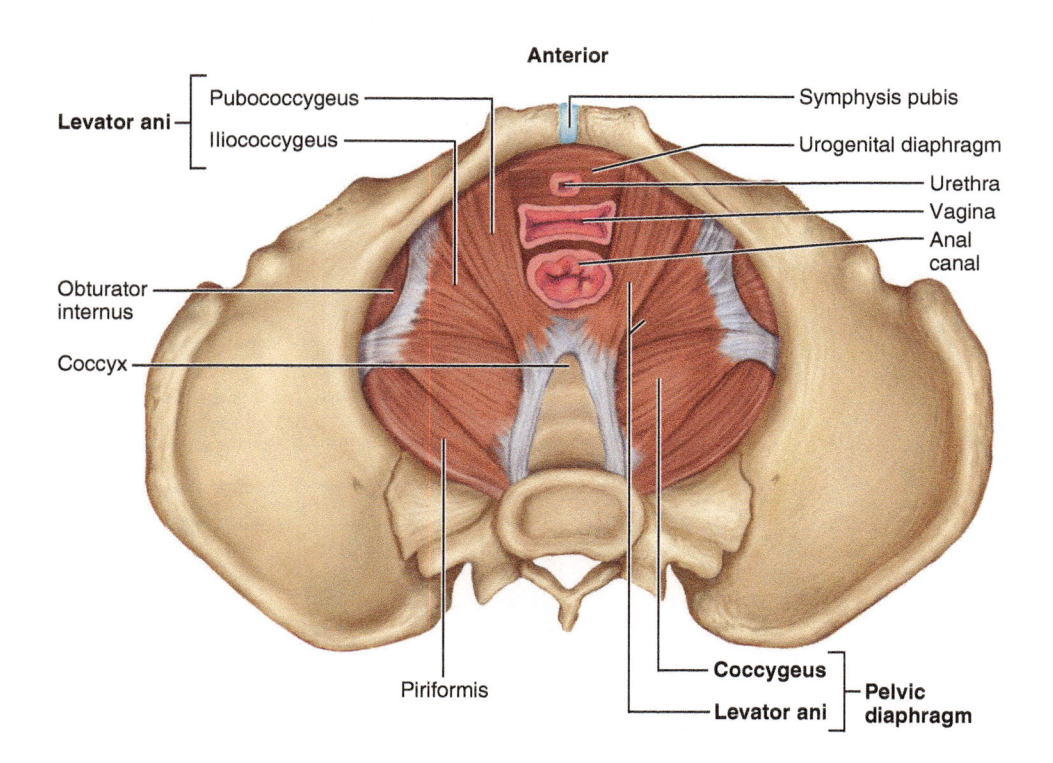

From *Human Anatomy 3.0*, Eighth Edition, by Elaine N. Marieb, Patricia Brady Wilhelm, and Jon B. Mallatt (2017), reproduced by permission of Pearson Education.

Figure 8.2 **Muscles of the Pelvic Floor and Perineum**

2. The **coccygeus muscle** lies posterior to the levator ani and anterior to the piriformis (see Fig. 8.2). The coccygeus originates at the ischium and inserts at the sacrum and coccyx. The coccygeus plays a strong role in assisting the levator ani in supporting the pelvic organs. Together the levator ani and coccygeus muscles form the **pelvic diaphragm**.

3. The **urogenital diaphragm** gives direct support to the urinary bladder (and in males the prostate gland). It spans between the left and right ischiopubic rami. The urethra and vagina (in females) pass through the urogenital diaphragm (see Fig. 9.2 and 9.3)

4. The **bulbospongiosus muscle**

    a. In males, the **bulbospongiosus muscle** encloses the bulb (base) of the penis. The actions of the bulbospongiosus in males are to maintain erection of the penis, aid in ejaculation of semen, and aid in ejection of urine from the urethra (Fig. 9.3).
    b. In females, the **bulbospongiosus muscle** is deep to the labia and covers the bulb of the vestibule. The bulb of the vestibule is the erectile tissue that surrounds the vaginal and urethral orifices (Fig. 9.2).

5. The **ischiocavernosus muscle** originates at the ischial tuberosity and inserts as a covering of the the crura ("legs") of the penis or clitoris.

6. The muscles of the pelvic diaphragm, the urogenital diaphragm, the bulbospongiosus and the ischiocavernosus receive motor innervation from the pudendal nerve and blood supply from the internal pudendal artery.

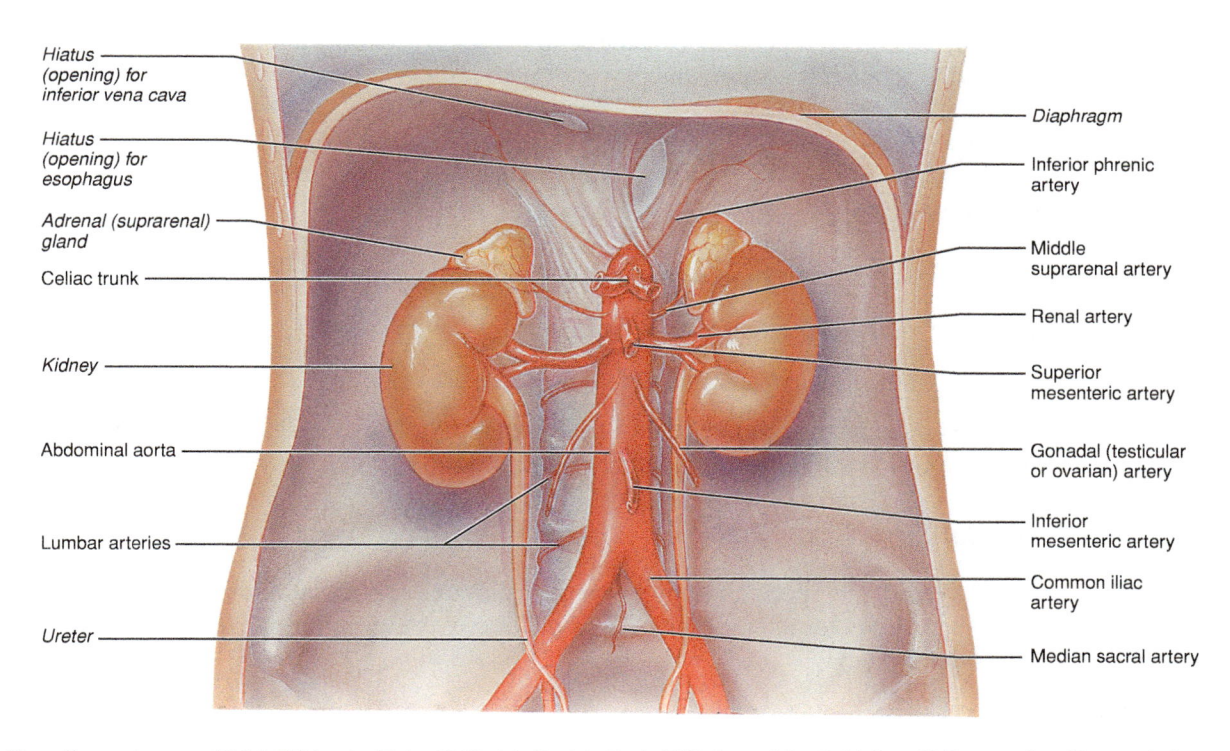

From *Human Anatomy*, Eighth Edition, by Elaine N. Marieb, Patricia Brady Wilhelm, and Jon B. Mallatt (2017), reproduced by permission of Pearson Education.

Figure 8.3   Major Branches of the Abdominal Aorta

IV. BLOOD VESSELS INFERIOR TO THE DIAPHRAGM

Branches from the Abdominal Aorta

The main branches arising from the abdominal aorta are the celiac, superior mesenteric, renal, gonadal and inferior mesenteric arteries. Each of these arteries supplies specific abdominal organs. Lumbar arteries supply the posterior abdominal wall. Branches that supply the liver, spleen and intestine are unilateral, and other branches are paired (left and right). The branches of the descending abdominal aorta are discussed in order of their branching from the abdominal aorta (Fig. 8.3).

1. The **celiac trunk** is the first major arterial branch from the descending abdominal aorta. It has branches to the liver, pancreas, stomach, gallbladder and part of the duodenum. Locate as many of these branches as possible on the cadaver or torso model.
2. The **superior mesenteric artery** is the second branch from the abdominal aorta and it supplies blood to the small intestine, part of the pancreas, ascending and transverse colon.
3. The paired **renal arteries** supply the kidneys and suprarenal (adrenal) glands.
4. **Gonadal arteries:**
   a. The paired **ovarian arteries** supply the ovaries in the female.
   b. The paired **testicular arteries** supply blood to the testes of the male.
5. The **inferior mesenteric artery** supplies the descending and sigmoid colon and rectum.
6. The **common iliac arteries** are the terminal branches of the descending abdominal aorta.

   Branches from the **common iliac arteries** include:
   a. The **external iliac arteries** continue as the **femoral arteries** in the thigh.
   b. The **internal iliac arteries** supply the pelvic organs and gluteal muscles.

Venous Drainage of Pelvis and Abdomen

Veins Draining the Pelvis

1. The **external iliac** and **internal iliac veins** join the common iliac veins.
2. The **common iliac veins** join the inferior vena cava.
3. The **renal veins** exit the kidneys and join the inferior vena cava.
4. The **gonadal** (testicular or ovarian) **veins** exit the testes or ovaries. The right gonadal vein drains into the inferior vena cava and the left gonadal drains into the left renal vein.

The Hepatic Portal System

The **hepatic portal system** is a special system of veins that drains specific abdominal organs. Not all veins draining the abdomen enter the inferior vena cava directly. Veins draining the digestive organs form the hepatic portal system.

The **hepatic portal system** carries blood between the capillaries of the gastrointestinal tract into capillaries in the liver before passing blood back to the systemic circuit. Freshly absorbed nutrients pass into the liver where they are either stored or modified.

1. The **splenic vein** brings blood from spleen, stomach and pancreas.

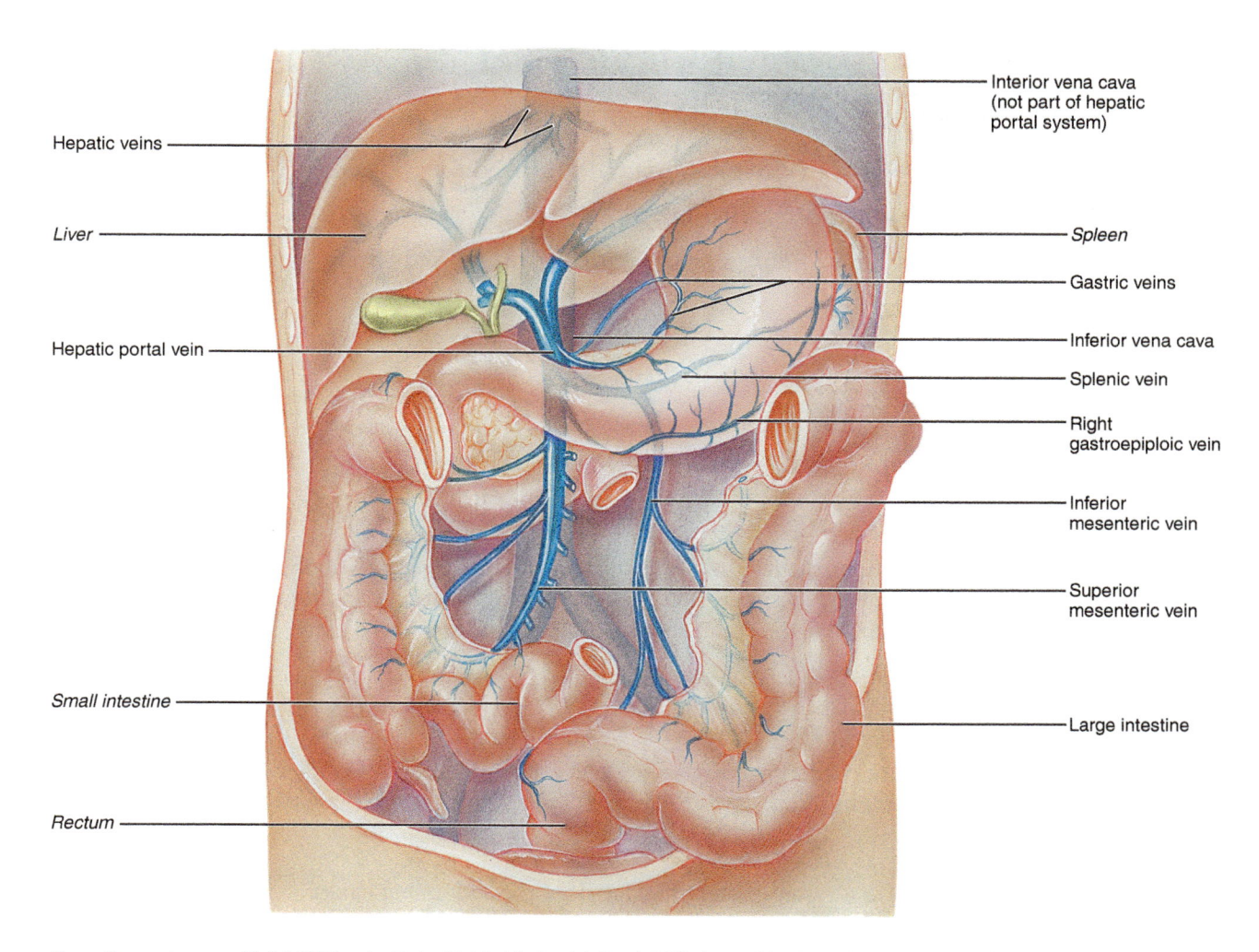

Figure 8.4 The Veins of the Hepatic Portal System

2. The **superior mesenteric vein** brings blood from the small intestine and stomach.
3. The **inferior mesenteric vein** brings blood back from the colon. The inferior mesenteric vein joins the splenic vein.
4. The **hepatic portal vein** forms from the union of **superior mesenteric** and the **splenic vein**. The hepatic portal vein then enters the liver.

The **hepatic vein** then drains blood *from* the liver into the inferior vena cava (Fig. 8.4).

V. NERVOUS INNERVATION OF ABDOMINAL AND PELVIC ORGANS.

Visceral organs of the abdominal and pelvic cavities receive motor innervation through the Autonomic Nervous System. This system was covered in chapter 5 and should be reviewed in the context of these organs.

VI. ORGANS OF THE DIGESTIVE TRACT & ACCESSORY ORGANS OF DIGESTION

ORGANS OF DIGESTION AND ASSOCIATED MEMBRANES

Histology of the Wall of the Digestive Tract

All regions of the digestive tract from esophagus to anus have the four primary components:

1. Mucosa
2. Submucosa
3. Muscularis externa
   a. Circular muscularis
   b. Longitudinal muscularis
4. Serosa

These components differ along the length of the digestive tract, particularly in the epithelial tissue type of their mucosal layer. The mucosa of the mouth, esophagus and anus is **stratified squamous epithelium**. The epithelium from the stomach through the distal end of the colon is **simple columnar epithelium**.

Membranes

Like the lungs and heart, the abdominal organs are enclosed in visceral membranes. They are important because the nervous innervation, blood supply and blood and lymphatic drainage pass between the membranes.

1. **Parietal peritoneum** is a serous membrane that lines the abdominal cavity.
2. **Visceral peritoneum** is a serous membrane that covers the abdominal organs.
3. The **greater omentum** is an apron-like structure made of peritoneum and fat, which covers the abdominal organs anteriorly. It is an extension of the visceral peritoneum from the greater curvature of the stomach and the transverse colon.

Stomach

The **stomach** is located just inferior to the diaphragm on the left side of the body. The stomach is continuous proximally with the **esophagus** and distally with the **duodenum**.

1. The **lesser curvature** is the short curve on the medial surface of the stomach. The **greater curvature** of the stomach is the longer curve located on the stomach's lateral surface.
2. The internal walls of the stomach are composed of folds called **rugae**.
3. The **cardiac sphincter** is a band of muscle encircling the junction between the **esophagus** and the **stomach**.
4. The **pyloric sphincter** is a band of muscle encircling the junction between the **stomach** and the **duodenum**.
5. The stomach aids in **mechanical breakdown** of foods and **chemical breakdown** of proteins.
6. Branches of the **celiac trunk** (artery) supply the stomach.

Small Intestine

The small intestine is the primary site for **digestion** and **absorption** of nutrients. The small intestine is divided into three anatomically distinct regions, the duodenum, jejunum and ileum. The duodenum, which is the first division of the small intestine, receives secretions of **bile** and **pancreatic fluid** that are essential to the digestion process.

1. The **duodenum** is the "C" shaped part of the small intestine. The duodenum is the shortest region of the small intestine. Part of the pancreas is nestled in the "C" of the duodenum.

2. The **jejunum** is convoluted and is continuous with the distal end of the duodenum.

3. The **ileum** extends between the jejunum and cecum. There is no distinct point of transition between the jejunum and ileum; the transition is seen as a gradual change in the structure of the mucosa. The ileum adjoins the cecum at the **iliocecal junction**.

4. The **superior mesenteric artery** supplies blood to the small intestine.

Colon (Large intestine)

The colon is continuous with the distal end of the small intestines. Important functions of the colon include **water reabsorption, bacterial production** of a few **B vitamins** and passing digested material toward the anus.

The colon has several unique external features.

- **Epiploic appendages** are small, finger-shaped fatty structures located along the length of the colon.
- The longitudinal layer of the muscularis external is reduced to three bands that run the length of the large intestine. These are the **tenia coli**.
- Contraction of the tenia coli gather the colon into pouches called **haustra**.

The haustra and tenia coli help pass digested material through the colon. The divisions of the colon are described below.

1. The **cecum** is a pouch at the beginning of the ascending colon. The **vermiform appendix** is attached at the cecum.

2. The **ascending colon** begins on the right side of the body at the cecum and continues to the right colic flexure, just beneath the liver.

3. The **transverse colon** is the horizontal portion of the colon between right and left colic flexures.

4. The **descending colon** begins at the left colic flexure and continues to the sigmoid colon.

5. The **sigmoid colon** begins close to the left iliac crest and then passes posterior to the urinary bladder.

6. The **rectum** is the straight part of the colon beginning at the distal end of the sigmoid colon and lying in the pelvis.

7. The **anal canal** is the final part of the colon, beginning at the distal end of the rectum and continuing to the "outside," the anus.

8. The **internal anal sphincter** is a modification of the circular muscularis. Its contraction is under involuntary control. When contracted, the internal anal sphincter inhibits defecation when one is under tension and prevents leakage of feces between bowel movements.

9. The **external anal sphincter** is a skeletal muscle under voluntary control. It is derived from the levator ani muscle. It contracts to inhibit defecation until an appropriate time.

10. The ascending and descending colon are attached to the posterior body wall by peritoneum. The transverse and sigmoid colons are enclosed in folds of peritoneum and have the ability to move.

ACCESSORY ORGANS OF DIGESTION

The accessory organs of digestion include the liver, gallbladder and pancreas. The "accessory" organs of digestion participate in digestion by secreting their substances into the gastrointestinal tract through ducts. (Fig. 8.5)

The Liver

1. The **liver** is located on the right side of the body inferior to the diaphragm. It performs hundreds of essential functions.

    a. The digestive function of the liver is to produce **bile**, which is a substance that emulsifies fats.
    b. Hepatic ducts transport **bile** out of the liver into the gallbladder. Bile exits the liver through the **common hepatic duct** and enters the gallbladder via the **cystic duct**. Bile is stored in the gallbladder until it is needed for digestion.
    c. The blood supply to the liver is the **proper hepatic artery**.
    d. The **hepatic portal vein** drains blood into the liver from the organs of the digestive system.

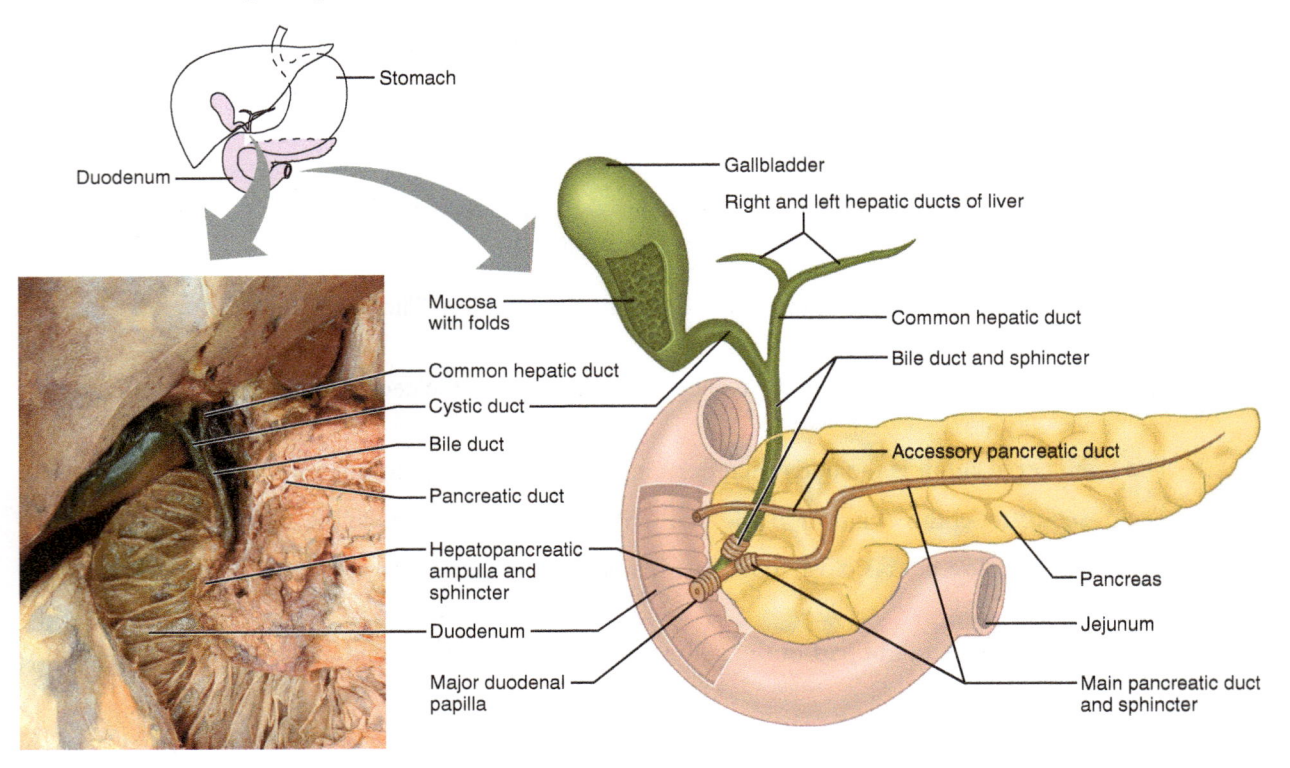

From *Human Anatomy*, Fifth Edition, by Elaine N. Marieb, Jon B. Mallatt, and Patricia Brady Wilhelm (2008), reproduced by permission of Pearson Education.

Figure 8.5 **The Duodenum and Related Organs.** For orientation, see the inset above. Note the various ducts opening into the duodenum from the pancreas, gallbladder, and liver. (In this figure, the gallbladder has been reflected upward.)

The Gallbladder

2. The **gallbladder** is a greenish sac that stores bile. It is located inferior to the right lobe of the liver. The cystic duct is a passage that allows bile to flow both into and out of the gallbladder. (Fig. 8.5)

   a. The **cystic duct** leaves the gallbladder and joins the common bile duct.
   b. The **common hepatic duct** exits the liver and joins the common bile duct.
   c. The **common bile duct** forms from the union of cystic and common hepatic ducts.
   d. The common bile duct enters the **duodenum** with the main pancreatic duct.

The Pancreas

3. The digestive function of the **pancreas** is to secrete digestive enzymes.

   a. The **main pancreatic duct** enters the duodenum with the common bile duct.
   b. Branches from the **celiac trunk** and superior mesenteric artery supply blood to the pancreas.

Lymphatic Organs in the Abdominal Cavity

1. Numerous lymph nodes are found in the abdominal cavity. Locate lymph nodes in the mesentery of the small intestine.

2. The **cisterna chyli** is an expanded chamber that collects lymph from the abdomen, pelvis and lower limbs. The cisterna chyli is continuous with the thoracic duct.

3. The **thoracic duct** carries lymph and travels cranially along the left side of the posterior chest wall. The thoracic duct enters the blood circulatory system and empties lymph into the junction of the **left internal jugular vein** and **left subclavian vein**.

4. The **spleen** functions as an organ of both **lymphatic** and **blood circulatory systems**.

VII. URINARY ORGANS

Gross Anatomy of the Kidney & Urinary Structures

The Kidneys

- The **kidneys** are located anterior and lateral to vertebrae T12–L3. Kidneys are "kidney bean-shaped" organs that are 10–15 cm (4–6 inches) in length (Fig. 8.3).
- Kidneys are located **retroperitoneally**. That is, they are located posterior to the parietal peritoneum.
- A thick layer adipose tissue surrounds both kidneys.
- The **hilus** is the indentation on the medial surface of the kidney through which the renal artery, nerves and lymph vessels enter, and the renal vein and ureter exit.
- The **suprarenal (adrenal) glands** rest on the superior pole of each kidney along the dorsal body wall. The suprarenal glands are endocrine glands.

Examine a frontal section of the kidney. Examine each of the following structures on preserved human kidneys and models.

1. The **renal capsule** is a fibrous covering surrounding each kidney.
2. The **cortex** is the brownish external layer of each kidney.
3. The **medulla** is the internal region of the kidney. It is sectioned into triangle-shaped structures known as the **pyramids of the medulla**. Pyramids of the kidney empty urine into minor calyces (singular = calyx) which, in turn empty into major calyces.
4. **Major calyces** empty their waste products into the renal pelvis.
5. The **renal pelvis** is a funnel-shaped structure that joins the ureter.
6. The **ureter** is a hollow, muscular tube that runs along the posterior body wall and connects each kidney with the urinary bladder.

The Urinary Bladder & Urethra

- The **urinary bladder** stores urine until it is voluntarily released. The urinary bladder is attached to the kidneys via the ureters.
- The **urethra** is the single tube that transports urine from the urinary bladder to the "outside."

1. The **female urethra** is about four centimeters long, extending from the base of the urinary bladder to the outside.
2. The **male urethra** is close to 20cm (8 inches) long and is named in three parts. At separate times, urine and semen pass through the male urethra. The three parts of the male urethra from internal to external are as follows:
   a. The **prostatic urethra** passes from the base of the urinary bladder through the prostate gland.
   b. The **membranous urethra** continues from the distal end of the prostatic urethra out of the pelvic cavity and passes through the pelvic floor. The membranous urethra is the shortest portion of the male urethra.
   c. The **penile urethra** (spongy urethra) continues from the distal end of the membranous urethra and passes through the corpus spongiosum of the penis to the outside.

MICROSCOPIC ANATOMY OF THE KIDNEY

The **nephron** is the functional unit of the kidney and consists of the **renal corpuscle** and **renal tubules**. Nephrons function to remove wastes from the blood. (Fig. 8.6)

1. **Renal corpuscles** are spherical and composed of the following parts.
   a. The **glomerular capsule** (Bowman's capsule) is the cup-shaped external portion of the renal corpuscle.
   b. The **glomerulus** is a tuft of capillaries enclosed by the glomerular capsule. It filters blood as it flows through the kidney. The filtrate passes into the capsular space of the glomular capsule, and then into the **proximal convoluted tubule**, which is the first portion of the renal tubule.
2. **Renal tubules** are subdivided according to function and location. Filtrate passes through the tubule and is modified by hormones. Beginning at the renal corpuscle, locate the following portions of the renal tubules on a model of the microscopic anatomy of the kidney.
   a. The **proximal convoluted tubule** is the twisting portion of the renal tubule extending from the glomerular capsule to the beginning of the descending limb of the loop of Henle (loop of the nephron).

Figure 8.6 The glomerular capsule of the kidney.

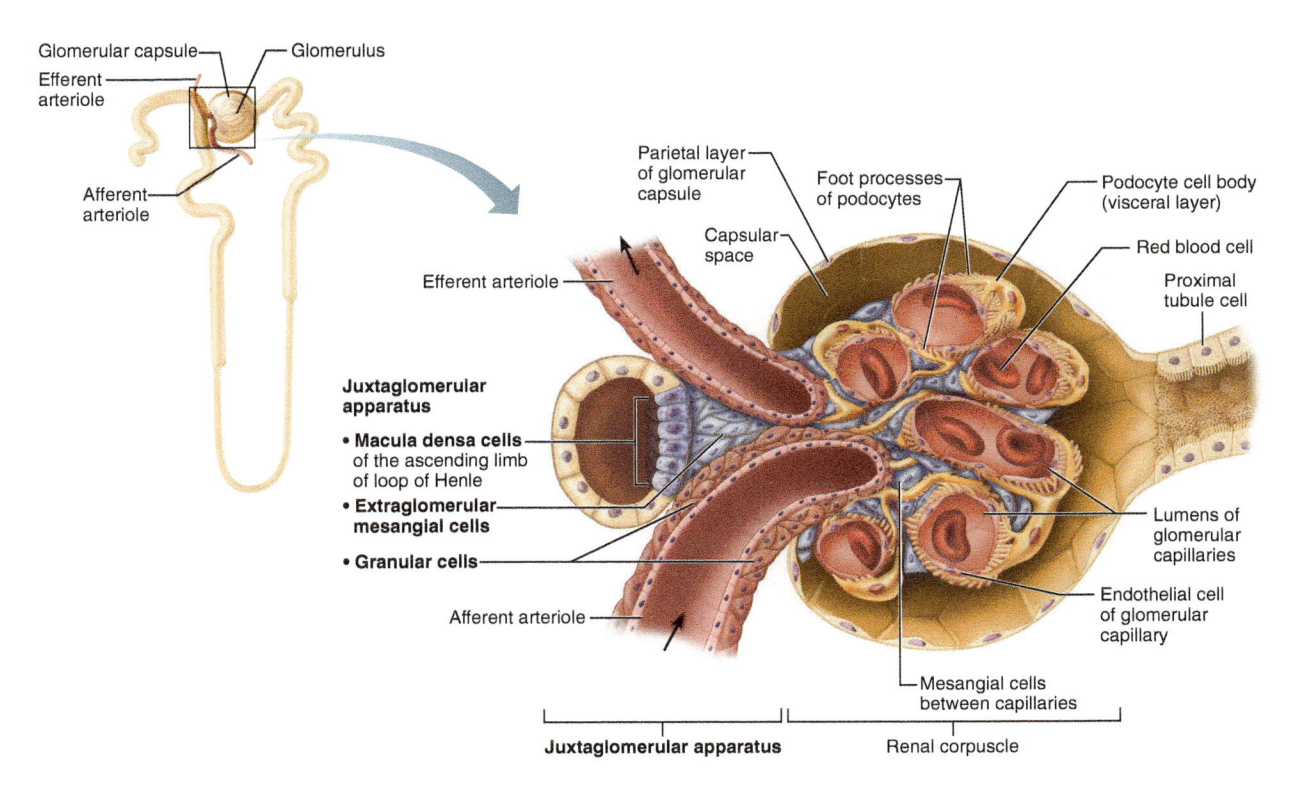

From *Human Anatomy*, Eighth Edition, by Elaine N. Marieb, Patricia Brady Wilhelm, and Jon B. Mallatt (2017), reproduced by permission of Pearson Education.

> b. The **Nephron loop** is divided into the ascending and descending limbs. The **Nephron loop** includes the thin descending limb and thick ascending limb.
> c. The **descending limb** enters the medulla of the kidney.
> d. The **ascending limb of loop of Henle** makes a sharp turn back toward the renal cortex. The **thin segment** is the portion of the loop of Henle in which the simple cuboidal epithelial tissue is very thin. It is interesting to note that the internal diameter of the thin segment is the same as in other regions of the tubule.
> e. The **distal convoluted tubule** is the twisted portion of the renal tubule beginning at the end of the loop of Henle. The distal convoluted tubule empties into a collecting duct. Many distal convoluted tubules empty into a single collecting duct.

3. Thousands of **collecting ducts** receive urine from the renal tubules and transport urine to the renal pelvis and then through the ureter.

4. The **renal artery** is the blood supply to the kidneys. Locate the renal artery and renal vein on a kidney or model of a kidney. Identify some of the blood vessels (macroscopic and microscopic) on a kidney model.

   a. Segmental arteries
   b. Interlobar arteries
   c. Afferent arteriole
   d. Glomerulus
   e. Efferent arteriole
   f. Capillaries and vasa recta
   g. Interlobar veins
   h. Segmental veins

CHAPTER EIGHT   *The Abdominopelvic Cavity: The Digestive & Urinary Systems*

Study and Review Questions – The Abdominal Cavity

CHAPTER EIGHT

Answers to these questions are found in Chapter Eight of this guide.

1. List three muscles of the lateral abdominal wall from external to internal.

   a. _____

   b. _____

   c. _____

2. Match the artery to the organ(s) it supplies. Match the artery in **column A** with the correct organ(s) in **column B**. Write the letter of your answer in the blank by the appropriate term in column A.

   Column A

   _____ Celiac trunk

   _____ Superior mesenteric artery

   _____ Renal artery

   _____ Gonadal artery

   _____ Inferior mesenteric artery

   Column B

   A. Testes or ovaries

   B. Colon

   C. Stomach, liver, and pancreas

   D. Small intestines.

   E. Kidneys

3. List the three major veins forming the **hepatic portal system** of veins.

   a. _____

   b. _____

   c. _____

4. What is the **pyloric sphincter**? _____

5. What is the primary function of the **small intestine**? _____

6. List three unique external features of the **colon**.

   a. _____

   b. _____

   c. _____

EXERCISES IN HUMAN ANATOMY

7. The **common bile duct** forms from the union of the _____ & _____ ducts.

8. Define retroperitoneal. _____

9. What organs are located **retroperitoneally**? _____ & _____

10. List the three parts of the male urethra and their location from internal to external.

    a. _____

    b. _____

    c. _____

11. What is the functional unit of the kidney? _____

    a. What structures is it composed of? _____

12. Trace the path of a drop of urine beginning at the glomerulus.

    _____
    _____
    _____
    _____
    _____

13. What is the digestive function of the liver?
    _____

14. What is the function of the external anal sphincter? What type of muscle is it?
    _____

NINE
Male & Female Reproductive Systems

MATERIALS

1. Male and female sagittal pelvis models
2. Preserved human uterus and testes and anatomical models
3. Photomicrographs

I. HISTOLOGY OF REPRODUCTIVE STRUCTURES

1. **Cross-section of ovary:**
   a. Follicles are structures that contain developing oocytes (egg cells) and are located within the ovary. (Fig. 9.1)
   b. A **primordial follicle** consists of a primary oocyte and the surrounding follicular epithelium. At the onset of the ovarian cycle, primordial follicles begin development into **primary follicles**.
   c. Observe the larger; more mature follicles as well as the smaller, less developed follicles.
   d. The less developed follicles are **primary** and **secondary follicles.** Mature follicles are known as **Graafian follicles.**

2. **Primordial follicles:**
   a. **Primordial follicles** have not been influenced by hormones to develop. Primordial follicles are the most numerous in the ovary.
   b. Females are born with close to 2 million primordial follicles, each containing a primary oocyte. By puberty only around 400,000 primordial follicles remain.
   c. A layer of **simple squamous epithelium** surrounds the primary oocyte. These are the follicular cells.

3. **Primordial & primary follicles:**
   a. Primordial follicles are small and undeveloped and have a squamous cell border.
   b. Primary follicles are larger than primordial follicles and have a **border of cuboidal follicular cells.**
   c. Beginning at puberty, hormones stimulate several primordial follicles to develop into **primary follicles** each month. Of the 400,000 available primordial follicles, only around 400 mature ova will be ovulated in a woman's lifetime.

4. **Primary follicle:**
   a. A single layer of **cuboidal follicular cells** surrounds primary follicles. Hormones stimulate primary follicles to begin developing.
   b. The **zona pellucida** separates the ovum from the surrounding follicular cells.
   c. **Follicular cells** supply the developing oocyte with both hormones and nutrients.

5. **Secondary follicle:**
   a. Each month, a few primary follicles will continue developing into **secondary follicles**; the remaining primary follicles will degenerate by a process called **atresia.**
   b. Secondary follicles have two or more layers of follicular cells surrounding the ovum.
   c. The **zona pellucida** is a glycoprotein layer between the oocyte and the granulosa (follicular) cells.
   d. The follicular cells secrete **estrogen** in the secondary follicle. **Estrogens** are the most important hormones prior to ovulation.
   e. Some follicular cells begin secreting fluid, which increases the size of the follicle. The ovum itself has not increased in size greatly.

6. **Mature follicle** (Tertiary follicle):
   a. The primary oocyte within the follicle has remained at an early stage *of meiosis I* until this time.
   b. Usually, only one follicle will develop completely to become a secondary oocyte each month.
   c. The secondary oocyte progresses through metaphase of meiosis II. The remainder of meiosis II will occur only if fertilization takes place.
   d. Follicular cells produce **estrogen** in the mature follicle.
   e. The fluid-filled **antrum** surrounds the ovum. This is the distinction of a Graffian (or tertiary) follicle.

7. **Corpus luteum:**
   a. After ovulation, the **corpus luteum** replaces the Graafian follicle. The corpus luteum consists of the remaining follicular cells.
   b. Both progesterone and estrogen are secreted by the corpus luteum. **Progesterone** is the primary hormone secreted after ovulation.
   c. If fertilization and implantation occur, the corpus luteum will be maintained for approximately 13 weeks until the placenta is fully functional.

8. **Corpus albicans:**
   a. The corpus luteum degrades into a **corpus albicans** if fertilization does not occur.
   b. The corpus albicans is scar tissue and does not release hormones.

9. **Uterine tube** (Fallopian tube):
   a. Note the **ciliated simple columnar epithelial tissue** lining the mucosa of the uterine tube.
   b. After menstruation the ciliated simple columnar cells become taller.
   c. After ovulation the ciliated simple columnar cells become shorter.

10. **Cross-section of a seminiferous tubule:**
    a. **Seminiferous tubules** are highly coiled tubes located with in the testes, in which sperm are produced. Mature sperm are found with their tails projecting into the lumen of the seminiferous tubules.
    b. A = basement membrane, B = spermatogonia, C = spermatocytes and D = spermatozoa.

11. **Leydig cells** (Interstitial cells) secrete **testosterone** and are located between the walls of seminiferous tubules.

12. **Cross-section of seminiferous tubule:** The more mature sperm have their tails in the lumen.

13. **Spermatozoa** (sperm): Observe the micrograph of human sperm and sperm within the seminiferous tubule.

14. **Penis in cross-section:**

    a. Two **corpora cavernosa** pass through the length of the penis. Corpora cavernosa are erectile tissues within the penis.
    b. The **corpus spongiosum** also courses through the penis. The corpus spongiosum is also erectile tissue and directly surrounds the length of the **spongy** (penile) **urethra**.

II. FEMALE REPRODUCTIVE SYSTEM

THE PERINEUM

The perineum (perineal region) is a diamond-shaped region outlined by the symphysis pubis, the two ischial tuberosities and the tip of the coccyx. The urogenital triangle contains the openings to the urethra and vagina.

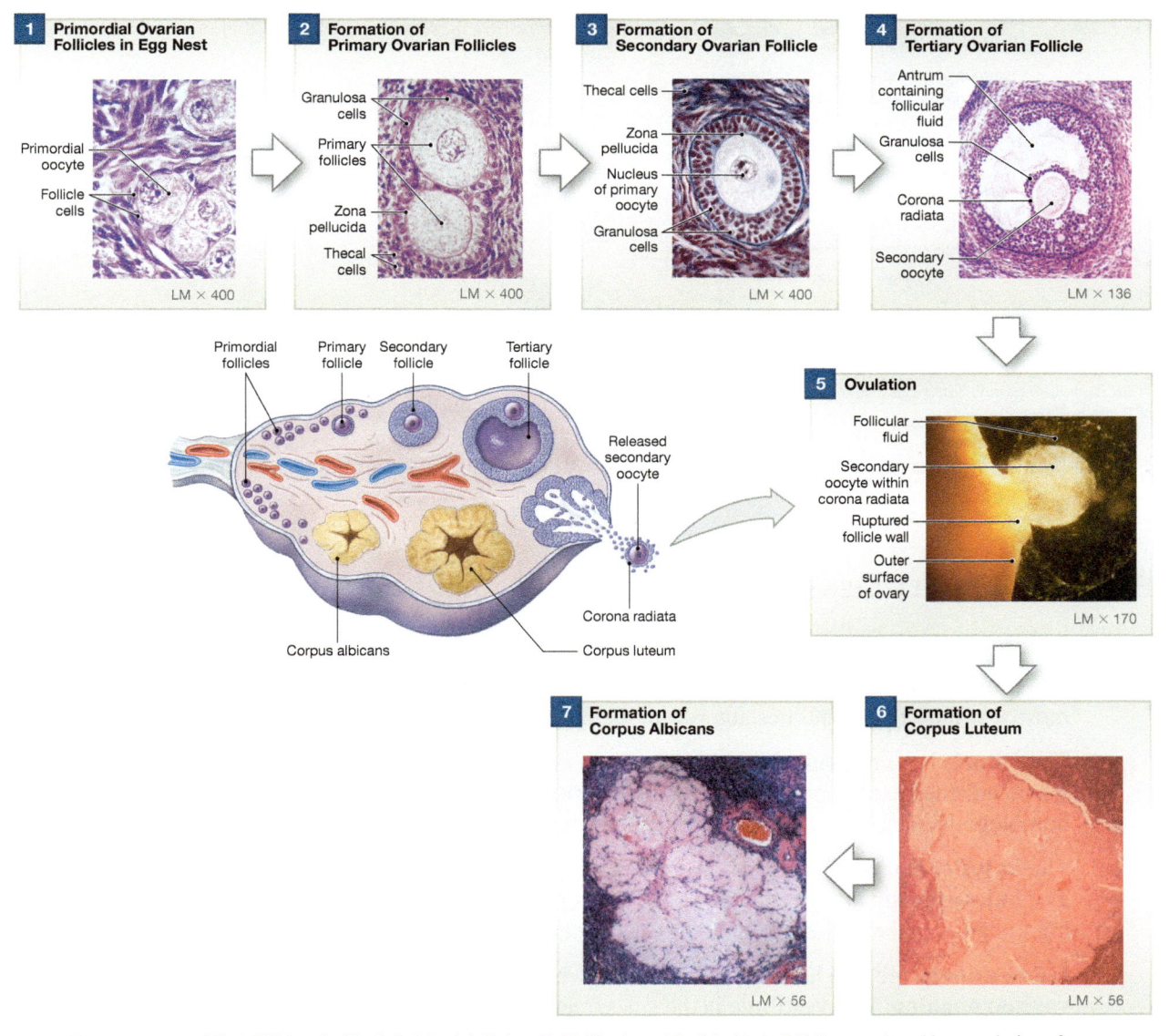

From *Human Anatomy*, Ninth Edition, by Frederic Martini, Robert B. Tallitsch, and Judi L. Nath (2018), reproduced by permission of Pearson Education.

Figure 9.1 **Histological Summary of the Ovarian Cycle.** Follicular development during the ovarian cycle.

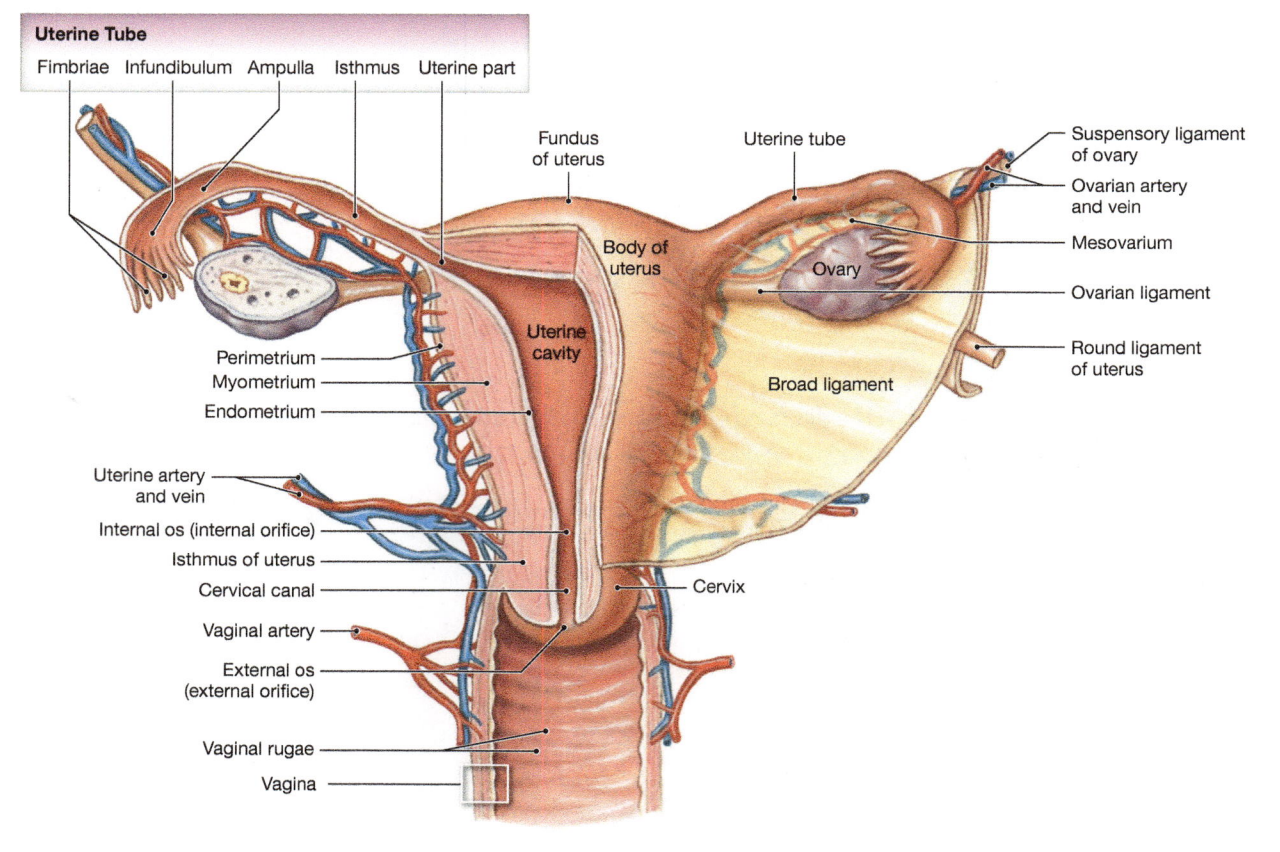

Posterior view of the uterus and stabilizing ligaments within the pelvic cavity

From *Human Anatomy*, Ninth Edition, by Frederic Martini, Robert B. Tallitsch, and Judi L. Nath (2018), reproduced by permission of Pearson Education.

Figure 9.2 **The Uterus.** Posterior view of the uterus and stabilizing ligaments within the pelvic cavity.

EXTERNAL FEMALE GENITALIA

The **vulva** comprises the external genitalia of the female. (Fig. 9.3)

1. The **mons pubis** is externally covered with pubic hair. Subcutaneously, the mons pubis consists mostly of fatty tissue and lies anterior to the pubic symphysis.

2. The **clitoris** is composed of erectile tissue and is partly covered by the ischiocavernosus muscle which attaches to the bone that forms the junction of the ischium and the pubis. The clitoris is homologous to the corpora cavernosa of the penis. (Fig. 9.3)

3. The **bulbs of the vestibule** are bodies of erectile tissue lying to either side of the vaginal orifice. The **bulbospongiosus** muscle covers the bulbs of the vestibule. The bulbs of the vestibule are homologous to the corpus spongiosum of the penis.

4. **Labia minora** are two hairless folds of skin, which enclose the external **urethral orifice** and **vaginal opening**. The **vestibule** is the space enclosed by the labia minora.

5. The **labia majora** are two, hair-covered folds of skin enclosing the labia minora. The labia majora are continuous with the mons pubis.

INTERNAL FEMALE REPRODUCTIVE STRUCTURES

The Vagina

The **vagina** opens inferiorly into the vestibule. The superior end of the vagina is continuous with the cervix (Fig. 9.2 & 9.3).

   a. The **vaginal opening** is posterior to the external urethral orifice and anterior to the anus.
   b. The vaginal **fornix** is the recess that surrounds the cervix where it joins to the superior end of the vagina.
   c. **Rugae** are transverse folds on the interior of the vaginal canal that allow for stretching of the vaginal epithelium.

The Uterus and Cervix

The **uterus** is a pear-shaped muscular organ. In its normal position it is **anteflexed**. That is, the uterus is folded anteriorly over the urinary bladder.

   a. The body of the uterus is the rounded, upper portion of the uterus
      - The **fundus** is the rounded portion of the body of the uterus. The fundus is the "top" of the uterus, but since the uterus is flexed forward, the fundus points anteriorly.
      - The **uterine tubes** attach below the fundus.
      - The **uterine cavity** is the space within the body of the uterus.

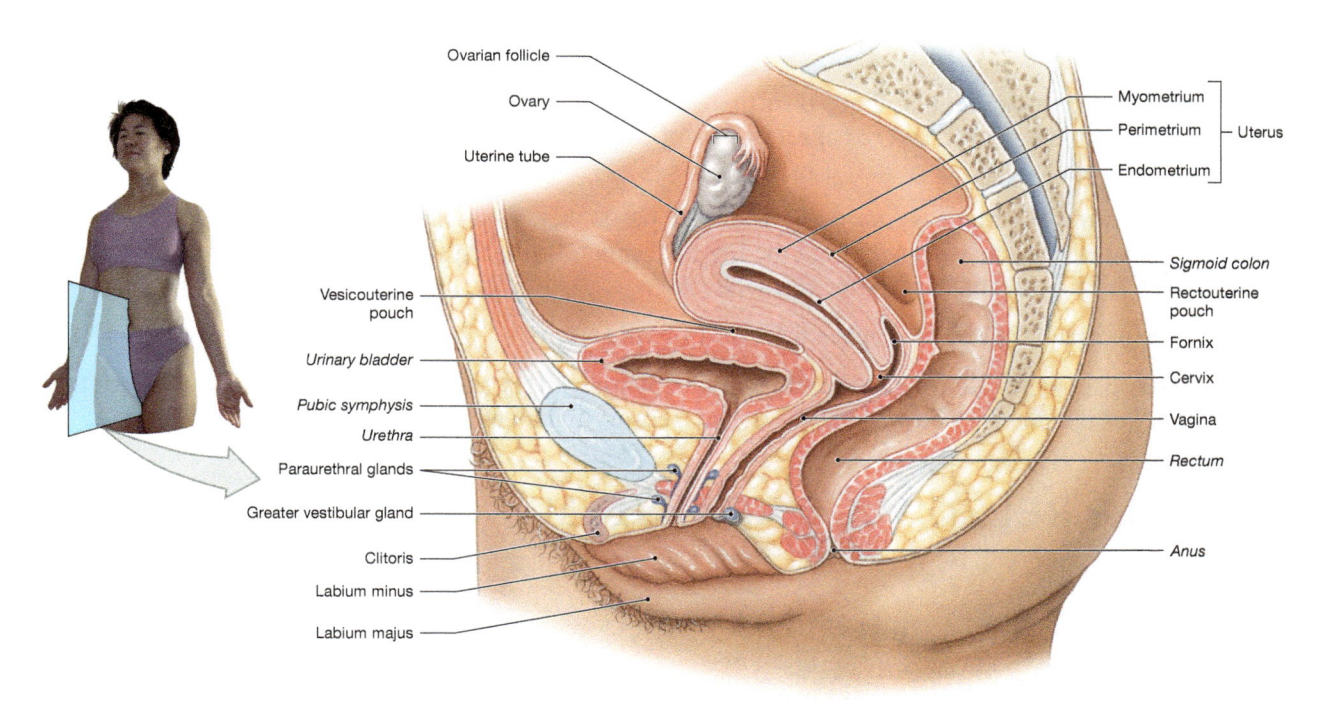

From *Human Anatomy*, Ninth Edition, by Frederic Martini, Robert B. Tallitsch, and Judi L. Nath (2018), reproduced by permission of Pearson Education.

Figure 9.3 The Female Reproductive System Sagittal section of female pelvis.

CHAPTER NINE   *Male & Female Reproductive Systems*

b. The **cervix** is the neck of the uterus at its inferior end protrudes into the superior end of the vagina.
- The **internal os** opens into the uterine cavity.
- The **external os** is the inferior opening of the cervix that communicates with the vagina.
- The **cervical canal** is the passageway that connects the external os and internal os.

The Uterine Tubes

Uterine tubes extend laterally from the uterus. They attract and transport ova from the ovaries toward the uterine cavity. Locate the parts of the uterine tube on preserved uteri and anatomical models.

1. **Fimbriae** are fringed edges of the infundibulum, which surround the ovaries.
2. The **infundibulum** is the dilated, distal end of the tube closest to the ovaries.
3. The **ampulla** is about midway along the uterine tube and continuous with the infundibulum. The ampulla is the usual location of fertilization.
4. The **isthmus** is the narrowed portion of the uterine tube directly attached to the uterus.
5. The **intramural** part of the uterine tubes pass through the wall of the uterus.

The Ovaries

The **ovaries** are small, rounded organs located within the pelvic cavity. Their functions include hormone secretion and oogenesis.

1. The ovaries are attached to the uterus by the **ovarian ligament**.
2. The **ovarian artery** supplies blood to the ovaries.

Ligaments

1. Folds of peritoneum that drape over the pelvic organs are referred to as ligaments. The **broad ligament** is a double-layered sheet of peritoneum extending from the sides of the uterus to the walls and floor of the pelvis. (Fig. 9.2)
2. The **round ligament** is a cord of connective tissue that runs within the layers of the broad ligament from the uterus through the inguinal canal. It is a remnant of embryonic development with no significant function in postnatal life.
3. The **ovarian ligament** attaches the ovaries to the uterus.
4. The **suspensory ligament** is found with the ovarian artery and vein and anchors the ovary to the wall of the pelvis. You will not see the suspensory ligament except on a female donor body.

III. MALE REPRODUCTIVE SYSTEM

EXTERNAL GENITALIA OF THE MALE

The Penis

1. The **root** of the penis attaches internally by ligaments to the ischium and the urogenital diaphragm.

2. The **body** of the penis is the elongated portion. It contains three erectile columns, which are composed of blood vessels, smooth muscle and elastic connective tissue. (Fig. 9.4)

   a. The **corpus spongiosum** of the penis is erectile tissue surrounding the length of the penile (spongy) urethra. The proximal part of the corpus spongiosum is covered by the bulbospongiosus muscle, and attaches to the inferior surface of the urogenital diaphragm.
   b. The **corpora cavernosa** of the penis (single = corpus cavernosum) are two separate columns of erectile tissue passing through the length of the penis, dorsal to the corpus spongiosum. The corpora cavernosa are attached at the root of the penis. The crura (or "legs") of the corpora cavernosa are enclosed by the ischiocavernosus muscles. They attach to the bone that forms the junction of the ischium and the pubis.

3. The **glans penis** is the expanded distal part of the corpus spongiosum.

The Scrotum

The **scrotum** is a skin-covered sac composed of several layers of muscle and connective tissue that contains the testicles. The **cremaster muscle** is a layer of skeletal muscle within the scrotum. Contraction of the cremaster muscle draws the testes closer to the body to help regulate the temperature of the testes.

1. **Testes** are egg-shaped organs within the scrotum. Testes are covered by peritoneum and fascia.

   a. **Seminiferous tubules** are highly coiled tubes within the testes. Sperm are manufactured in the seminiferous tubules.

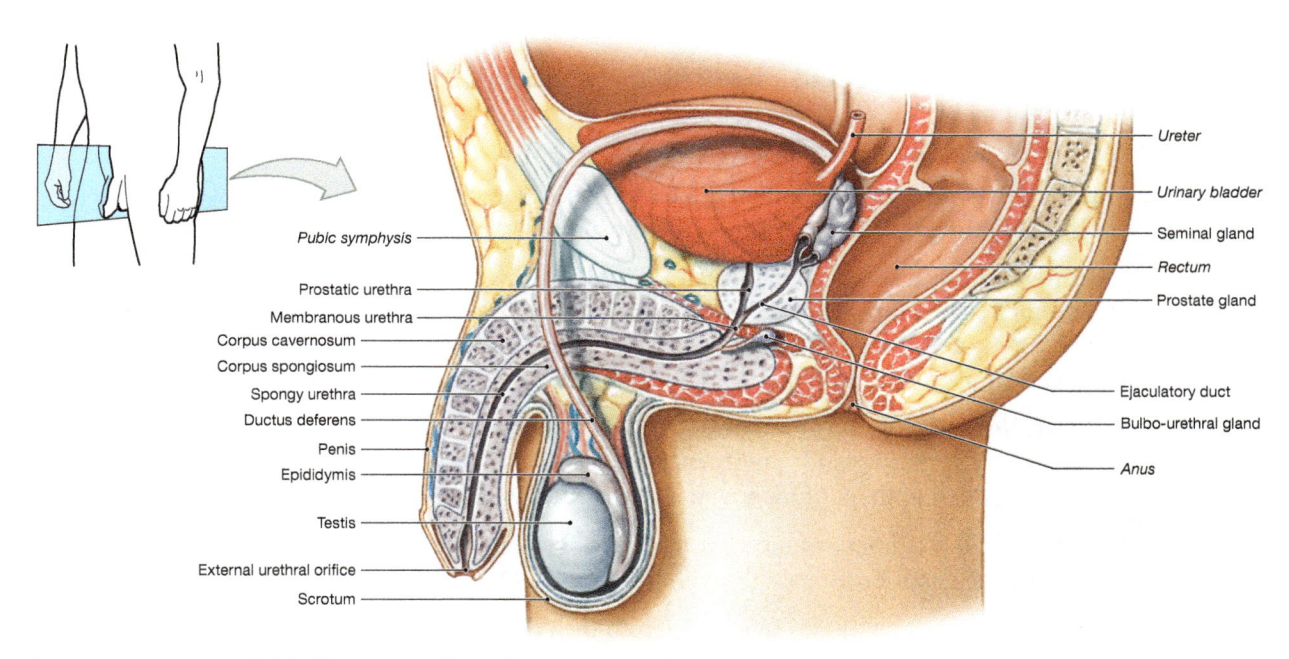

From *Human Anatomy*, Ninth Edition, by Frederic Martini, Robert B. Tallitsch, and Judi L. Nath (2018), reproduced by permission of Pearson Education.

Figure 9.4 **The Male Reproductive System** The male reproductive system as seen in sagittal section. The diagrammatic view shows several intact organs on the left.

CHAPTER NINE   *Male & Female Reproductive Systems*

b. Seminiferous tubules unite to eventually form the **ducts of the epididymis**.
   c. **Interstitial cells**, which produce **testosterone**, are located in the space between the seminiferous tubules.
2. The **epididymis** is a comma-shaped structure, which rests on the superior and lateral surfaces of the testis.
   a. The duct of the epididymis is continuous with the **ductus deferens**.
   b. Sperm mature and gain motility in the epididymis.

The Spermatic Cord

The **spermatic cord** passes through the inguinal canal, which is a passageway through the abdominal wall. It is covered externally by fascial layers derived from the abdominal wall. Structures located within the spermatic cord include:

1. The **ductus deferens** courses from the epididymis through the spermatic cord and then through the inguinal canal. The ductus deferens is the tube through which sperm travel towards the urethra.
2. The **testicular artery** provides the blood supply to the testes.
3. The **pampiniform plexus** of veins drains into the **testicular vein**.
4. **Lymph vessels** and **nerves** are located within the spermatic cord.

INTERNAL MALE REPRODUCTIVE STRUCTURES

1. The **ductus deferens** courses through the spermatic cord, through the abdominal wall and then posteriorly and laterally over the urinary bladder to the seminal vesicles.
2. **Seminal glands** (or seminal vesicles) secrete approximately 60–65% of the fluid portion of semen. The seminal vesicles are located at the posterior surface of the urinary bladder. The seminal vesicles resemble a honeycomb in cross-section.
3. **Ejaculatory ducts** receive the seminal glands and the ductus deferens. Ejaculatory ducts enter the **prostatic urethra** by passing through the prostate gland.
4. The **prostate gland** is a small, round organ located just inferior to the male urinary bladder. The prostatic urethra passes through the prostate. At separate times, urine or semen passes through the prostatic urethra. Prostatic fluid is slightly acidic and contributes to sperm motility. Prostatic secretions contribute about 25% of seminal fluid.
5. The **bulbourethral glands** are small pea-sized glands located to either side of the membranous urethra. The ducts of these glands empty into the penile (spongy) urethra. The bulbourethral glands secrete a small amount of clear ejaculatory fluid, which cleanses the male urethra.
6. The male **urethra** is a continuous tube from urinary bladder to the external urethral orifice. At separate times, urine and semen pass through the urethra. The three parts of the male urethra are:
   a. The **prostatic urethra** passes inferiorly from the base of the bladder through the prostate gland.
   b. The **membranous urethra** continues from the prostatic urethra out of the pelvic cavity and passes through the urogenital diaphragm.
   c. The **penile urethra** (spongy urethra) continues from the membranous urethra and passes through the corpus spongiosum of the penis to the "outside."

Study and Review Questions – The Reproductive System

CHAPTER NINE

Answers to these questions are found in Chapter Nine of this guide.

1. Describe the attachments and location of the clitoris. _____
_____

2. The labia minora enclose both the _____ & _____ openings.

3. The normal position of the uterus is _____ over the urinary bladder.

4. Match the part of the uterine tube with its description. Match the structure in **column A** with the correct description in **column B**. Write the letter of your answer in the blank by the appropriate term in column A.

   Column A   **Column B**

   _____ Intramural   A. Fringed edges of the infundibulum

   _____ Fimbriae   B. Narrow portion of the tube, directly attached to the uterus

   _____ Ampulla   C. Dilated, distal end of the tube

   _____ Infundibulum   D. Usual location of fertilization

   _____ Isthmus   E. Within the wall of the uterus

5. Describe the cervix and name the recesses that surround it where it joins to the superior end of the vagina. _____
_____

6. Describe the **corpora cavernosa** and their function. _____

7. Where is the **cremaster muscle** located and what is its function? _____

8. What happens to sperm in the epididymis? _____

9. List three structures located in the **spermatic cord**.

   a. _____

   b. _____

   c. _____

10. List three glands that contribute to the **seminal fluid**.

    a. _____

    b. _____

    c. _____

11. Where along the uterine tube is the usual site of fertilization? _____ .

12. Where are the **bulbourethral glands** and what is the role of their secretions? _____
    _____ .

13. Which bodies of erectile tissue in the female have similar structure and embryonic origins to the penis? _____
    _____ .

14. What are each of the boundaries of the **perineum**? _____
    _____ .

15. What is the function/action of the bulbospongiosus muscle in males? _____
    _____ .

16. What is the epithelial lining of the vagina? Why is this type of epithelium appropriate for this organ? _____
    _____ .